362.196 TRA.

DATE DUE			
14/2			

Outcome Measurement in Mental Health

Outcome Measurement in Mental Health

Theory and Practice

Edited by
Tom Trauer

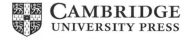

CAMBRIDGE UNIVERSITY PRESS
Cambridge, New York, Melbourne, Madrid, Cape Town, Singapore, São Paulo, Delhi, Dubai, Tokyo

Cambridge University Press
The Edinburgh Building, Cambridge CB2 8RU, UK

Published in the United States of America by
Cambridge University Press, New York

www.cambridge.org
Information on this title:
www.cambridge.org/9780521118347

First published 2010

Printed in the United Kingdom at the University Press, Cambridge

A catalogue record for this publication is available from the British Library

Library of Congress Cataloguing in Publication data

Outcome measurement in mental health : theory and practice / edited by Tom Trauer.
  p. ; cm.
Includes bibliographical references and index.
ISBN 978-0-521-11834-7 (hardback)
1. Mental health services–Evaluation. 2. Outcome assessment (Medical care)
I. Trauer, Tom, 1944–II. Title.
[DNLM: 1. Mental Disorders–therapy. 2. Mental Health Services–organization & administration. 3. Quality Assurance, Health Care–methods. 4. Treatment Outcome. WM 400 O94 2010]

RA790.5.O98 2010
362.196′89–dc22   2010009144

ISBN 978-0-521-11834-7 Hardback

Contents

Contents

Contributors

Sylke Andreas
Department of Medical Psychology,
University Medical Centre
Hamburg-Eppendorf,
Hamburg, Germany

Thomas Becker
Professor, Department of Psychiatry II,
University of Ulm,
Günzburg, Germany

Peter Brann
Director, Research and Evaluation,
Senior Psychologist, Eastern Health
CAMHS, and
Honorary Lecturer, Department of
Psychological Medicine,
Monash University,
Melbourne, Australia

Tom Callaly
Professor and Executive Director and
Clinical Director,
Mental Health, Drugs and Alcohol,
Barwon Health, and
School of Medicine, Deakin University,
Victoria, Australia

Tim Coombs
Training and Service Development,
Australian Mental Health Outcomes and
Classification Network
(AMHOCN),
NSW Institute of Psychiatry,
Parramatta, New South Wales,
Australia

Mark Deady
Research Officer,
National Drug and Alcohol Research
Centre,
University of New South Wales,
Sydney, Australia

James Healy
Manager, Ohio Consumer
Outcomes System,
Office of Research and Evaluation,
Ohio Department of Mental Health,
Ohio, United States of America

Rowena Jacobs
Senior Research Fellow,
Centre for Health Economics,
University of York,
York, United Kingdom

Michael J. Lambert
Professor, Department of Psychology,
Susa Young Gates University
Professor,
Brigham Young University,
Provo, Utah, United States of America

Regina McDonald
Area Clinical Nurse Consultant,
Specialist Mental Health Services for Older
People,
Braeside Hospital and Sydney South West
Area Health Service,
Sydney, Australia

Rod McKay
Senior Staff Specialist,
Specialist Mental Health Services for Older
People, Braeside Hospital, and
Conjoint Senior Lecturer,
School of Public Health and
Community Medicine,
University of New South Wales,
Sydney, Australia

Graham Mellsop
Professor of Psychiatry,
Waikato Clinical School,
University of Auckland,
Auckland, New Zealand

Allen Morris-Yates
Director, Centralised Data Management Service,
Private Mental Health Alliance,
Australia

Tricia Nagel
Associate Professor and Consultant Psychiatrist,
Top End Mental Health Services, and
Head, Healing and Resilience Division,
Menzies School of Health Research,
Darwin, Australia

Andrew C. Page
Professor, Clinical Psychology Unit,
School of Psychology,
University of Western Australia,
Perth, Australia

Jane Pirkis
Professor and Director,
Centre for Health Policy, Programs and Economics,
Melbourne School of Population Health,
University of Melbourne,
Victoria, Australia

Bernd Puschner
Department of Psychiatry II,
University of Ulm,
Günzburg, Germany

Dee Roth
Chief of the Office of Research and Evaluation,
Ohio Department of Mental Health,
Ohio, United States of America

Mirella Ruggeri
Professor of Psychiatry,
Section of Psychiatry and Clinical Psychology,
Department of Medicine and Public Health,
University of Verona,
Verona, Italy

Torleif Ruud
Professor, Institute of Psychiatry,
University of Oslo, and
Department of Research and Development,
Akershus University Hospital,
Norway

Holger Schulz
Department of Medical Psychology,
University Medical Centre Hamburg-Eppendorf,
Hamburg, Germany

Mike Slade
Reader in Health Services Research,
Institute of Psychiatry,
King's College London,
London, United Kingdom

David Smith
Project Manager,
Community Mental Health Common Assessment Project,
Senior Managing Consultant, Blue Pebble Consulting,
Toronto, Ontario, Canada

Mark Smith
Clinical Lead Specialist,
Te Pou, New Zealand

Maree Teesson
Professor and NHMRC Senior Research Fellow,
Assistant Director, National Drug and Alcohol Research Centre,
University of New South Wales,
Sydney, Australia

Glen Tobias
State Manager, Victoria,
Neami Limited,
Fairfield, Victoria, Australia

Tom Trauer
Professor, Department of Psychiatry, The University of Melbourne, and
School of Psychology and Psychiatry,
Monash University, and
St Vincent's Hospital Mental Health Service, Melbourne,
Australia

Foreword

Outcomes measurement (OM) in medicine has been around, as an ideal, since Codman's "End Result Idea" in the early 1900s. Astonishingly, it has lain dormant almost all of the time since. I've been active in this field for just over twelve years, but in that time it has developed very rapidly. This book marks a crucial phase in its evolution - a coming of age in mental health, arguably its most problematic arena. Across the world, as it shows, many local and regional mental health services (like South Verona in Italy) have reached different stages of implementation and some larger units (like Ohio in the US and Ontario in Canada, again at very different stages) have also taken a methodical approach. But in two countries (Australia and New Zealand) there is national implementation of OM in mental health services. Of these Australia is by far the most advanced; a beacon to the rest of us. This book is therefore quite rightly dominated by Australian authors. Let me adopt an Australasian forthrightness. Anyone can write a book on the theory of OM in mental health and stuff it with the psychometrics of research scales or the philosophy of causality. Anyone can carry out surveys of non-participants' views of OM, and especially why OM can't be done in mental health, ignoring the words of the sage: "口头说该事无法完成的人不应当阻挠别人完成它" (the person who says something cannot be done should not interrupt the person doing it). This book, full of excellent advice about how to implement, sustain and develop OM programmes in mental health, has contributors who are actually doing it. And only Tom Trauer, internationally acknowledged leader of the mental health OM community, could have edited it. For these reasons alone I am certain that this book will swiftly become the standard text.

I use the present tense; OM is never finally "implemented" – it is a process, and all the sites described in this book are at different stages on sometimes different paths. Why do I talk of evolution? Tautologically, only those programmes that have the right attributes to survive will do so. As Tom Trauer himself describes, enthusiastic champions may be necessary at the start but they are not sufficient. It is certain that many local OM initiatives have started, blossomed and then died without trace, perhaps when the champions moved on. But when a well established and documented whole state OM system begins to crumble like that in Ohio, starkly described here by James Healy and Dee Roth, we should all be asking the question: what are the attributes of an OM system that survives? There is a view that OM has not yet proved itself - that it is a luxury of some sort. There is also more or less hostility to OM from various quarters; why else would it have taken so long for such an obvious development? (Tom has long compared OM with the development of the mercury thermometer, without which we would still be talking of unquantifiable "fever".) When the cold winds of recession blow, as they have particularly in Ohio, those hostile to OM leap forward and cry "it's all very nice but we can't afford it!" But the truth is that medicine in general, and mental health services in particular, cannot afford not to embrace OM, thus allowing us to move beyond whimsy and prejudice to ecologically valid knowledge of effectiveness.

If you are curious about OM, I am sure you will relish this book. And if you are involved in OM already you are certain to find here new suggestions for development; it covers every sort of service and client group. In particular, you will surely find new attributes that might help your OM system survive and flourish in what is once again becoming a precarious world for the systematic understanding of effectiveness.

Alastair Macdonald MD, FRCPsych
Chair, Clinical Outcomes Group
South London & Maudsley NHS Foundation Trust
London, UK

Chapter

1

Introduction

Tom Trauer

In this introductory chapter I shall cover the historical and theoretical background to outcome measurement in mental health, provide a road map to the contents of this book, and express my appreciation to contributors. The final chapter will aim to draw conclusions from what has been presented and give some pointers to the future.

Preliminaries

Before embarking on the main aims of this chapter, I pause to note and explain some conventions I shall adopt. This book is about Outcome Measurement, but this is not a universally agreed term. Some have written about Outcome Assessment (Close-Goedjen and Saunders, 2002), others of Outcome Management (Andrews and Page, 2005, Miller et al., 2005, Puschner et al., 2009) and others of Outcome Evaluation (Ciarlo, 1982, Speer, 1998). While recognizing differences in nuance, we shall treat these terms as interchangeable for the most part, and talk of Outcome Measurement (OM) by default. To some degree, the different terminologies reflect the fact that OM, like the term outcome itself, has no firm or formal definition. At this stage, we may say that OM concerns the use, in a systematic and ongoing way, of standard instruments that assess aspects of mental health for the purpose of promoting the care of service recipients.

Background

In this section we shall survey the history and theoretical underpinnings of outcome measurement (OM) in mental health. An appreciation of the background of a subject can illuminate its current status. Given that OM can be a time-consuming and costly business, it would be short-sighted not to take the opportunity to learn from the experience of people in other countries and in other times, always remembering that 'Those who cannot remember the past are condemned to repeat it' (Santayana, 1905).

When did OM in mental health begin? Certainly OM in health services has been around for a long time. In 1987 there was published an article entitled 'Outcome assessment 70 years later: are we ready?' (Schroeder, 1987); this provocative title alluded to origins in attempts to get surgeons and hospitals to publicize the results of their operations in the early twentieth century. The earliest publication in my personal mental health OM database is 1980, when McPheeters (1980) discussed the use of several commonly used scales to evaluate the community impact of mental health services. Shortly thereafter, Ciarlo (1982) wrote about the arrival of client outcome evaluation, noting that 'Increasingly, these officials [program managers and funders] are becoming concerned with more than just the numbers and targets of services delivered, and the cost involved, and are looking for evidence of positive outcome or impact on clients to justify program implementation and maintenance'. Outcomes evaluation offered a route to accountability through performance measurement and quality assurance.

Outcome Measurement in Mental Health: Theory and Practice, ed. Tom Trauer. Published by Cambridge University Press.
© Cambridge University Press 2010.

These ideas produced several reactions, one of which sounds eerily contemporary: Newman (1982) noted the importance of good computer technology and for the data to be fed back to clinicians rapidly, and he also warned of a potential problem with practitioner compliance. He cited evidence that 'both level of functioning and treatment selection judgements increase in reliability when staff have had more training . . . and experience in using a level of functioning scale as an ordinary part of their clinical assessment and communication'.

One of the most influential events around that time was the annual Shattuck lecture, hosted by the venerable Massachusetts Medical Society and reported in its journal, the prestigious *New England Journal of Medicine*. In 1988 the title was 'Outcomes Management – A technology of experience'. In his address, Paul Ellwood (1988) called for the evaluation of medical services to move away from a focus on expenditure and towards enhanced quality of life. He spoke of a 'common patient-understood language of health outcomes' and a national database containing clinical, financial and outcomes information, which would 'routinely and systematically measure the functioning and well-being of patients, along with the disease specific clinical outcomes, at appropriate times'. Two years later, Epstein (1990), commenting on Ellwood's clarion call, asked whether outcomes management was the third revolution in medical care, the first two having been the Era of Expansion and the Era of Cost Containment, according to Relman (1988). Noting that Ellwood was a champion of the HMO (Health Maintenance Organization), Epstein identified the origins of the outcomes movement in cost containment, competition between providers, and the wide geographic variations in the use of certain medical procedures. A similar point was made by Mirin and Namerow (1991): 'Concern about the spiralling cost of mental health care has increased the need for reliable data about the outcomes of such care'.

Our foray into some of the early history of OM has revealed that practically all of that work was from the United States of America. This may simply be a reflection of the dominance of the USA of the medical literature, and maybe of medical innovation, but it may also relate to the economic climate in which health care, including mental health care, operated, and continues to operate. Health care costs in the USA are among the highest of developed nations, and it is clear that a large part of the early motivation for OM was economic.

The rise of Outcome Measurement

Since its origins in the 1980s, OM has expanded rapidly. The idea has spread internationally, and one section of this book contains accounts of how it is currently manifested in Australia, Canada, Germany, Italy, New Zealand, Norway, the United Kingdom and the USA. At this point it is worth noting that this set of countries is not meant to suggest that OM doesn't exist in some form in other countries; the countries reported herein represent those where OM has been most clearly developed and where it has been best reported. Furthermore, even within the countries that are represented by chapters, OM practices are not necessarily uniformly distributed. For example, the Canada chapter reports developments in the province of Ontario, and the Italy chapter focuses largely on work done in Verona.

The rise of OM can also be seen from the growth of the OM literature. Two literature searches were undertaken of the PsycInfo and Medline databases of the period 1988 to 2007 inclusive. One search was on the terms Psychiatry or Mental Health, and the other was on those terms and Outcome. Figure 1.1 shows the results.

It can be seen that, between 1988 and 1990, about 5% of citations matching Psychiatry or Mental Health also matched Outcome as a search term. This had risen to about 10% by 1995, and has been consistently above 15% since 2000. Of course, not all of the citations matching

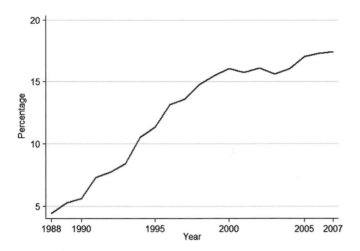

Figure 1.1 Percentage of citations on Psychiatry or Mental Health that were also about Outcome, 1988 to 2007.

Outcomes were concerned with the narrower concept of OM as understood here, but it is nevertheless clear that there has been a steadily increasing focus on outcome in the mental health literature.

What is an outcome?

Having established that there has been steadily increasing interest in outcome, we now turn to the more difficult question of what outcome actually means in the present context. At one level, everyone knows what an outcome is – it is a result, effect or product, usually of some action. The idea of an outcome as a consequence of action is echoed in the most widely cited definition of outcome in mental health: 'the effect on a patient's health status that is attributable to an intervention' (Andrews et al., 1994). The straightforwardness of this definition has no doubt contributed to its popularity. However, a number of commentators have suggested that things may not be so simple.

It may appear that the minimum requirement for an outcome is that something must have changed. However, it has pointed out that 'Maintaining a patient's health status may in some circumstances be considered a positive outcome' (Jacobs, 2009, p. 3). This is especially pertinent for consumers with enduring, or even deteriorating, conditions, who are not realistically expected to make significant gains. Even when changes on measures are obtained, there can be technical issues with judging whether a change in the score yielded by an instrument corresponds with a change in the consumer. This issue is considered in greater depth in the chapter on assessing change, but the point here is that some judgement needs to be made as to whether a change in score is merely random, clinically trivial fluctuation, or measurement imprecision, or a true and significant change in health status. One useful perspective on the centrality of change was proposed by Eagar (2002), who distinguished between 'before and after' and 'with and without'. The former ('before and after') models the outcome as the change in scores before and after an intervention. But, as Eagar argues, the 'with and without' approach is 'of particular relevance to chronic diseases where the goal of the intervention may be to maintain current health status … which would be rated as a good outcome if the alternative were a possible decline' (p. 143).

The requirement for a change to be attributable to an intervention has attracted a number of reservations. It has been noted that 'Although routine measurement of outcomes will tell us something about what is being achieved by health care, the difficult question is one of attribution. . . . Methodological flaws in routine outcomes data preclude strong assertions on attribution' (Davies and Crombie, 1997). That an intervention precedes a change does not mean that it must have caused it. In focus groups conducted by Stedman et al. (1997), consumers and service providers expressed concern over 'the extrapolation of data collected on these measures to judgements concerning the effectiveness of service provision. That is, attributing change in a person's mental health condition to the efficacy of treatment' (p. 93); a similar point was made by Rissel et al. (1996). Stedman et al. felt that 'to reduce the emphasis on attribution may assist the promotion of the use of routine consumer outcomes measurement' (p. 93). Proof of causality in the human sciences is difficult; the strongest evidence comes from randomized controlled trials, and only a handful of such studies have been conducted in the OM field. Some 'outcomes' may be largely a product of self-help, or of informal, non-professional care, and others could occur after no obvious intervention, i.e. spontaneous remission. Even when appropriate, targeted treatment appears to work, one cannot always be sure who should take the credit; to paraphrase the sixteenth-century physician Ambroise Paré 'I treated him, but God healed him' (Strauss, 1968, p. 627). Trauer (1998) has suggested that when the focus of the outcome is the intervention itself, attribution may be straightforward ('The operation was a success'); it is when the focus is on the consumer ('She is less depressed') that attribution becomes problematic. He therefore suggested that the requirement for attribution be omitted from the definition of outcome. An attribution-free definition of outcomes was put forward by Charlwood et al. (1999, p. 3): '. . . changes in health, health related status or risk factors affecting health, or lack of change when change is expected'.

Another component of the Andrews et al. definition of outcome to come under scrutiny is the intervention. Sonnanburg (1996) pointed out the difficulty of knowing what are the real change agents since there are so many influences in real life. I (Trauer, 1998) noted that even standard mental health care comprises many components, such as medication, psychological therapy and case management, so 'Since we generally cannot disentangle the active ingredients of therapy, we cannot unequivocally specify the intervention'. I went on to suggest that 'This problem is resolved if we break the link with interventions and regard outcome as, say, the change in health status between two points in time. The two points need not be random, but can have particular significance in the patient's career, such as pre-operation and post-operation, or admission and discharge. The establishment of a causal connection between any change in health status and the intervening activity then becomes an empirical question which can be studied scientifically'.

The last issue relating to the understanding of outcome that we shall consider here is that of mixed outcomes. It is by no means unusual for some things to get better while other things are getting worse. I (Trauer, 1998) gave the examples of psychotic symptoms reducing at the expense of side-effects, and hospitalization increasing safety at the expense of independence. Detailed assessments of the different elements of symptoms, functioning and experience can track their separate movements. Aggregated scores, on the other hand, may have improved reliability, but will lose much of the nuances; also, summing improvements and deteriorations in multi-item scales can lead to 'cancelling out', which will give a false impression of less change than actually occurred.

Why measure outcomes?

In this section we shall review some of the models and principles that have been put forward as to why outcomes should be measured. As was suggested earlier, all stakeholders in the health care enterprise have a natural interest in outcome (although what they mean by that term may differ in certain important ways). Therefore, why go to the extra expense and trouble in subjecting outcomes to measurement?

(a) The information needs of managers

In a section entitled 'What Performance Areas Does a Manager Need to Know About', Leginski et al. (1989, p. 23) enunciated their informational needs thus:

> *Who* receives *what* from *whom* at what *cost* and with what *effect*.

The italicized words represent the informational domains. 'Who' refers to the consumers; a service will need to know how many of them there are, plus certain basic demographic and clinical (e.g. diagnostic) details. This information is generally readily available through the medical records system, or equivalent. Sometimes the 'who' may refer to the population served, as in a catchment area, and sometimes the people served include carers and/or family members, as in child and adolescent services. Generally, however, the 'who' information is not problematic. The 'what' refers to the services provided, in the sense of elements such as inpatient beds, residential places, day programmes, outpatient clinics, case management, emergency teams, and maybe additional specialist teams. The 'what' may include property, such as buildings and equipment. Mostly, these elements are easy to catalogue since they describe the settings where services are delivered. Services are not always direct to identified consumers; in preventive work, such as community consultation, and health promotion, the activity is directed to individuals and organizations other than registered service recipients. Nevertheless, as with the 'who', this element is relatively straightforward. The 'from whom' refers to the staff. Leginski et al. advise that this should be all staff working in the organization, not just the direct care component. For the clinicians, however, this will include the mix of professions, perhaps supplemented by details of their levels of training, qualifications and experience. For the sake of judging how well the clinical staff reflect the composition of the consumers served, one might also be interested in further descriptions, such as age, gender and ethnic background. 'At what cost' is obviously the available budget, an element that most managers are only too acutely aware of.

It is with the last element of the group, 'with what effect', that measured outcomes are concerned. As Leginski et al. say in their chapter on assessing impact, 'Assuming that managers within the organization have ample information on the other components of this knowledge model, i.e. clientele, services, finances and staff, it is quite logical for them to pose the question, So what?' (p. 89). Indeed, they go further and assert that 'Managers have a responsibility to assess'.

This formulation has the value of showing, in a succinct way, the relationship of outcomes to other fundamental aspects of complex human services. In addition, it alerts one to the need to take clientele, services, finances and staff into account when evaluating the performance of a service. The Leginski model has proved attractive as explaining the rationale of outcome measurement in Australia; it has been cited in the informational priorities in the Second National Mental Health Plan (Department of Health and Aged Care, 1999) and in the model for outcome measurement in private psychiatric hospitals in Australia (Morris-Yates and The Strategic Planning Group for Private Psychiatric Services Data Collection and Analysis Working Group, 2000).

(b) Assisting with decision-making

While there may be legitimate interest in quantifying the magnitude of treatment effects in scientific studies, one clear reason for measuring outcomes has been to provide a guide for action. Sutherland and Till (1993) distinguish three levels of decision-making: micro (clinical), meso (agency, institutional or regional) and macro/meta (governmental). Stedman et al. (1997, p. 12) suggested the following kinds of decision associated with each level: 'What treatment goals are necessary to meet the needs of this individual?' (clinical); 'What are the best treatment approaches for addressing the needs of this group of people?' (agency); and 'What are the best treatment approaches for meeting the needs of this population of people?' (governmental).

There are many expressions of the intention or hope that the measurement of outcomes will assist decision-makers in some way. Ellwood (1988) envisaged opportunities for each decision-maker to have access to the analyses that are relevant to the choices they must make. Benjamin et al. (1995, p. AS299) said that 'outcomes research is meant to be used to make better decisions about health care in the context of social, political, economic, and regulatory forces'. Mirin and Namerow (1991) saw the study of outcomes as rationalizing clinical decision-making, a view challenged by Gale (1997) on the grounds that services do not have sufficient control over all the relevant functions and factors. So important is this purpose that Speer and Newman (1996) went so far as to propose that relevance for decision-makers must take priority over scientific rigour. This is similar to the position characterized by Iezzoni (1994): 'Given the dearth of information currently available about the relative merits of health care providers, one needs to start somewhere, even if the data are not perfect'.

For the most part, these early expectations related to decision-making at the agency and governmental level, and were expressed in quite general terms, with little detail as to what those outcome-based decisions might be. One example was offered by Bilbrey and Bilbrey (1995), who interviewed 49 health care payors. They identified the selection of which providers to make contracts with as the primary type of decision that would be most influenced by outcomes data. At that time, this primary strength of outcomes data for purchasers of services was also one of the primary threats to the providers; Iezzoni (1994, p. 350), in her list of common concerns of providers, included that 'These imperfect data may be used wrongly to threaten providers or make punitive decisions (e.g., withdrawing third-party reimbursements)'.

In parallel with meso- and macro-level uses, outcomes information is expected to have decision-making uses at the micro, or individual, clinical, level. Slade (2002) identified 'the ongoing measurement and use of outcome data to inform decisions about whether to continue, change or curtail treatment' as a central purpose. The notion of ongoing measurement implies that it is the trajectory that these measurements reveal that will form the basis of action on the part of the clinicians. This is at the heart of the system developed by Michael Lambert and colleagues, and detailed in his chapter in this book. Lueger et al. (2001) talk of the 'expected treatment response' as the predicted path of progress, against which the actual path can be compared. This leads directly to the concepts of 'on track' and 'off track' (Lambert et al., 2001), which can be communicated immediately to the clinician, along with suggestions for corrective action. This is particularly valuable in the early identification of consumers at risk for treatment failure, a risk that therapists systematically underestimate (Hannan et al., 2005).

There are examples of outcome measures obtained at single points in time being used in assisting with decisions in the individual case. Prowse and Coombs (2009) described the use of high or low severity scores on the Health of the Nation Outcome Scales (HoNOS, Wing et al., 1998) to suggest transfer to (respectively) more or less intensive forms of care. Prowse and Hunter (2008) used a measure of functioning and disability (the Life Skills Profile, LSP, Rosen et al., 1989, 2006) to assist in choosing the form of psychological treatment for consumers with Borderline Personality Disorder. Slattery and Anstey (2008) described the discussion of HoNOS results in multidisciplinary team meetings as contributing to the development of consumer care plans and assessing readiness for discharge. It is also proper to acknowledge that there have been some doubts expressed over the suitability of outcome measures to guide treatment decisions. Iezzoni (1994) has noted that 'Most existing severity measures were intended to be used across groups of patients and are not well suited to making inferences about individual case' (p. 202). Others (e.g. Gifford, 1996) have questioned whether measures on standard instruments are sufficiently sensitive to the unique qualities and needs of consumers.

(c) Incorporating the consumer's perspective

Part of the impetus for outcome measurement came from the recognition of the importance of the consumer perspective in the treatment process. This is of course true in all aspects of health care, but no less so in mental health, where many of the issues and problems are not readily visible to clinicians, who are especially reliant on personal reports from service recipients. While much of the rationale for outcome measurement has revolved around the needs of funders, managers and clinicians, the increasingly prominent and effective consumer constituency, as well as many non-consumers, have pointed out that the service recipients, and their interests, should be central to the outcome measurement enterprise. Sometimes the motivation appears to be that involving the consumer aids the objectives of the provider; Eisen et al. (1991) have suggested that patients can be recruited as evaluators of their own progress, and their satisfaction with services received can be an indicator of acceptability. Other possible benefits of including the consumer's point of view can be the enhancement of the clinician–consumer relationship. Greenhalgh et al. (2005, p. 834), however, have reviewed evidence suggesting that while feedback of quality of life scores to clinicians may increase their discussion within sessions, it generally does not influence (clinicians') decisions concerning treatment.

There is abundant evidence that consumers' priorities in mental health care are often at some variance with those of providers, hence when we speak of outcomes there can be the unspoken question: 'According to whom?'. Very broadly, clinicians tend to prioritize symptoms and functioning, while consumers, and often their family members and carers as well, prioritize clear information and involvement in decision-making (Graham et al., 2001, Noble and Douglas, 2004). Unfortunately, there is now considerable evidence that clinicians tend to consistently misread their consumers' wants, while confidently believing that they appreciate them accurately (Noble et al., 1999, Trauer and Callaly, 2002).

Even when the relevant parties agree on what the important problems are, consumers can, and do, argue that their evaluations are the more valid – in effect, they are the 'experts by experience' (Faulkner, 1998). This issue becomes even more acute when trying to judge the outcomes of consumers who belong to certain ethnic and cultural subpopulations, which may hold quite different conceptions of health and illness from the mainstream (e.g. Maori, Durie and Kingi, 1997). There exists wide variation in the extent to which the consumer perspective is formally incorporated into outcome systems; some systems rely exclusively or predominantly on consumer self-report (see chapters by Michael Lambert and by Jim Healy and

Dee Roth in this book), while others are more heavily weighted toward clinician-completed measures, such as the HoNOS.

About this book

Any new book needs to justify its existence. There are already several excellent, substantial and authoritative works on outcome measurement, such as Sederer and Dickey (1996), Lyons et al. (1997), Speer (1998), Tansella and Thornicroft (2001) and IsHak et al. (2002). But these works all appeared some time ago and, as was shown earlier, much has happened in the field of outcome measurement since then. In addition, much of the more recent work has been done in Australasia. So one of the purposes of this book has been to bring some of the more recent developments together into a single source.

It is apparent from the table of contents that this book is organized into three main sections. The first presents implementations of outcome measurement in large jurisdictions, countries or (American) states. The objective here is to demonstrate how the same concept can be manifested in different settings, and how the principles are realized differently according to national policy, local leadership and the economic and cultural organization of health, and mental health, services. The jurisdictions represented are those that are best known to myself through the literature and through personal contacts. The absence of a country or region should not be taken to mean that outcome measurement does not happen there; indeed, there are a number of such local implementations of outcome measurement, but generally at a relatively small and limited level, making it difficult to justify a full treatment in this book.

Outcome measurement cannot be undertaken in an identical fashion in all parts of a mental health system; it must be adapted to the specific requirements of the population served. The second section comprises chapters describing how outcome measurement has been and can be delivered in three main age categories (Child and Adolescent, Adult and Older Persons), as well as to indigenous consumers, and those in private hospitals, non-government services (NGOs) and drug and alcohol services.

The third section deals with several central themes in most of which there is as yet no clear consensus. The 'applications and utility' chapter presents examples of what outcome measurement has to offer to various stakeholders, followed by a chapter reviewing stakeholders' attitudes and opinions in relation to OM. The 'assessment of change' chapter deals with some of the issues involved in the judgement of individual and group change. A chapter is devoted to training and workforces issues, and another presents an overview of the domains that are covered by some of the leading instruments; the section concludes with a chapter on outcome measurement from an economics point of view.

It will be apparent that there is no chapter written by a service recipient; all of the contributions are from people with predominantly clinical and/or academic backgrounds. The book is primarily intended for a clinical, managerial and academic readership, and the selection of content and authors reflects this.

The previous paragraph spoke of the service recipients. This raises the question of what is the respectful and proper way to describe those who receive mental health services. Patient, consumer, user and survivor are just some of the terms that have been used, and there are sometimes strong preferences and aversions to some of them among different stakeholders in different countries. In some countries there are national conventions: the common usage in mental health services in Australia and New Zealand is 'consumer', and in the United Kingdom it is 'user'. In this book, contributors have been free to choose their own terminology. Being from Australia, I have used 'consumer' in this chapter.

References

Andrews, G. and Page, A. C. (2005). Outcome measurement, outcome management and monitoring. *Australian and New Zealand Journal of Psychiatry*, **39**, 649–51.

Andrews, G., Peters, L. and Teesson, M. (1994). *The Measurement of Consumer Outcome in Mental Health: a Report to the National Mental Health Information Strategy Committee*. Sydney: Clinical Research Unit for Anxiety Disorders.

Benjamin, K. L., Perfetto, E. M. and Greene, R. J. (1995). Public policy and the application of outcomes assessments: paradigms versus politics. *Medical Care*, **33**, AS299–AS306.

Bilbrey, J. and Bilbrey, P. (1995). Judging, trusting, and utilizing outcomes data: a survey of behavioral healthcare payors. *Behavioral Healthcare Tomorrow*, **4**(July/August), 62–5.

Charlwood, P., Mason, A., Goldacre, M., Cleary, R. and Wilkinson, E. (1999). *Health Outcome Indicators: Severe Mental Illness*. Report of a working group to the Department of Health, Oxford.

Ciarlo, J. A. (1982). Accountability revisited: the arrival of client outcome evaluation. *Evaluation and Program Planning*, **5**, 31–6.

Close-Goedjen, J. L. and Saunders, S. M. (2002). The effect of technical support on clinician attitudes toward an outcome assessment instrument. *Journal of Behavioral Health Services & Research*, **29**, 99–108.

Davies, H. T. O. and Crombie, I. K. (1997). Interpreting health outcomes. *Journal of Evaluation in Clinical Practice*, **3**, 187–99.

Department of Health and Aged Care (1999). *Mental Health Information Development: National Information Priorities and Strategies under the Second National Mental Health Plan 1998–2003* (First Edition), Canberra.

Durie, M. and Kingi, T. K. (1997). *A Framework for Measuring Maori Mental Health Outcomes*. A report prepared for the Ministry of Health, Palmerston North.

Eagar, K. (2002). An overview of health outcomes measurement in Australia. *Mental Health Research & Development Strategy: Outcomes Conference*. Wellington, New Zealand.

Eisen, S. V., Grob, M. C. and Dill, D. L. (1991). Outcome measurement: tapping the patient's perspective. In S. M. Mirin, J. T. Gossett and M. C. Grob, eds., *Psychiatric Treatment: Advances in Outcome Research*. Washington DC: American Psychiatric Press.

Ellwood, P. M. (1988). Shattuck Lecture: Outcomes Management – A technology of experience. *New England Journal of Medicine*, **318**, 1549–56.

Epstein, A. M. (1990). The outcomes movement – will it get us where we want to go? *New England Journal of Medicine*, **323**, 266–70.

Faulkner, A. (1998). Experts by experience. *Mental Health Nursing*, **18**, 6–8.

Gale, L. (1997). Why a traditional health outcomes approach will fail in health care and a possible solution. *Australian Health Review*, **20**, 3–15.

Gifford, F. (1996). Outcomes research and practice guidelines. *Hastings Center Report*, **26**, 38–44.

Graham, C., Coombs, T., Buckingham, W., et al. (2001). *Consumer Perspectives of Future Directions for Outcome Self-Assessment*. Report of the Consumer Consultation Project, Wollongong.

Greenhalgh, J., Long, A. F. and Flynn, R. (2005). The use of patient reported outcome measures in routine clinical practice: lack of impact or lack of theory? *Social Science & Medicine*, **60**, 833–43.

Hannan, C., Lambert, M. J., Harmon, C., et al. (2005). A lab test and algorithms for identifying clients at risk for treatment failure. *Journal of Clinical Psychology*, **61**, 155–63.

Iezzoni, L. I. (ed.) (1994). *Risk Adjustment for Measuring Health Care Outcomes*. Ann Arbor, MI: Health Administration Press.

IsHak, W., Burt, T. and Sederer, L. (eds.) (2002). *Outcome Measurement in Mental Illness. A*

Critical Review. Washington DC: American Psychiatric Press.

Jacobs, R. (2009). *Investigating Patient Outcome Measures in Mental Health*. York: Centre for Health Economics, University of York.

Lambert, M. J., Hansen, N. B. and Finch, A. E. (2001). Patient focused research: using patient outcome data to enhance treatment effects. *Journal of Consulting and Clinical Psychology*, **69**, 159–72.

Leginski, W. A., Croze, C., Driggers, J., et al. (1989). Data Standards for Mental Health Decision Support Systems. *A Report of the Task Force to Revise the Data Content and System Guidelines of the Mental Health Statistics Improvement Program*. Washington DC.

Lueger, R. J., Howard, K. I., Martinovich, Z., et al. (2001). Assessing treatment progress of individual patients using expected treatment response models. *Journal of Consulting and Clinical Psychology*, **69**, 150–8.

Lyons, J. S., Howard, K. I., O'Mahoney, M. T. and Lish, J. D. (1997). *The Measurement and Management of Clinical Outcomes in Mental Health*. New York: John Wiley and Sons.

McPheeters, H. L. (1980). Measurement of mental health program outcomes. *New Directions for Program Evaluation*, **6**, 53–63.

Miller, S. D., Duncan, B. L., Sorrell, R. and Brown, G. S. (2005). The partners for change outcome management system. *Journal of Clinical Psychology*, **61**, 199–208.

Mirin, S. M. and Namerow, M. J. (1991). Why study treatment outcome? *Hospital and Community Psychiatry*, **42**, 1007–13.

Morris-Yates, A. and The Strategic Planning Group for Private Psychiatric Services Data Collection and Analysis Working Group (2000). *A National Model for the Collection and Analysis of a Minimum Data Set with Outcome Measurement for Private, Hospital-based, Psychiatric Services*. Canberra: Commonwealth of Australia.

Newman, F. L. (1982). Outcome assessment in evaluation and treatment research; a response to Ciarlo and Hargreaves (1982). *Evaluation and Program Planning*, **5**, 359–62.

Noble, L. M. and Douglas, B. C. (2004). What users and relatives want from mental health services. *Current Opinion in Psychiatry*, **17**, 289–96.

Noble, L. M., Douglas, B. C. and Newman, S. P. (1999). What do patients want and do we want to know? A review of patients' requests of psychiatric services. *Acta Psychiatrica Scandinavica*, **100**, 321–7.

Prowse, L. and Coombs, T. (2009). The use of the Health of the Nation Outcome Scales (HoNOS) to inform discharge and transfer decisions in community mental health services. *Australian Health Review*, **33**, 13–18.

Prowse, L. and Hunter, S. (2008). Using the LSP to inform programme decisions for individuals with Borderline Personality Disorder. *Australian and New Zealand Journal of Psychiatry*, **42**, A16.

Puschner, B., Schofer, D., Knaup, C. and Becker, T. (2009). Outcome management in in-patient psychiatric care. *Acta Psychiatrica Scandinavica*, **120**, 308–19.

Relman, A. S. (1988). Assessment and Accountability. *New England Journal of Medicine*, **319**, 1220–2.

Rissel, C., Ward, J. and Sainsbury, P. (1996). An outcomes approach to population health at the local level in NSW: practical problems and potential solutions. *Australian Health Review*, **19**, 23–39.

Rosen, A., Hadzi-Pavlovic, D. and Parker, G. (1989). The Life Skills Profile: a measure assessing function and disability in schizophrenia. *Schizophrenia Bulletin*, **15**, 325–37.

Rosen, A., Hadzi-Pavlovic, D., Parker, G. and Trauer, T. (2006). *The Life Skills Profile: Background, Items and Scoring for the LSP-39, LSP-20 and the LSP-16*, Sydney, available at: http://www.blackdoginstitute.org.au/docs/LifeSkillsProfile.pdf.

Santayana, G. (1905). *The Life of Reason*.

Schroeder, S. A. (1987). Outcome assessment 70 years later: are we ready? *New England Journal of Medicine*, **316**, 160–2.

Sederer, L. I. and Dickey, B. (Eds.) (1996). *Outcomes Assessment in Clinical Practice*. London: Williams & Wilkins.

Slade, M. (2002). The use of patient-level outcomes to inform treatment. *Epidemiologia e Psichiatria Sociale*, **11**, 20–7.

Slattery, T. and Anstey, S. (2008). Clinical utility of HoNOS in an inpatient setting. *Australian and New Zealand Journal of Psychiatry*, **42**, A6.

Sonnanburg, K. (1996). Meaningful measurement in psychotherapy. *Psychotherapy*, **33**, 160–70.

Speer, D. C. (1998). *Mental Health Outcome Evaluation*. San Diego, CA: Academic Press.

Speer, D. C. and Newman, F. L. (1996). Mental health services outcome evaluation. *Clinical Psychology: Science and Practice*, **3**, 105–29.

Stedman, T., Yellowlees, P., Mellsop, G., Clarke, R. and Drake, S. (1997). *Measuring Consumer Outcomes in Mental Health*. Canberra: Department of Health and Aged Care.

Strauss, M. B. (Ed.) (1968). *Familiar Medical Quotations*. Boston: Little Brown.

Sutherland, H. J. and Till, J. E. (1993). Quality of life assessments and levels of decision making: differentiating objectives. *Quality of Life Research* (2005) **14**, 297–303.

Tansella, M. and Thornicroft, G. (eds.) (2001). *Mental Health Outcome Measures*. London: Gaskell.

Trauer, T. (1998). Issues in the assessment of outcome in mental health. *Australian and New Zealand Journal of Psychiatry*, **32**, 337–43.

Trauer, T. and Callaly, T. (2002). Concordance between mentally ill clients and their case managers using the Health of the Nation Outcome Scales (HoNOS). *Australasian Psychiatry*, **10**, 24–8.

Wing, J. K., Beevor, A. S., Curtis, R. H., et al. (1998). Health of the Nation Outcome Scales (HoNOS). Research and Development. *British Journal of Psychiatry*, **172**, 11–18.

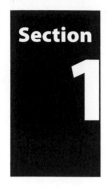

Section 1

Outcome Measurement around the World

Mental health outcome measurement in Australia

Jane Pirkis and Tom Callaly

Australia is regarded as a world leader in routine outcome measurement in mental health services (Slade, 2002), having been the first to undertake such an exercise on a national scale. A number of other countries have since gone down a similar track. This chapter describes Australia's experiences in this area, with a view to offering some lessons for other countries attempting similar exercises. The chapter begins with a history of the mental health outcome movement in Australia, and then describes the current state of play, both nationally and by way of an example of best practice at a local level. It considers whether we've got it right and what future steps might be taken to consolidate our current efforts. The chapter is primarily concerned with Australia's public mental health sector, but makes brief reference to developments in the private mental health sector as well.

History of mental health outcome measurement in Australia

Mental health outcome measurement has been firmly on the agenda in Australia since the inception of the National Mental Health Strategy in 1992. In that year, Health Ministers agreed to the National Mental Health Policy, which emphasized service quality and effectiveness. One of its specific objectives was: 'To institute regular review of client outcomes of services provided to persons with serious mental health problems and mental disorders as a central component of mental health service delivery' (Australian Health Ministers, 1992b).

Translating this policy objective into on-the-ground practice has been no small undertaking. At the time, the slate was relatively blank. There were no international precedents to draw upon, since no other country had implemented routine outcome measurement on a national scale. It was not clear what outcome measures might be appropriate and, even if it had been, most services would not have had the capacity to collect outcome data in a manner than could inform clinical care.

In response to this lack of direction, several major research and development activities were funded in the mid-1990s under the first five-year National Mental Health Plan (1992 to 1997) (Australian Health Ministers, 1992a), which operationalized the National Mental Health Strategy. A review was undertaken of potential outcome measures which might be suitable for use with adults (Andrews et al., 1994), and a subset of the identified instruments were tested in a field trial (Stedman et al., 1997). A similar programme of work was also instigated with respect to outcome measures for children and adolescents (Bickman et al., 1999). At the same time, a national casemix-development project known as the Mental Health Classification and Service Costs (MH-CASC) project was conducted (Burgess et al., 1999). The MH-CASC project established a protocol to collect data from 21 sites across Australia, using a number of the outcome measures identified in the reviews and field trials.

Australia also looked to its overseas counterparts during this period, some of whom were going down a similar track with regard to routine outcome measurement. For example,

Outcome Measurement in Mental Health: Theory and Practice, ed. Tom Trauer. Published by Cambridge University Press.
© Cambridge University Press 2010.

Professor John Wing from the Royal College of Psychiatrists in London came to Australia to offer his expertise both to the review of adult outcome measures and to the MH-CASC project. The Health of the Nation Outcome Scales (HoNOS) (Wing et al., 1998), developed by Wing, was increasingly gaining favour as a candidate instrument for measuring outcomes for adults. Wing was able to provide advice about the use of this measure from its preliminary roll-out as a routine measure in the United Kingdom.

In addition, momentum was increasing at a state and territory level. Victoria took the lead in 1996, trialling the HoNOS in five area mental health services. The trial was designed to examine the utility of the instrument as a routine outcome measure, and to help establish an ethos of routine outcome data collection and analysis. Clinical staff at each of the five services took part in extensive training. These staff rated 2,137 consumers attending these services in April of the study year, and followed around half of them up over the next 3 months. The trials indicated that routine outcome measurement was possible, and pointed to various strengths and weaknesses of the HoNOS as a measure (Trauer et al., 1999).

Nineteen ninety-eight saw a renewal of the National Mental Health Strategy under the Second National Mental Health Plan (1998–2003) (Australian Health Ministers, 1998), and a shift in emphasis from research and development activities to the development of infrastructure and resources. In 1999, a statement of information development priorities (Department of Health and Aged Care, 1999) was released, and this was accompanied by formal Information Development Agreements between the Australian Government and each of the state and territory governments. Under these agreements, states and territories were bound to introduce consumer outcome measurement as a core component of routine service delivery and submit outcome measurement ratings to the Australian Government routinely. In return, the Australian Government undertook to provide national leadership. This involved offering funding to states and territories to develop comprehensive, local clinical information systems and train their respective clinical workforces; establishing three national expert groups (adult, child/adolescent and older persons) to advise on the implementation and use of routine outcome data in mental health services; and putting in place arrangements to receive, process, analyse and report on outcome data submitted by states and territories.

By 2003, the commitments made by the respective parties under the Information Development Agreements were bearing fruit. States and territories had begun to routinely submit de-identified, consumer-level outcome data (referred to as the National Outcomes and Casemix Collection, or NOCC) (Department of Health and Ageing, 2003). These outcome data were, in turn, being submitted to states and territories by area mental health services which collected the data according to the NOCC protocol (described in more detail below) (Department of Health and Ageing, 2003). All states and territories had established data-collection systems (albeit with varying degrees of sophistication), and all had trained significant numbers of their clinical workforces (Pirkis et al., 2005). The policy momentum continued to be maintained with the release of the Third National Mental Health Plan (Australian Health Ministers, 2003), which included as one of its stated goals: 'Comprehensive implementation and further development of routine consumer outcome measures in mental health'.

At the same time, as promised, the Australian Government had rolled out substantial funding to states and territories to build infrastructure and train the clinical workforce, and had established all three of the expert groups. It had also contracted a consortium known as the Australian Mental Health Outcomes and Classification Network (AMHOCN) to provide national leadership in the field by pursuing a work programme centred on the data submitted by states and territories. The work programme had three components: data management;

analysis and reporting; and training and service development (Pirkis et al., 2005). More detail about AMHOCN and related national activities can be found at http://www.amhocn.org (accessed 1 March 2010).

Mental health outcome measurement in Australia today

Today, all public-sector mental inpatient and community mental health services collect outcome data according to the NOCC protocol and submit it to their state or territory health departments, who, in turn, submit it to AMHOCN (Department of Health and Ageing, 2003). The NOCC protocol requires that clinician-rated and consumer-rated measures are administered during given 'episodes of care', at particular 'collection occasions'. An episode is defined as '... a more or less continuous period of contact between a consumer and a mental health service organisation that occurs within the one mental health service setting [e.g. inpatient or community]' (Department of Health and Ageing, 2003). Collection occasions occur at set points and for different reasons: admission (new referral; transfer from other setting; other), at review (91 days; other), and at discharge (no further care; change of setting; death; other). The specific measures vary by the target age group of a given setting, and are summarized in Table 2.1.

Since 2003, ongoing efforts have been made by individuals, services, state and territory governments and the Australian Government to embed routine outcome measurement in the culture of service delivery. For example, AMHOCN has endeavoured to increase the clinical relevance of outcome measurement to those working in the field. AMHOCN has developed a web-based Decision Support Tool (wDST) which enables clinicians to compare their own consumers against normative data from Australia as a whole. AMHOCN is also working on a library of clinical prompts, which would offer specific advice to junior clinicians confronted with a consumer with a particular pattern of scores on any of the NOCC measures (McKay et al., 2008).

Training and support for clinicians has gone well beyond one-off education sessions. In addition to offering face-to-face training, AMHOCN has now developed a range of online training options and materials, produces a regular newsletter and fosters ongoing discussion through a forum. The focus of the training has shifted too; whereas it was once about the nuts and bolts of how to administer the NOCC suite of measures, it now goes beyond this to focus on the clinical utility of outcome measurement. Further detail about the training and service development activities of AMHOCN can be found elsewhere in this volume.

Analysis and reporting of routine outcome data have gradually become more sophisticated. Considerable effort has been put into issues such as the meaning of 'clinically significant change' and how best to measure such change (Burgess et al., 2009a, 2009b,). In addition, there has been a move from the presentation of standard reports to a more flexible report portal which allows users to navigate directly to the specific table of interest. More advanced 'data cube' technology has also been developed which enables users to interrogate outcome data in the manner most relevant to them.

Have we got it right?

Australia's activity with regard to routine outcome measurement is advanced by international standards, but the question still remains as to whether we've got it right. The national outcome data have been used to demonstrate that, in the main, consumers in contact with public-sector mental health services get better (Burgess et al., 2006). In other words, the outcome data are

Table 2.1 Administration of outcome measures according to the NOCC protocol

		Inpatient			Community residential			Ambulatory		
		Admission	Review	Discharge	Admission	Review	Discharge	Admission	Review	Discharge
Children and adolescents	HoNOSCA	●	●	●	●	●	●	●	●	●
	CGAS	●	●	●	●	●	●	●	●	●
	FIHS	·	●	·	·	●	●	·	●	●
	Principal and additional diagnoses	·	●	●	·	●	●	·	●	●
	Mental health legal status	·	●	●	·	●	●	·	●	●
Adults	HoNOS	●	●	●	●	●	●	●	●	●
	LSP-16	·	●	·	●	●	●	·	●	●
	Consumer self-report	·	·	·	●	●	●	●	●	●
	Principal and additional diagnoses	·	●	●	·	●	●	●	●	●
	Focus of care	·	·	·	·	·	·	·	●	●
	Mental health legal status	·	●	●	·	●	●	·	●	●

Older persons										
HoNOS 65+	●	●	·	●	●	●	●	●	●	●
LSP-16	·	·	·	●	●	·	●	●	●	·
RUG-ADL	●	●	·	·	●	●	·	·	●	·
Consumer self-report	·	·	●	·	●	·	●	●	●	·
Principal and additional diagnoses	·	●	·	·	●	·	●	●	●	●
Focus of care	·	·	·	·	·	·	·	·	●	●
Mental health legal status	·	●	·	·	●	·	●	●	●	●

HoNOS: Health of the Nation Outcome Scales – Clinician-rated (Wing et al., 1998).
LSP-16: Life Skills Profile 16 – Clinician-rated (Parker et al., 1991).
MHI: Mental Health Inventory – Consumer-rated (Veit and Ware, 1983).
BASIS-32: Behaviour and Symptom Identification Scale – Consumer-rated (Eisen et al., 2000).
K-10+: Kessler 10 Plus – Consumer-rated (Kessler et al., 2002).
HoNOSCA: Health of the Nation Outcome Scales for Children and Adolescents – Clinician-rated (Gowers et al., 1999).
CGAS: Children's Global Assessment Scale – Clinician-rated (Schaffer et al., 1983).
SDQ: Strengths and Difficulties Questionnaire (Goodman, 1997).
HoNOS65+: Health of the Nation Outcome Scales 65+ (Clinician-rated) (Burns et al., 1999).
RUG-ADL: Resource Utilisation Groups – Activities of Daily Living (Clinician-rated) (Fries et al., 1994).

Table adapted from Department of Health and Ageing (2003).

being used for the purpose that was originally envisaged under the National Mental Health Policy which related to monitoring the quality and effectiveness of services.

Having said this, the completion rates for outcome measures vary. In the 2006/07 financial year (the year for which the most recent reliable data are available), data were available from a total of 336,492 collection occasions across all target age groups and mental health service settings (Burgess and Pirkis, 2008). The completeness of the outcome measures rated at these collection occasions was high for the HoNOS family of measures, but lower for other clinician-rated measures and particularly low for consumer-rated measures (see Table 2.2) (Burgess and Pirkis, 2008).

Australian clinicians and consumers have expressed a range of views about the benefits and disadvantages of routine outcome measurement (a comprehensive review of the international literature on stakeholders' views of routine outcome measurement can be found elsewhere in this volume). A narrative review of a number of studies examining the attitudes of clinicians to routine outcome measurement in Australia identified some common concerns in relation to the psychometric properties and relevance of the instruments themselves, the availability of appropriate information technology, the time demands imposed, a suspicion of the underlying motivations behind the roll-out of routine outcome measurement, and their own competence and confidence in using outcome data (Callaly et al., 2006). This is not to say that all clinicians share these concerns; in fact views are quite mixed. A recent qualitative study of the attitudes of 83 clinicians from one Australian service found roughly equal numbers of positive and negative observations about the value of the existing suite of outcome measures (Callaly et al., 2006). Consumers also hold a range of views, many of which are positive. A recent study involving structured interviews with 50 consumers from one Victorian service found that consumers generally saw the benefits of routine outcome measurement and believed that it leads to improved care, particularly in circumstances where it encourages dialogue between clinicians and consumers (Guthrie et al., 2008).

Best practice at a local level: supporting the inclusion of a consumer-rated measure in routine clinical practice

An example of best practice in terms of embedding routine outcome measurement in clinical practice comes from Barwon Health: Mental Health, in Victoria. Barwon Health has been supporting the inclusion of outcome measure ratings in everyday clinical practice since 1996, when it was one of the five pilot agencies to trial the use of HoNOS in Victoria (see above). Barwon Health provides a comprehensive range of mental health services for a population of approximately 270,000 living in and around the city of Geelong. Early on, there was a realization that outcome measurement needed to be embedded in routine paperwork and that immediate feedback to clinicians was important if there was to be a chance of including discussion about ratings in everyday clinical practice. Software was developed by Barwon Health to collect data and give graphical feedback which enabled clinicians to compare current ratings for a given consumer with previous ratings for that consumer, and with ratings for others being cared for by the service.

Since 1996, consumers have been included in planning and they have consistently emphasized the view that the consumer-rated measure (the Behaviour and Symptom Identification Scale, or BASIS-32 (Eisen et al., 2000), in Victoria) is the measure that can be most valuable, from the consumer's perspective, in supporting improved dialogue between the consumer and the clinician. In planning, the leadership at Barwon Health have emphasized the

Table 2.2 Percentage of collection occasions at which outcome data were collected under the NOCC protocol, 2006/07

		Inpatient			Community residential			Ambulatory		
		Admission	Review	Discharge	Admission	Review	Discharge	Admission	Review	Discharge
Adults	HoNOS	89	83	84	90	95	70	87	91	59
	LSP-16	N/A	N/A	N/A	25	89	40	N/A	82	43
	MHI or BASIS-32 or K-10+	N/A	N/A	N/A	42	56	22	25	28	7
Children and adolescents	HoNOSCA	86	86	78	91	90	42	91	86	55
	CGAS	85	83	N/A	85	95	N/A	91	88	N/A
	SDQ-PC[a]	58	85	15	30	33	0	51	27	9
	SDQ-PY[b]	20	12	5	58	6	5	43	20	6
	SDQ-YR[c]	15	16	5	58	6	16	42	20	6
Older persons	HoNOS65+	92	97	89	86	98	57	94	95	82
	LSP-16	N/A	N/A	N/A	28	96	40	N/A	78	63
	RUG-ADL	85	73	N/A	79	90	N/A	N/A	N/A	N/A
	MHI or BASIS-32 or K-10+	N/A	N/A	N/A	26	23	4	10	14	5

Table adapted from Burgess and Pirkis (2008).
[a]Parent-rated version of the SDQ for children aged 4–10 years.
[b]Parent-rated version of the SDQ for adolescents aged 11–17 years.
[c]Consumer-rated version of the SDQ for adolescents aged 11–17 years.

consumer-rated measure. The patient records system has been redesigned to ensure that a record is kept of whether the clinician offers the consumer the BASIS-32 to complete, whether this offer is accepted by the consumer and, if not, the consumer's reasons for choosing not to complete the measure. This dimension of dialogue with consumers is emphasized in staff orientation and ongoing education. In addition, written material is given to each consumer advising him or her of the opportunity to be involved in giving feedback to their clinician using the consumer-rated outcome measure. Posters have been placed in all consumer areas advising them of this opportunity. The result is that 60–70% of all consumers across the service, including older consumers, complete the BASIS-32 – a figure considerably higher than that found nationally (see Table 2.2).

Where to from here?

Continued investment in routine outcome measurement is required in order for Australia to capitalize on the achievements made so far. Under the Second National Mental Health Plan, the Australian Government provided $37 million to states and territories for routine outcome measurement; under the Third National Mental Health Plan, it provided a further $15 million, with the requirement that recipient jurisdictions had to match each dollar they received. Ongoing backing of a similar magnitude will be necessary to ensure that routine outcome measurement doesn't falter.

The outcome measurement enterprise must be given the opportunity to continue to evolve if it is to achieve maximum value. In particular, further emphasis must be given to ensuring its clinical utility at a local level (Callaly and Hallebone, 2001). AMHOCN has made inroads in this regard with, for example, the wDST, the preliminary development of the library of clinical prompts, and training initiatives that focus on how outcome data can inform clinical practice. More needs to be done, however, in order to address the criticism made by some commentators that services are not yet using outcome data to guide treatment options and other clinical decisions (Andrews and Page, 2005).

Outcome measurement has not yet achieved its goal of providing a means by which services can compare themselves with their peers with a view to learning from each other. AMHOCN has taken some steps in this regard, exploring methods of grouping services into peer categories and means of catering for the case complexity of individual consumers, in order to facilitate like-with-like comparisons and benchmarking exercises (Burgess and Pirkis, 2009). Again, further work is required in this area in order for outcome measurement to provide the necessary information to improve overall service quality.

It is also timely to review some of the existing 'givens' that underpin mental health outcome measurement in Australia. For example, the NOCC suite of measures should be revisited to ensure that the outcomes being measured are those which are of the greatest importance to stakeholders. Consideration should also be given to whether these measures cater for the diversity of the Australian population. For example, there is a question as to whether they are appropriate for consumers from culturally and linguistically diverse backgrounds. Some forays have been made into this area (Queensland Transcultural Mental Health Centre, 2005), but there is still much to be done. Similarly, the appropriateness of the measures for consumers of Aboriginal and Torres Strait Islander descent requires further attention. Again, some efforts have been made in this regard (described in Chapter 14 by Tricia Nagel and Tom Trauer), but much remains to be tackled. The idea of adding a carer measure to the NOCC suite should also be further explored (Dare et al., 2007).

A comment on mental health outcome measurement in the private sector

The majority of this chapter has focused on mental health outcome measurement in Australia's public-sector mental health services which are the responsibility of state and territory governments and are free at the point of contact to consumers. Before concluding, it is worth making a comment on mental health outcome measurement in Australia's private sector, and specifically in private hospitals which offer mental health services. These are run by private organizations and their services may be paid for by a combination of public and private health insurance and out-of-pocket payments by consumers.

Like the public sector, the private sector is also investing in mental health outcome measurement. The Private Mental Health Alliance, a collaboration between the major stakeholders who fund and provide mental health services in the private sector, is responsible for this. Over three-quarters of private hospitals with psychiatric beds are collecting the clinician-rated HoNOS and the consumer-rated Mental Health Questionnaire (MHQ-14) (Ware and Sherbourne, 1992) at admission and discharge, according to a protocol outlined in the National Model for the Collection and Analysis of a Minimum Data Set with Outcome Measures for Private Hospital-based Psychiatric Services (Morris-Yates and The Strategic Planning Group for Private Psychiatric Services Data Collection and Analysis Working Group, 2000). Data are entered into a system known as the Centralized Data Management Service, and reported back to the hospitals and to private health insurers on a quarterly basis. Further detail on the activities of the private sector in this area can be found in Chapter 15 by Allen Morris-Yates and Andrew Page.

Conclusion

To conclude, Australia has made great strides in introducing routine outcome measurement to public-sector inpatient and community services across the nation. Australia's experiences provide some lessons for other countries undertaking a similar exercise. Embedding routine outcome measurement into service culture does not happen overnight: it is an evolutionary process. It cannot happen without appropriate policy direction, sufficient resourcing and strong leadership. Perhaps most importantly, it must be valued by clinicians and consumers. If these conditions are in place, routine outcome measurement can strengthen service quality.

Acknowledgements

The authors would like to thank Bill Buckingham, Philip Burgess and Tim Coombs for offering advice on this chapter.

References

Andrews, G. and Page, A. C. (2005). Outcome measurement, outcome management and monitoring. *Australian and New Zealand Journal of Psychiatry*, **39**, 649–51.

Andrews, G., Peters, L. and Teesson, M. (1994). *The Measurement of Consumer Outcome in Mental Health: a Report to the National* *Mental Health Information Strategy Committee*. Sydney: Clinical Research Unit for Anxiety Disorders.

Australian Health Ministers (1992a). *National Mental Health Plan*. Canberra: Australian Government Publishing Service.

Australian Health Ministers (1992b). *National Mental Health Policy*. Canberra: Australian Government Publishing Service.

Australian Health Ministers (1998). *Second National Mental Health Plan*. Canberra.

Australian Health Ministers (2003). *National Mental Health Plan 2003–2008*. Canberra.

Bickman, L., Nurcombe, B., Townsend, C., et al. (1999). *Consumer Measurement Systems for Child and Adolescent Mental Health*. Canberra: Department of Health and Aged Care.

Burgess, P. and Pirkis, J. (2008). *Overview of 2006–2007 MH-NOCC Data: Technical and Conceptual Issues*. Brisbane.

Burgess, P. and Pirkis, J. (2009). *Case Complexity Adjustment and Mental Health Outcomes: Conceptual issues*. Brisbane: Australian Mental Health Outcomes and Classification Network.

Burgess, P., Pirkis, J., Buckingham, W., Eagar, K. and Solomon, S. (1999). Developing a casemix classification for mental health. *Casemix Quarterly*, **1**, 4–20.

Burgess, P., Pirkis, J. and Coombs, T. (2006). Do adults in contact with Australia's public sector mental health services get better? *Australia and New Zealand Health Policy*, **3**, 9.

Burgess, P., Pirkis, J. and Coombs, T. (2009a). Modelling candidate effectiveness indicators for mental health services. *Australian and New Zealand Journal of Psychiatry*, **43**, 531–8.

Burgess, P., Trauer, T., Coombs, T., McKay, R. and Pirkis, J. (2009b). What does 'clinical significance' mean in the context of the Health of the Nation Outcome Scales? *Australasian Psychiatry*, **17**, 141–8.

Burns, A., Beevor, A., Lelliott, P., et al. (1999). Health of the Nation Outcome Scales for elderly people (HoNOS 65+). Glossary for HoNOS 65+ score sheet. *British Journal of Psychiatry*, **174**, 435–8.

Callaly, T. and Hallebone, E. L. (2001). Introducing the routine use of outcomes measurement to mental health services. *Australian Health Review*, **24**, 43–50.

Callaly, T., Hyland, M., Coombs, T. and Trauer, T. (2006). Routine outcome measurement in public mental health – results of a clinician survey. *Australian Health Review*, **30**, 164–73.

Dare, A., Hardy, J., Burgess, P., et al. (2007). *Carer Outcome Measurement in Mental Health Services: Scoping the Field*. Melbourne/Brisbane/Sydney.

Department of Health and Aged Care (1999). *Mental Health Information Development: National Information Priorities and Strategies under the Second National Mental Health Plan 1998–2003*, 1st edn. Canberra.

Department of Health and Ageing (2003). *Mental Health National Outcomes and Casemix Collection: Technical Specification of State and Territory Reporting Requirements for the Outcomes and Casemix components of 'Agreed Data' (Version 1.50)*. Canberra.

Eisen, S. V., Dickey, B. and Sederer, L. I. (2000). A self-report symptom and problem rating scale to increase inpatients' involvement in treatment. *Psychiatric Services*, **51**, 349–53.

Fries, B. E., Schneider, D. P., Foley, W. J., et al. (1994). Refining a case-mix measure for nursing homes: resource utilization groups (RUG-III). *Medical Care*, **32**, 668–85.

Goodman, R. (1997). The Strengths and Difficulties Questionnaire: a research note. *Journal of Child Psychology and Psychiatry*, **38**, 581–6.

Gowers, S. G., Harrington, R. C., Whitton, A., et al. (1999). Brief scale for measuring the outcomes of emotional and behavioural disorders in children. Health of the Nation Outcome Scales for Children and Adolescents (HoNOSCA). *British Journal of Psychiatry*, **174**, 413–16.

Guthrie, D., McIntosh, M., Callaly, T., Trauer, T. and Coombs, T. (2008). Consumer attitudes towards the use of routine outcome measures in a public mental health service: a consumer-driven study. *International Journal of Mental Health Nursing*, **17**, 92–7.

Kessler, R. C., Andrews, G., Colpe, L. J., et al. (2002). Short screening scales to monitor population prevalences and trends in non-specific psychological distress. *Psychological Medicine*, **32**, 959–76.

McKay, R., Coombs, T., Burgess, P., et al. (2008). Development of Clinical Prompts to Enhance Decision Support Tools Related to the National Outcomes and Casemix Collection (Version 1.0), Brisbane/Sydney/Melbourne.

Morris-Yates, A. and The Strategic Planning Group for Private Psychiatric Services Data Collection and Analysis Working Group (2000). *A National Model for the Collection and Analysis of a Minimum Data Set with Outcome Measurement for Private, Hospital-based, Psychiatric Services.* Canberra: Commonwealth of Australia.

Parker, G., Rosen, A., Emdur, N. and Hadzi-Pavlovic, D. (1991). The Life Skills Profile: psychometric properties of a measure assessing function and disability in schizophrenia. *Acta Psychiatrica Scandinavica*, **83**, 145–52.

Pirkis, J., Burgess, P., Coombs, T., et al. (2005). Routine measurement of outcomes in Australia's public sector mental health services. *Australia and New Zealand Health Policy*, **2**, 8.

Queensland Transcultural Mental Health Centre (2005). *Transcultural Applications of Mental Health Outcome Measures.* Brisbane.

Schaffer, D., Gould, M. S., Brasic, J., et al. (1983). A children's global assessment scale (CGAS). *Archives of General Psychiatry*, **40**, 1228–31.

Slade, M. (2002). Routine outcome assessment in mental health services. *Psychological Medicine*, **32**, 1339–43.

Stedman, T., Yellowlees, P., Mellsop, G., Clarke, R. and Drake, S. (1997). *Measuring Consumer Outcomes in Mental Health: Field Testing of Selected Measures of Consumer Outcomes in Mental Health.* Canberra: Department of Health and Aged Care.

Trauer, T., Callaly, T., Hantz, P., et al. (1999). Health of the Nation Outcome Scales (HoNOS): results of the Victorian field trial. *British Journal of Psychiatry*, **174**, 380–8.

Veit, C. T. and Ware, J. E. (1983). The structure of psychological distress and well-being in general populations. *Journal of Consulting and Clinical Psychology*, **51**, 730–42.

Ware, J. E. and Sherbourne, C. D. (1992). The MOS 36-item Short Form Health Status Survey (SF-36): I. Conceptual framework and item selection. *Medical Care*, **30**, 473–83.

Wing, J. K., Beevor, A. S., Curtis, R. H., et al. (1998). Health of the Nation Outcome Scales (HoNOS). Research and Development. *British Journal of Psychiatry*, **172**, 11–18.

Outcome Measurement around the World

Outcome measures in New Zealand

Graham Mellsop and Mark Smith

Introduction

New Zealand is a relatively small country, with approximately four million people, and is ethnically diverse, with 15% Maori, 5% Pacific Island, 70% European and 10% other – including a sizable Asian population. Although New Zealand has a strong tradition of publicly funded mental health services, much of this is delivered through non-government organizations (NGOs). Approximately 30% of New Zealand's services are delivered in this way, compared with 5% in Australia.

This chapter will provide a chronology of the development of outcome measurement in New Zealand. It will indicate the way that this development has been implemented and the strategies for developing utility from this outcome information. We will also indicate anticipated future directions in outcome measurement and the overall strengths and weaknesses of the New Zealand experience.

The chronology

While clinicians and service users have always had an interest in the outcome of their interactions (Mellsop and Wilson, 2006), in New Zealand that area has been the focus of particular leadership, policy and mental health service activities in the last 10 years (Peters, 1994, Mental Health Commission, 1998, Mellsop and O'Brien, 1999, Krieble, 2003, Eagar et al., 2004, Trauer et al., 2006). The commitment of the Mental Health community in New Zealand was first translated into action when the Ministry of Health funded the national Classification and Outcome Study (CAOS). While the first aim of this large study of approximately 18,000 episodes of care was to develop a national casemix classification (Gaines et al., 2003), the second aim was to implement the routine use of selected outcome measures in the one-third of New Zealand's psychiatric services which participated during a six-month study period in 2002 (Eagar et al., 2004, 2005). For that study the choice of outcome measures was heavily influenced by previous Australian work (Andrews et al., 1994, Stedman et al., 1997, Buckingham et al., 1998). The most central measure used was the Health of the Nation Outcome Scales (HoNOS, Wing et al., 1998).

That large and rich database resulted in a number of feedback exercises conducted under the auspices of the Mental Health Standard Measures of Assessment and Recovery (MH-SMART) Programme, which is now called Te Pou (or the National Centre for Mental Health Research, Information and Workforce Development) as well as some separate analyses which utilized the outcome measurement data (Eagar et al., 2004, 2005, Trauer et al., 2006, Mellsop and Smith, 2008, Mellsop et al., 2008).

Under Ministry of Health leadership, the particular post-CAOS development was the decision to have a National Outcome Usage Plan, which would be known as MH-SMART (see above). The first major principle adopted by the relevant working party was to speak of

Outcome Measurement in Mental Health: Theory and Practice, ed. Tom Trauer. Published by Cambridge University Press.

standardized assessments, rather than outcome measures. A commitment was developed to the concept that routine use of standardized and quantified assessments would allow status comparisons over time and so be usable as measures of progress or outcome.

The planning processes for MH-SMART also specified that over a period of years, New Zealand would implement the usage of five different outcome domains:

1. *A measure of symptomatology.* HoNOS was chosen as the preferred measure and later in its various other forms, such as for children, older persons, forensic and intellectually disabled.

2. *A Maori culturally specific measure.* Considerable resources have been put into developing an instrument (Hua Oranga, Kingi and Durie, 2000) which has two particular, novel, characteristics. Firstly it allows for a triangulation through three versions, completed by the consumer, the family and the clinician. Secondly it covers a broader range of consumer characteristics, including cultural-specific issues, functionality, spirituality and physical health. This is all explicitly within the framing of the Maori concept of health (Durie, 1994).

3. *An alcohol and drug tool.* The Alcohol and Drug Outcome Project Tool (known as ADOPT ii) is specific to the needs of drug and alcohol services. This outcome measurement tool has been specifically developed by New Zealand researchers. Adopt ii is the revised version of an earlier Adopt i version. This has completed the research phase though still technically under development, and will be known as ADOM (alcohol and drug outcome measurement).

4. *A consumer-completed instrument.* The New Zealand-based consumer review group, after an exhaustive international literature review, concluded there were no instruments available which covered the 12 domains they regarded as essential (Gordon et al., 2004). Subsequently, a related group drafted a very comprehensive instrument (Taku Reo – Taku Mauri Ora; My voice my life) which covers the 12 domains. Development of this instrument continues.

5. *A measure of functioning.* This has proved to be very contentious. New Zealand consumers were resistant to using Life Skills Profile (LSP-16), which had been developed and used in Australia (Rosen et al., 1989, Buckingham et al., 1998). A final decision has not yet been made, but an investigative group specified the domains that should be covered and recommended the Personal and Social Performance scale (PSP, Morosini et al., 2000) as the best available compromise (Lutchman et al., 2007). It was considered potentially easier to persuade clinicians to use this measure, as it was similar to the more widely used GAF of DSM-IV (Mellsop et al., 2007), without the references to psychopathology. One of the currently unresolved issues in New Zealand is whether there can be one recommended measure of functioning or whether there needs to be several recommended for use depending on the context.

The implementation

For most of the new millennium there has been a national structure designed to oversee the introduction of the standardized assessment measures and their development. It has continued to be overseen and directed at a policy level and financed at a budgetary level by the Ministry of Health, with Te Pou as the implementation arm (see Te Pou website, www.tepou.co.nz). The Ministry and Te Pou see their roles as complementary. They have put in place and utilized a national network of resource people, called Site Co-ordinators, in each of the 21 District Health Boards (DHBs). The availability of these site co-ordinators has been crucial to obtaining relatively high compliance rates with HoNOS collections.

There are a number of other implementation strategies which have been adopted in New Zealand. These are:

(a) *An outcome test project.* Starting in 2006, Te Pou developed a test project for outcomes data collecting HoNOS, HoNOSCA and HoNOS 65+ data. This involved working closely with six District Health Boards, latterly five. *SMART on line* was an online mechanism by which outcomes data were passed on to Te Pou. This approach generated a number of standard outcome reports (see the section on 'Developing utility').

(b) *Ongoing training in outcomes.* Te Pou have continued to provide basic MH-SMART training using a centralized 'Train the Trainer' model, in conjunction with refresher training and latterly online training in HoNOS.

(c) *Attempting to obtain wide stakeholder buy-in.* One of the defining approaches adopted by New Zealand has been the attempt to obtain wide stakeholder buy-in. This has particularly been sought in relation to cultural protocols (tikanga), and the clinical, managerial, service user and families' perspectives. This has met with mixed success, as will be discussed later.

Developing utility

New Zealand has attempted to provide utility to its outcome measurement by four main approaches. This is still work in progress. Much of its eventual success will depend on the outcome reports and the explanatory and interpretive material around these being made widely available.

(a) The mental health information system has been revamped to include outcomes information in conjunction with activity information, in line with the national mental health information strategy and implementation plan (Ministry of Health, 2005, 2006). This new mental health information system – called PRIMHD (Programme for the Implementation of Mental Health Data) – replaced MHINC (Mental Health Information National Collection) and went live on 1 July 2008. The PRIMHD reports, which will include outcomes data analyses, will, it is hoped, have significant utility for the sector.

(b) Te Pou has developed an outcomes analytical tool, initially called the Decision Support System (DSS) but now rebranded as the MHOSys (Mental Health Outcomes System) tool. This sophisticated electronic tool is able to sort and order outcome information in many different ways as a means of generating outcome reports. The standard outcome reports developed in the outcomes test project used a number of reporting areas: number and percentage of service users with clinically significant items (where clinically significant is defined as any item rating at 2 or above on the HoNOS(CA) outcome measure scales), total scores, subscales and an index of severity. With the development of PRIMHD the standing reports developed using MHOSys in Te Pou will be moved to the Ministry for standard order reports. There is, however, the possibility that ad hoc reporting will continue using MHOSys.

(c) There has been an attempt to provide national training in information utility aimed at the clinical level. This training has focused on providing context to the training, explaining the content of PRIMHD, showing how outcome measures, such as HoNOS, could be integrated into clinical teams and providing training in understanding graphs, tables and statistics. Te Pou (see www.tepou.co.nz) has developed a trainers' forum for trainers to continue to be resourced outside the training sessions and various e-tools, such as access to an Outcome Graph Builder (OGB) for developing simple graphs based on HoNOS, HoNOSCA and HoNOS 65+ data.

(d) Connected to the need to obtain good stakeholder buy-in, there has been a strong emphasis upon working with Maori and ensuring that training vignettes and material accurately reflects Maori protocol, customs and beliefs.

Future developments

Further developments for outcome measurement in New Zealand are planned. We will mention four:

(a) *PRIMHD reporting.* At the time of writing the Ministry of Health and Te Pou have developed eight standard outcome reports based on HoNOS, HoNOSCA and HoNOS 65+ data inputs. These outcome reports consist of compliance/validation reports, total score reports, percentage and number of service users with clinically significant items reports, clinically significant items based on the sub-scales and index of severity reports. There are plans to disseminate these reports through the Ministry and Te Pou websites as they become available. There are also plans to produce integrated outcome and activity reports – for example – on seclusion activity data and standardized assessment data when this becomes possible.

(b) *Introduction of further measures.* New Zealand intends to introduce further measures over the next few years, in line with the different outcome domains referred to above.

(c) *Benchmarking and casemix.* New Zealand intends to use outcome reporting for casemix and benchmarking purposes. Initially the plan is to perform casemix analyses on outcome (standardized assessment) data obtained from the test project, but eventually the plan would be to undertake casemix adjustment of PRIMHD data, using the 42-class system developed in the CAOS study (Eagar et al., 2004). Such casemix work will make possible the benchmarking of data from across the country to compare DHB and service performance, using the Key Performance Indicators (Counties Manukau District Health Board, 2007).

(d) *Dashboard reporting.* New Zealand is keen to develop clinical dashboard reporting (where a clinical dashboard is a 'visual interface that provides at-a-glance views into key measures relevant to a particular objective or business process. Dashboards contain predetermined conclusions that relieve the end user from performing their own analysis') (Alexander, 2008) at all the information levels as a way of presenting information in ways which are user-friendly and approachable for service users, clinicians and managers. New Zealand has developed a Data Use Guidelines document, which makes this recommendation. This document is available from the Te Pou website.

Strengths and weaknesses of the New Zealand experience

The main strength of the New Zealand experience is that there has been an attempt to provide standardized assessments which engage with the mental health sector. This engagement has seen cultural-, service- and clinician-specific attempts to provide utility for outcome meas-urement. Additionally the use of key Site Co-ordinators to provide leadership at a local level in terms of outcomes has proven to be indispensable. However, the results have fallen well short of the aims, hopes and expectations, for three particular reasons.

First, the appropriate information technology (IT) infrastructure for saving the data and providing feedback in a timely and effective fashion for utilization and service continuous improvement activities has so far often not been in place. The lack of IT infrastructure has probably been a significant contributor to the low priority given to HoNOS form completion by clinicians.

Second, there has been a high degree of clinician (particularly psychiatrist) resistance. This has not been helped by the variability in quality and quantity of relevant education.

Third, many of New Zealand's mental health service providers now give limited feedback at a service level on HoNOS score changes for adult mental health service users but there is no agreed national software. Essentially this has meant not only much slower progress than initially envisaged, but a significant loss of the initial goodwill demonstrated in the CAOS study, where completion rates for the outcome measures were of the order of 96%. Now completion rates are more in the 10–80% range, depending on service type. The lack of closure on choice of cultural measure, consumer-rated measure or functionality measure is also a source of frustration to the national oversight of the MH-SMART Programme, but quite probably a relief to the service providers, who are often heard expressing the view that they are increasingly distracted in their work by the proliferation of form-filling, which they see as providing little benefit to service users' progress through the mental health systems.

Conclusion

New Zealand has had a nationally led project which has been policy, rather than legislatively, driven. Its particular (positive) idiosyncrasy has been the commitment to the standardized assessment concept, rather than the problematic word of 'outcomes'. It has had a national plan and continues to have an evolving, national co-ordinating structure (see Te Pou website, www.tepou.co.nz).

Delivery, consistent with the initial aims of utilizing the standardized assessments for quality improvement activities, has been particularly inhibited by the lack of national or locally available IT support systems. Clinical staff participation, in the sense of formal assessment completion rates, has been significantly sub-optimal. That issue is only likely to be improved by co-ordinated education, appropriate IT infrastructure support, and clinical leadership on the essential contributions of the MH-SMART approach to improving mental health services effectiveness and efficiency.

References

Alexander, M. (2008). *Excel 2007-Dashboards & Reports for Dummies*. Oxford: John Wiley.

Andrews, G., Peters, L. and Teesson, M. (1994). *The Measurement of Consumer Outcome in Mental Health: a Report to the National Mental Health Information Strategy Committee*. Sydney: Clinical Research Unit for Anxiety Disorders.

Buckingham, W., Burgess, P., Solomon, S., Pirkis, J. and Eagar, K. (1998). *Developing a Casemix Classification for Mental Health Services*. Canberra: Department of Health and Ageing.

Counties Manukau District Health Board (2007). *Report on The key Performance Indicator Framework for New Zealand Mental Health and Addiction Services*. Counties Manukau, New Zealand: Counties Manukau District Health Board.

Durie, M. (1994). *Maori Health Perspectives. Maori Health Development*. Auckland: Oxford University Press.

Eagar, K., Gaines, P., Burgess, P., et al. (2004). Developing a New Zealand casemix classification for Mental Health Services. *World Psychiatry*, 172–7.

Eagar, K., Trauer, T. and Mellsop, G. (2005). Performance of routine outcome measures in adult mental health care. *Australian and New Zealand Journal of Psychiatry*, **39**, 713–18.

Gaines, P., Bower, A., Buckingham, W., et al. (2003). *New Zealand Mental Health Classification and Outcomes Study: Final Report.* Auckland: Health Research Council of New Zealand.

Gordon, S., Ellis, P., Haggerty, C., et al. (2004). *Preliminary work towards the development of a self-assessed measure of consumer outcome.* Auckland: Health Research Council of New Zealand.

Kingi, T. K. and Durie, M. (2000). *'Hua Oranga' A Maori Measure of Mental Health Outcome.* Palmerston North: Te Pūmanawa Hauora, School of Māori Studies, Massey University.

Krieble, T. (2003). *Towards an outcome-based mental health policy for New Zealand. Australasian Psychiatry*, **11**, S78–S82.

Lutchman, R., Tait, H., Aitchison, R. and Mellsop, G. W. (2007). In search of a standardised comprehensive assessment of functionality. *New Zealand Journal of Occupational Therapy*, **54**, 33–8.

Mellsop, G. and Smith, B. (2008). Reflections on masculinity, culture and the diagnosis of depression. *Australian and New Zealand Journal of Psychiatry*, **41**, 850–3.

Mellsop, G. and Wilson, J. (2006). Outcome measures in mental health services: Humpty Dumpty is alive and well. *Australasian Psychiatry*, **14**, 137–40.

Mellsop, G. W. and O'Brien, G. (1999). *Outcomes Summary Report.* Mental Health Research and Development Strategy Project Report to the Health Research Council of New Zealand. Wellington, New Zealand.

Mellsop, G. W., Robinson, G. and Dutu, G. (2007). New Zealand psychiatrist views on global features of ICD-10 and DSM-IV.

Australian and New Zealand Journal of Psychiatry, **41**, 157–65.

Mellsop, G. W., Dutu, G. and El Badri, S. (2008). CAOS contribution to understanding cultural/ethnic differences in the prevalence of bipolar affective disorder in New Zealand. *Australian and New Zealand Journal of Psychiatry*, **41**, 392–6.

Mental Health Commission (1998). *Blueprint for Mental Health Services for New Zealand.* Wellington: Mental Health Commission.

Ministry of Health (2005). *National mental health information strategy.* Wellington: Ministry of Health.

Ministry of Health (2006). *National mental health implementation plan*, Wellington: Ministry of Health.

Morosini, P. -L., Magliano, L., Brambilla, L., Ugolini, S. and Pioli, R. (2000). Development, reliability and acceptability of a new version of the DSMIV Social and Occupational Functioning Assessment Scale (SOFAS) to assess routine social funtioning. *Acta Psychiatrica Scandinavica*, **101**, 323–9.

Peters, J. (1994). *Performance and outcome indicators in mental health service: A review of the literature. A report prepared for the Ministry of Health.* Wellington: Ministry of Health.

Rosen, A., Hadzi-Pavlovic, D. and Parker, G. (1989). The Life Skills Profile: a measure assessing function and disability in schizophrenia. *Schizophrenia Bulletin*, **15**, 325–37.

Stedman, T., Yellowlees, P., Mellsop, G., Clarke, R. and Drake, S. (1997). *Measuring Consumer Outcomes in Mental Health.* Canberra: Department of Health and Aged Care.

Trauer, T., Eagar, K. and Mellsop, G. (2006). Ethnicity, deprivation and mental health outcomes. *Australian Health Review*, **30**, 310–21.

Wing, J. K., Beevor, A. S., Curtis, R. H., et al. (1998). Health of the Nation Outcome Scales (HoNOS). Research and Development. *British Journal of Psychiatry*, **172**, 11–18.

Outcome measurement in England

Mike Slade

History and legislative framework

Since the inception of the National Health Service (NHS) in 1948, a key policy driver has been establishing the value-for-money offered from this centrally funded service. This has happened in stages, mapping on to a focus on inputs, processes and outcomes (Thornicroft and Tansella, 1999).

For the first 40 years of the NHS, effort was focused on establishing the inputs. Inputs involved considering the actual expenditure, with the goal of allocating resources to match supply with demand through the use of deprivation indices, initially based on general practitioner consensus about patient characteristics predictive of psychiatric admission (Jarman, 1983), and more recently on statistical models quantifying the relationship between social variables measured in censuses and service use (Glover et al., 1998). However, the organization of the NHS until 1991 was into 14 regional-level health care authorities with a strategic rather than managerial remit (Slade and Glover, 2001). This changed in the early 1990s, with the imposition of the market structure onto the NHS, involving the devolution to more local authorities of administrative and financial responsibility, and the forcible introduction of general management. The result of this upheaval was a new focus on productivity.

A defining piece of legislation was the NHS and Community Care Act (Department of Health, 1990) which was passed into law in 1990, and came into force in 1993. The act introduced an internal market into the supply of healthcare, positioning the state as an enabler rather than a supplier of health and social care provision. Furthermore, the Act imposed a duty on Local Authorities to assess people for social care and support, thus ensuring that people with mental health problems can access a full range of community care for both health and social needs. This approach was reinforced in the Mental Health National Service Framework (1999) (Department of Health, 1999), which set standards for seven areas of mental health services for adults of working age (i.e. aged 16–65). Other legislation mandated that specific types of teams be introduced nationally, such as the 335 crisis response teams required by the NHS Plan (2000) (Department of Health, 2000). The consequent focus since the 1990s has been on the structures and processes which allow an internal market to operate, integrated health and social care to be provided, and specific types of mandated teams to be available.

Outcome measurement in England

Only in the past decade has outcome – *the effect on patients' health status that is attributable to an intervention* (Andrews et al., 1994) – become a major focus of effort. The Children's National Service Framework identifies the need for routine evaluation in Child and Adolescent Mental Health Services (CAMHS), and the CAMHS Outcome Research Consortium (CORC) is a voluntary collaboration of CAMHS who have agreed common measures, a protocol and common dataset (www.corc.uk.net). The agreed measures are the Strengths and Difficulties

Outcome Measurement in Mental Health: Theory and Practice, ed. Tom Trauer. Published by Cambridge University Press.
© Cambridge University Press 2010.

Questionnaire (SDQ) completed by referred children aged 11–16 and parents of children aged 3–16 before the first meeting and at 6 months after their first appointment, the Children's Global Assessment Scale (C-GAS), completed by clinicians for all age groups after the first meeting and 6 months later, and the Commission for Health Improvement (CHI) experience of service questionnaire (ESQ), completed by everyone aged 9 and over at 6 months after the first appointment (Care Services Improvement Partnership, 2006).

For adults, there has been a growing focus on central collection of minimum outcome data (Glover, 1997), leading to an information strategy specific to mental health (Department of Health, 2001). This underpinned the Mental Health Minimum Dataset, which was introduced in 2000 and became mandatory in 2003. This introduced a requirement for quarterly returns from all adult and older adult mental health services, structured around the clinical process – what is termed a mental health care spell (MHCS) – and with mandatory use of the Health of the Nation Outcome Scales (HoNOS, Wing et al., 1998) (or HoNOS 65+ for older adults) with all patients. The returns need to provide (for each MHCS of each patient) the date and rating of the first, worst, best and most recent HoNOS administration. The aim was explicit: 'The prime purpose of the data set is to provide local clinicians and managers with better quality information for clinical audit, and service planning and management' (www.ic.nhs.uk/services/datasets/dataset-list/mental-health).

In retrospect, there are a number of problems with this approach.

1. No funding was allocated – implementation was to be undertaken within existing service provider resources.
2. The MHMDS was in addition to, rather than replacing, other national reporting requirements: 'the collection of the Mental Health Minimum Data Set does not replace any other collection of mental health data such as the Admitted Patient Care Commissioning Data Set Type Detained and/or Long Term Psychiatric Census, which should continue to be collected' (www.ic.nhs.uk/services/datasets/dataset-list/mental-health).
3. Whilst HoNOS training was mandatory for anyone using the measure, there was no national training strategy. Provider services were expected to develop in-house training capacity, and cascade training throughout the organization. Implementation was predictably patchy, of uneven quality and not always sustained.
4. There was no central information technology (IT) strategy. Mental health providers use a wide variety of information systems, so resources were needed from each service to develop and evaluate IT systems which supported rather than hindered outcome measurement.
5. The decision to use HoNOS was made centrally using an undisclosed process which did not involve widespread consultation. This meant that the people who had to do the work – mental health professionals who were being asked to complete the HoNOS – had no sense of ownership of the initiative.
6. The broader health and social care economy is in constant flux, making this or any other initiative difficult to sustain. This inevitably leads in large systems to un-joined-up thinking, with one policy initiative having unintended consequences for another. For example, mental health services have increasingly been attaining 'Foundation Trust' status, with increasing autonomy in their clinical and financial operations. What has never been clear is the extent to which MHMDS requirements apply to Foundation Trusts, and this ambiguity has engendered a sense that HoNOS completion is 'yesterday's target'.
7. Perhaps most compellingly, the aim of the MHMDS (as stated earlier) did not mesh with the basic orientation of most clinicians. Whereas managers, service planners and

policy-makers are highly interested in aggregated population-level information, most clinicians are highly interested in individual patient care. When research suggesting limited inter-rater reliability for HoNOS emerged (Amin et al., 1999, Brooks, 2000, Rock and Preston, 2001), and when HoNOS was found not, in general, to be useful for informing clinical decision-making, implementation was always going to be problematic.

There are no published data on MHMDS completion levels for HoNOS in either academic journals or the MHDMS web-site (www.mhmdsonline.ic.nhs.uk). Apart from a few local initiatives led by HoNOS champions (Macdonald, 2002), the full roll-out of HoNOS has not been successful.

Recent initiatives

In the light of this emerging experience, the Care Services Improvement Partnership (CSIP) – an arms-length Government body which provides guidance to the field – established an outcomes initiative. This involved pilot studies in four provider services between 2002 and 2003. In addition to HoNOS, they evaluated the use of the Carers and Users Experience of Services (CUES) (Lelliott et al., 2001), the Functional Analysis of Care Environments (FACE) (Clifford, 1999) and the Manchester Short Assessment of quality of life (MANSA) (Priebe et al., 1999). Following the pilot studies, an Outcomes Reference Group was established, which published the results of the pilot study in 2005 (National Institute for Mental Health in England, 2005). The results were not encouraging: 'The main barrier to successful implementation identified by the Reference Group was the need to gain the positive engagement of the service users, carers and clinicians. These key groups are most likely to engage with the initiative where they have a clear understanding of the benefits of outcome measurement to themselves and services as a whole'. In response, the Reference Group proposed a Benefits Pyramid, shown in Figure 4.1.

This pyramid has, however, had little impact on routine clinical practice, and outcome measurement remains an unco-ordinated and fragmented activity. Two themes are becoming apparent.

First, some measures which are helpful for informing clinical care are being adopted in provider services, notwithstanding the central guidance emphasizing HoNOS. For example, the Clinical Outcomes in Routine Evaluation – Outcome Measure (CORE-OM) (Evans et al., 2000) is becoming widely used as an evaluation of psychological therapy services. Similarly, the Camberwell Assessment of Need (Phelan et al., 1995, Slade et al., 1999) is being adopted by many individual services, for example as part of the Gloucester Caseload Project (Macpherson et al., 2003, 2007).

Second, a key emerging driver of behaviour is the commissioning arrangements – the agreements between Primary Care Trusts (PCTs) (who receive money from central Government to buy services to meet local mental health needs) and Mental Health Trusts (who provide services). The demands arising from centrally driven initiatives such as MHMDS are in practice being trumped by contracts with PCTs. Mental health services are not commissioned on the basis of outcome measurement (let alone improvement), as PCTs have other priorities. Since there are no financially adverse consequences following from non-compliance with MHMDS requirements, HoNOS completion rates have never come close to their goal of characterizing health gain at a national level. Outcome-focused commissioning is beginning to emerge as a priority (Slade, 2006).

Two specific types of outcome commissioning are being proposed. The Commission for Social Care Inspection has developed an outcomes framework for performance assessment of

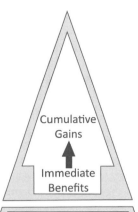

Cumulative
Gains

Immediate
Benefits

Level 4: Benchmarking
Aim: Comparing outcomes
for services and trusts against
nationally derived benchmark
data to refocus services
Application: Assessing the
effectiveness of services nationally

Requirements for Level 4
• Development of normative data of
sufficient quality, history and breadth (to
include contextual data) on non-treatment
factors influencing outcomes
• Developing expert peer groups to pool
expertise in interpreting OM data

Level 3: Service & Treatment Management
Aim: Using OM data to inform provision of services
and assess treatment of patients within trusts
Application: Assessing the effectiveness of treatments and
services within a trust

Requirements for Level 3
• Contextual data to include type of intervention and diagnosis
• Rapid feedback of data to inform interventions within a course
of treatment
• Interpreting OM reports to devise appropriate enhancements
in practice and service delivery

Level 2: Monitoring Data
Aim: Profiling services and assessing needs at trust level
Application: Enables comparisons of needs across teams within a trust

Requirements for Level 2
• Quality checks on data including review of data by those providing ratings
• Production of timely and accessible reports
• Ability to aggregate data across the trust

Level 1: Measurement
Aim: Collecting OM data and achieving good completion rates from the targeted population
Application: Provides tool for comparing individual patient and clinician perceptions about treatment
outcomes

The Mental Health Outcome Measurement Initiative

Figure 4.1 The benefits pyramid.

adult social care services (Commission for Social Care Inspection, 2006). This proposes that performance be assessed in relation to nine key standards: Improving Health and Emotional Well-being; Improved Quality of Life; Making a Positive Contribution; Increased Choice and Control; Freedom from Discrimination; Economic Well-being; Maintaining Personal Dignity and Respect; Leadership; and Commissioning and Use of Resources. The National Social Inclusion Programme has also developed an outcome framework for mental health services (National Social Inclusion Programme, 2009). It identifies key domains for outcome assessment as Community Participation, Social Networks, Employment, Education and Training, Physical health, Mental Well-being, Independent living, and Personalisation and choice. Key service outcome indicators are service user satisfaction, service user involvement and diversity. Identified outcome measures are the Recovery star (www.mhpf.org.uk/recoveryStarApproach.asp), the Outcomes star (www.homelessoutcomes.org.uk) and the Inclusion web (www.ndt.org.uk).

Research into outcome measurement

One contribution of England is the evaluation of routine outcome assessment as an intervention, using randomized controlled trial designs. Several studies have now been completed, which we briefly review.

Marshall and colleagues used the Cardinal Needs Schedule (CNS, Marshall et al., 1995) in a single-blind cluster-randomized trial. They compared outcomes across three arms: 18 professionals received feedback from the CNS on all 88 of their patients, 36 professionals received feedback from the CNS on half of their 140 patients, and 18 professionals received no feedback on their 76 patients. They found that this approach to standardized needs assessment did not substantially enhance care planning, although giving professionals some experience of feedback from a standardized assessment of need did improve satisfaction for some patients.

Ashaye and colleagues investigated the Camberwell Assessment of Need for the Elderly (CANE, Reynolds et al., 2000) in a randomized controlled trial (Ashaye et al., 2003). They compared outcome for 54 day hospital patients assessed with CANE which was then fed back to staff, with 58 patients who were not assessed. They found no difference in social disability (assessed using HoNOS) or unmet needs (assessed using CANE) at follow-up.

Priebe and colleagues evaluated a computer-mediated intervention to structure patient–clinician dialogue in a multi-national cluster-randomized controlled trial (Priebe et al., 2007). Every 2 months for a year, a total of 64 clinicians with 271 patients used the DIALOG intervention, which involved asking patients to rate their satisfaction with eight life domains (mental health, physical health, accommodation, job situation, leisure activities, friendships, relationship with family/partner, personal safety) and three treatment domains (practical help, psychological help and medication), followed by a question on whether the patient wanted any additional or different help in the given domain. If the patient answered yes, the type of the requested additional or different support was recorded. They were compared with 70 clinicians with 236 patients who did not receive the DIALOG intervention analyses. Patients receiving the DIALOG intervention had better subjective quality of life, fewer unmet needs and higher treatment satisfaction after 12 months.

Finally, Slade and colleagues investigated the use of routine outcome assessment in an epidemiologically representative randomized control trial (Slade et al., 2006b). The intervention was based on a predefined model (Slade, 2002), and involved asking 101 patients and their matched staff to complete separate monthly postal questionnaires, and to receive 3-monthly postal feedback. Their outcomes were compared with 59 staff–patient pairs where the patient received treatment as usual. No difference was found for subjective outcomes of unmet needs or quality of life, but the intervention reduced psychiatric inpatient days (3.5 vs.16.4 mean days, bootstrapped 95% CI 1.6–25.7), and hence service use costs were £2,586 (95% CI 102–5,391) less for intervention-group patients. Net benefit analysis indicated that the intervention was cost-effective. Premorbid IQ was a moderator of intervention effectiveness (Slade et al., 2006a).

The future

At the time of writing, there is no clear direction for development of outcomes measurement in England. There are clear incentives in a taxpayer-funded system to establish value for money. However, the leap from efficacy to effectiveness has not been easy to make. Clinicians do not find high value in filling in forms about their patients, and there has been no substantial initiative around patient-rated outcome measurement.

That said, there are positive signs. First, the developing emphasis on social inclusion and recovery may provide an ideological platform around which people both using and working in mental health services can meet (Shepherd et al., 2008, Slade, 2009). This may counter-balance some of the previous focus on measures which are of high policy and manager relevance but less importance to staff and patients. Second, there is an emerging consensus about the pool of outcome measures to draw from. In 2008 the National Institute for Mental Health in England published an outcomes compendium of 69 measures (National Institute for Mental Health in England, 2008). Five measures were recommended for assessing general health care needs under the Health Care and Needs Assessment heading: CAN (Slade et al., 2002), CUES (Lelliott et al., 2001), FACE (Clifford, 1999), HoNOS (Wing et al., 1998) and the Threshold Assessment Grid (TAG) (Slade et al., 2000, 2002). Finally, the NHS Connecting for Health Programme (www.connectingforhealth.nhs.uk) may prove to be the national IT solution which is needed before consistent use of outcome measures in mental health services becomes a reality in England.

References

Amin, S., Singh, S. P., Croudace, T., et al. (1999). Evaluating the Health of the Nation Outcome Scales: reliability and validity in a three-year follow-up of first-onset psychosis. *British Journal of Psychiatry*, **174**, 399–403.

Andrews, G., Peters, L. and Teesson, M. (1994). *The Measurement of Consumer Outcome in Mental Health: A Report to the National Mental Health Information Strategy Committee*. Canberra.

Ashaye, O. A., Livingston, G. and Orrell, M. W. (2003). Does standardized needs assessment improve the outcome of psychiatric day hospital care for older people? A randomized controlled trial. *Aging & Mental Health*, **7**, 195–9.

Brooks, R. (2000). The reliability and validity of the Health of the Nation Outcome Scales: validation in relation to patient derived measures. *Australian and New Zealand Journal of Psychiatry*, **34**, 504–11.

Care Services Improvement Partnership (2006). *Measuring health and care outcomes in mental health. Communications Update*. London: Department of Health.

Clifford, P. (1999). The FACE Recording and Measurement System: a scientific approach to person-based information. *Bulletin of the Menninger Clinic*, **63**, 305–31.

Commission for Social Care Inspection (2006). *A New Outcomes Framework for Performance Assessment of Adult Social Care. 2006–2007 Consultation document*. Leeds: CSCI.

Department of Health (1990). *National Health Service and Community Care Act*. London: The Stationery Office.

Department of Health (1999). *Mental Health National Service Framework*. London: The Stationery Office.

Department of Health (2000). *The NHS Plan*. London: HMSO.

Department of Health (2001). *Mental Health Information Strategy*. London: The Stationery Office.

Evans, C., Mellor-Clark, J., Margison, F., et al. (2000). CORE: clinical outcomes in routine evaluation. *Journal of Mental Health*, **9**, 247–55.

Glover, G. (1997). The development of a new minimum data set for specialist mental health. *Health Trends*, **29**, 48–51.

Glover, G. R., Robin, E., Emami, J. and Arabscheibani, G. R. (1998). A needs index for mental health care. *Social Psychiatry and Psychiatric Epidemiology*, **33**, 89–96.

Jarman, B. (1983). Identification of underprivileged areas. *British Medical Journal*, **286**, 1705–9.

Lelliott, P., Beevor, A., Hogman, G., et al. (2001). Carers' and Users' Expectations of Services – User version (CUES – U): a new instrument to measure the experience of users of mental health services. *British Journal of Psychiatry*, **179**, 67–72.

Macdonald, A. J. D. (2002). The usefulness of aggregate routine clinical outcomes data: the example of HoNOS65+. *Journal of Mental Health*, **11**, 645–56.

Macpherson, R., Haynes, R., Summerfield, L., Foy, C. and Slade, M. (2003). From research to practice: a local mental health services needs assessment. *Social Psychiatry and Psychiatric Epidemiology*, **38**, 276–81.

Macpherson, R., Gregory, N., Slade, M. and Foy, C. (2007). Factors associated with changing patient needs in an assertive outreach team. *International Journal of Social Psychiatry*, **53**, 389–96.

Marshall, M., Hogg, L., Gath, D. H. and Lockwood, A. (1995). The Cardinal Needs Schedule: a modified version of the MRC Needs for Care Schedule. *Psychological Medicine*, **25**, 605–17.

National Institute for Mental Health in England (2005). *Outcomes Measures Implementation Best Practice Guidance*. Leeds: NIMHE.

National Institute for Mental Health in England (2008). *Outcomes Compendium*. Birmingham: National Institute for Mental Health in England (NIMHE).

National Social Inclusion Programme (2009). *Outcomes Framework for Mental Health Services*. London: NSIP.

Phelan, M., Slade, M., Thornicroft, G., et al. (1995). The Camberwell Assessment of Need: the validity and reliability of an instrument to assess the needs of people with severe mental illness. *British Journal of Psychiatry*, **167**, 589–95.

Priebe, S., Huxley, P., Knight, S. and Evans, S. (1999). Application and results of the Manchester Short Assessment of quality of life. *International Journal of Social Psychiatry*, **45**, 7–12.

Priebe, S., McCabe, R., Bullenkamp, J., et al. (2007). Structured patient-clinician communication and 1-year outcome in community mental healthcare Cluster randomised controlled trial. *British Journal of Psychiatry*, **191**, 420–6.

Reynolds, T., Thornicroft, G., Abas, M., et al. (2000). Camberwell Assessment of Need for the Elderly (CANE); development, validity, and reliability. *British Journal of Psychiatry*, **176**, 444–52.

Rock, D. and Preston, N. (2001). HoNOS: is there any point in training clinicians? *Journal of Psychiatric and Mental Health Nursing*, **8**, 405–9.

Shepherd, G., Boardman, J. and Slade, M. (2008). *Making recovery a reality. Briefing Paper*. London: Sainsbury Centre for Mental Health.

Slade, M. (2002). Routine outcome assessment in mental health services. *Psychological Medicine*, **32**, 1339–43.

Slade, M. (2006). Commissioning outcome-focussed mental health services. *Mental Health Review*, **3**, 31–6.

Slade, M. (2009). *Personal Recovery and Mental Illness. A Guide for Mental Health*

Professionals. Cambridge: Cambridge University Press.,

Slade, M. and Glover, G. (2001). *The needs of people with mental disorders.* In G. Thornicroft and G. Szmukler, eds., *Textbook of Community Psychiatry.* Oxford: Oxford University Press.

Slade, M., Thornicroft, G., Loftus, L., Phelan, M. and Wykes, T. (1999). *CAN: Camberwell Assessment of Need: A comprehensive assessment tool for people with severe mental illness.* London: Gaskell.

Slade, M., Powell, R., Rosen, A. and Strathdee, G. (2000). Threshold Assessment Grid (TAG): the development of a valid and brief scale to assess the severity of mental illness. *Social Psychiatry and Psychiatric Epidemiology*, **35**, 78–85.

Slade, M., Cahill, S., Kelsey, W., Powell, R. and Strathdee, G. (2002). Threshold 2: the reliability, validity and sensitivity to change

of the Threshold Assessment Grid (TAG). *Acta Psychiatrica Scandinavica*, **106**, 453–60.

Slade, M., Leese, M., Gillard, M., Kuipers, E. and Thornicroft, G. (2006a). Pre-morbid IQ and response to routine outcome assessment. *Psychological Medicine*, **36**, 1183–91.

Slade, M., McCrone, P., Kuipers, E., et al. (2006b). Use of standardised outcome measures in adult mental health services: Randomised controlled trial. *British Journal of Psychiatry*, **189**, 330–6.

Thornicroft, G. and Tansella, M. (1999). *The Mental Health Matrix.* Cambridge: Cambridge University Press.

Wing, J. K., Beevor, A. S., Curtis, R. H., et al. (1998). Health of the Nation Outcome Scales (HoNOS). Research and development. *British Journal of Psychiatry*, **172**, 11–18.

5 Outcomes measurement in Ohio and the United States

James Healy and Dee Roth

Introduction

The history of mental health treatment outcomes measurement (OM) in the United States is complex, defying a simple telling due to the diversity of systems that exists today. While other states have created outcomes systems of their own, this chapter briefly describes the Federal OM requirements that set a floor for states and describes Ohio's own approach to OM.

OM history in Ohio and the USA

Behavioural health OM has played a strong role in research and has evolved as part of the overall development and evolution of human services. Attkisson and Broskowski (1978) show strongly developed models for conducting evaluations including OM. However, the implementation of evaluations within services agencies was sporadic throughout the 1980s. Federal community mental health centres (CMHCs) had evaluation requirements but this comprised a small percentage of state services. Federal Medicaid funds have only been tied to certification by state mental health authorities, whose requirements differed widely.

In 1988, Ohio instituted a services evaluation rule that was a comprehensive set of prescriptive steps to measure clinical outcomes, satisfaction, sentinel events, service rates and other processes across various populations. The Ohio Department of Mental Health (ODMH) developed further advice on how to implement the rule for use by boards and provider agencies. The supervision of the rule was left to local boards, which varied in their enforcement efforts from no enforcement, to enforcement of select parts of the rule. At the same time, local mental health boards were responsible for the determination of cost-effectiveness of services, but this rule has generally not been followed.

The 1990s brought forces for reform of OM. Nationally, a drive for accountability for government spending crystallized in the Government Performance Results Act of 1993 that pushed government at all levels to measure performance. Efforts to reform health care loomed large, providing a sense of urgency about OM. Scarce resources in Ohio's public mental health system increased the need to determine what worked. Local county efforts to develop standard OM for their area would have required some providers to measure outcomes in multiple ways. One of the local efforts led to a lawsuit over the use of outcomes data in making financial decisions. To address these factors, in 1996 ODMH convened a diverse, multi-stakeholder Outcomes Task Force (OTF) made up of mental health service consumers, agency staff, local mental health board staff, ODMH staff and academics to develop a standardized outcomes reporting system. Setting a model for subsequent outcomes work groups, the OTF used a consensus-building model for decision-making that forced many compromises, but grudging acceptance for an outcomes system. The 18 months of the OTF work coincided with the development of the recovery movement, and reflected many of the recovery principles. The OTF envisioned outcomes to be a driver of treatment planning (especially to include

Outcome Measurement in Mental Health: Theory and Practice, ed. Tom Trauer. Published by Cambridge University Press.
© Cambridge University Press 2010.

consumer voice in treatment), to measure quality improvement impact and to provide accountability for expenditures. The final report of the OTF, Vital Signs (Ohio Mental Health Outcomes Task Force, 1998), included vision and values, outcomes statements and selected instruments. Ohio settled on four domains of measurement: clinical status (symptom distress), functional status, quality of life (life satisfaction, fulfillment and empowerment) and safety/health.

An extensive pilot followed. These efforts led to the replacement of the youth instruments with the recently validated Ohio Scales for Youth. An OM database that allowed agencies data entry and basic clinical reporting was developed. At the end of the pilot, $3 million dollars for incentives were used to stimulate the uptake of the still voluntary Outcomes System, allowing 200 agencies to purchase necessary tools.

Meanwhile, the state replaced a grant-funding mechanism with a fee-for-service claims reporting system. Implementing this system enabled maximal claiming for federal Medicaid money. This was desirable, as state mental health funding fell behind inflation. However, Medicaid set a rate ceiling for all funds that has not been raised since 1999. This had the effect of driving out all activities not directly related to billing for services, including many quality-related activities. In response to this and other pressures, ODMH engaged in a regulatory relief effort that exchanged most of the felt-to-be-burdensome department regulations – including the services evaluation rule – for a system based upon deemed status and the retention of a few core reporting rules. Deemed status requires that agencies be accredited by one of three national accrediting bodies. One of the core rules ODMH kept was an OM rule requiring agencies to collect and report standard outcomes data, and to show evidence of the use of outcomes data in treatment planning and in quality improvement.

At the federal level, block grant dollars were tied to reporting on the National Outcomes Measures (NOMs), which come from the Substance Abuse and Mental Health Services Administration (SAMHSA). Ohio used parts of its outcomes data and data from other sources to fulfill NOM report requirements. The NOMs that are required continue to evolve, with more measures requiring within-subject change over time. Table 5.1 outlines the NOMs as they are currently structured. More details about these measures are available at http://www. nationaloutcomemeasures.samhsa.gov/

In 2002, ODMH launched the Statewide Outcomes Data Reports Workgroup (SODRW), which established some basic outcomes reports that should be produced. The group recommended standard reports that should be produced every 6 months, as well as topical reports that would 'drill-down' on various areas that would be produced every 6 months. The most important product of the group was the specifications for the Outcomes Data Mart, a flexible, open, web-based outcomes reporting system that allows anyone to produce reports on scales or items from any of the instruments. Reports can be run at an agency, board area or state level, and can be restricted or broken out on a variety of demographic information. The primary specification for the Outcomes Data Mart was ease-of-use. To that end, users need only make selections from a set of pull-down menus to create a report. This system has enabled a significant number of agencies to fulfil accreditation requirements through the reports that are created, and has provided numerous benchmarks.

In 2005, ODMH launched a review of the OM system by asking another multi-constituency work group to recommend improvements. The Outcomes System Quality Improvement Group (OSQIG) worked for 18 months and addressed over 300 comments, issues and requests that ODMH had collected from the community since 1998. The group made 18 recommendations that simplified, clarified and/or improved the clinical utility of the system. The first recommendation was that no instruments be changed prior to May 2008 that would require changes to

Table 5.1 National Outcomes Measures – USA

NOMS Category	Measures required
1. Increased Access to Services	Based on consumer with billed services
2. Reduced Utilization of Psychiatric Inpatient Beds	Decreased rate of readmission to state psychiatric hospitals within 30 days, and within 180 days
3. Use of Evidence-Based Practices	Number of clients receiving Evidence-Based Practices (EBP)
4. Client Perception of Care	Reporting positively about access, general satisfaction, perception of outcomes, participation in treatment planning by adults and youth
5. Increased/Retained Employment or Return to/Stay in School	Percent of consumers competitively employed
	Percent of consumers reporting improvement return to/stay in school
6. Decreased Criminal Justice Involvement	Rate of arrests for adults and youth
7. Increased Stability in Housing	Percent of consumers who are homeless or living in shelters
8. Increased Social Supports/Social Connectedness	Social Support in adults and youth
9. Improved Level of Functioning	Functioning in adults and youth

data flow or collection software. Because OSQIG was a sitting committee when the requirement to show use of outcomes data approached, the committee was asked for input. The group wanted a menu of options, a reliance on existing documentation such as reports used for accreditation, and relatively low thresholds. ODMH came up with a menu of options that included items that the OSQIG group felt would need to be completed in order to use outcomes well. OSQIG's final report (2006) identified five 'bigger-than-outcomes' factors that shaped the Outcomes System (an appendix to the OSQIG final report addresses these factors and ways to address them in detail). These factors are outlined later in the 'Obstacles' section.

In 2007, ODMH chartered another work group, called Outcomes System Quality Improvement Group-Instruments (OSQIG-I), to review the instruments for changes. The group began with over 150 suggestions, comments and issues related to the instruments, and generated another 100 when it asked its members to gather further concerns. Ironically, the single most-stated concern was about the burden of the Outcomes System, but the most common suggestion was for the addition of specific items or constructs to measure. OSQIG-I held off most suggestions for adding items, and reduced the number of items on all instruments. The group worked for 18 months, with ODMH staff performing extensive research and analysis to support the meetings.

On the adult consumer instrument, several major changes were made. The first shortened the Symptom Distress scale from 15 to 10 items, which still retained a 0.92 correlation with the Symptom Checklist-90 (SCL-90, Derogatis, 1983). The second reduced the Making Decisions Empowerment Scale from 28 to 15 items. Factor analysis of the 28-item version failed to confirm the factor structure reported by Rogers et al. (1997). Our analysis, with 44,000 records included, found that the Righteous Anger subscale had a small negative correlation with the overall Empowerment scale. The correlation between the Self-Esteem and Optimism subscales was 0.94. Based upon analyses and further discussion, the Optimism and Righteous Anger subscales were dropped and the remaining subscales further refined. A possible source of the difference between Rogers et al.'s findings and ours was that their work was based upon participants in consumer-operated services, whereas our data included consumers of all types of services.

Prior to revision of the adult provider instrument, the Community Functioning scale was the only 'home-made' scale in all the instruments, and had Cronbach's alpha reliability estimates between 0.69, and 0.71, near or below the standard of 0.70 that OSQIG had set. In an excellent review of the state of the art in measuring functioning in adults with severe mental illness, Bellack et al. (2007) point out the many difficulties of constructing a brief, single factor scale. Our experience bore this out. Our scale measured social involvement, daily living skills, role performance, problem behaviors and dangerous behaviors, and so included critical aspects of functioning. The group made several changes to the Community Functioning scale, which may have improved the scale's reliability somewhat, but no one in the OSQIG-I group felt that we had solved the problem of measuring community functioning for adults with serious mental disorder.

OSQIG-I made little change to the Ohio Scales for Youth (Parent, Worker and Youth versions), as they were widely reputed to be about the right length and content. All three versions contain a Problem Severity and a Functioning scale, each with 20 identically worded items. The Parent and Youth instruments share two four-item scales that measure Hopefulness and Satisfaction (with therapeutic alliance). Three items were re-worded on the Parent and Worker versions that had lower response rates for young children. The Restrictiveness of Living Arrangement Scale, or ROLES (Hawkins et al., 1992), living arrangement categories were reduced from 23 to 16. The largest change made was the addition of a Family Quality of Life scale to the Parent and Youth versions. This addition was hotly debated. Many felt that family quality of life was outside the purview of mental health treatment focus – explicitly so, since Medicaid rules require that the services address the needs of the individual rather than the family. However, OSQIG-I voted to add the scale because of the criticality of the family's well-being to the health and welfare of the youth in treatment.

Two OSQIG-I recommendations cut across all instruments. The first was the decision to remove all information that was reported elsewhere, such as some basic demographic information reported in claims data. This decision made sense, but it was recognized that this raised the level of effort required for some agencies to combine demographic and outcomes data for analysis. The other recommendation was that other, non-outcomes data be reported to ODMH that was necessary to properly interpret outcomes data. For example, information about a youth's mental retardation is necessary to fully understand the youth's outcomes on the Functioning scale.

Toward the end of the OSQIG-I's tenure, Ohio's recession deepened and revenues dwindled, leading to calls for further streamlining of administrative overhead, and outcomes was deemed to be one of the most burdensome processes required of agencies. Objectively, this was demonstrably not the case, as the clinical documentation process was at least 50-times more burdensome, but many of the clinical documentation rules resided at the federal level or were otherwise outside the control of ODMH to change. Perhaps more importantly, clinical documentation was the means by which agencies demonstrated medical necessity and thereby established the billability of services. ODMH gathered input from agencies, boards and consumers about the perceived benefits and cost-effectiveness of the Outcomes System. Not surprisingly, the Outcomes System did not fare as well with providers, but did better with boards and consumers. This is discussed later in the 'What constituents think' section.

In September of 2008, in response to the deepening budget crisis, ODMH made outcomes reporting voluntary, and established another work group (called Measuring Outcomes

Table 5.2 Benefits addressed through the Outcomes System

- Provides data for agency care management and treatment planning, agency clinical supervision and agency quality improvement
- Addresses needs inherent in person-centred treatment models
- Meets other funders' needs for consumer outcomes data
- Provides data for planning and analysis at agency, board and state levels
- Provides data to document medical necessity
- Provides data to track whether recovery is really taking place
- Replaced earlier, more burdensome, Service Evaluation Rule
- Meets some or all Outcomes Measurements standards of The Joint Commission, Council on Accreditation and Council on Accreditation Rehabilitation Facilities
- Top performing agencies report outcomes and provide additional information for accreditations requirements in at least the following standards: Service Delivery/Provision of Care; Performance/Quality Improvement; Individual Planning; Ethics, Rights & Responsibilities; Risk Prevention & Management, Governance/Leadership/Organizational Leadership
- Provides data for Board-Area Service Utilization Review
- Provides data for Board-Area Quality Improvement
- Provides data to assist Boards with duties required by Ohio Revised Code 340, including: (1) review and evaluation of services; (2) assessment of cost-effectiveness; (3) programme development/needs assessment; and (4) conducting studies for the promotion of mental health
- Meets accountability requirements for other ODMH programs (e.g. Block Grant, TSIG)
- Meets needs of ODMH Balanced Score Card
- Incorporated into Medicaid Business Plan
- Creates a common data standard for service research, lowering the cost of research
- Provides data for statewide benchmarking
- Provides data for statewide quality improvement
- Contributed to the National Alliance for the Mentally Ill's B+ rating of Ohio's public mental health system
- Staff moving from agency to agency already know Outcomes System
- Economies of scale in development of information systems, procedures, training materials, etc.

Efficiently, or MOE) tasked with reducing the burden of measuring outcomes by 50% at all levels, and recommending major changes to the system including even complete replacement of the current instruments. The change to voluntary status resulted in approximately 50% reduction in the number of administrations reporting to ODMH, and has caused the outcomes data use review process necessary for certification to cease entirely.

As of this writing in early 2009, the work of the MOE group continues. It is unknown what the result will be, but one test of the new system will be to compare how well the new streamlined system achieves the benefits outlined in Table 5.2, which were delivered by the current system.

Ohio's legislative framework for OM

Effective September 2003, Ohio Administrative Code 5122–28–04, the Outcomes Rule, directed agencies to collect and submit Outcomes System data to ODMH, and to show evidence of the use of outcomes in treatment planning and in quality improvement. The Rule directs that the operational details shall be spelled out in the Outcomes Procedural Manual. This has allowed changes to be made to the Outcomes System without going through the administrative rule revision process, though no changes have been made to the Outcomes System without review by a multi-constituency work group. The actual operations of the Outcomes System would be difficult to incorporate fully in a rule as the manual is currently over 200 pages and has had 10 editions.

Compliance with the Rule is measured in two ways. Data reporting is measured in missing-data reports that establish expected numbers of consumers that should have outcomes data reported, and the actual number of consumers for whom outcomes data have been reported. Compliance with data use has been handled with a 'desk audit', where agencies submit documentation of data use. The standards set for evidencing use of data were based upon a menu of data use options.

ODMH obtained acceptance of its instruments from all three accrediting bodies during the pilot, and mapped ways in which the outcomes data could be used to fulfil core accrediting requirements, yet many agencies struggled with accreditation for the first time while trying to implement the Outcomes System.

Funding for OM system

Aside from the initial outcomes incentive grants, agencies and boards have been expected to fund outcomes start-up and ongoing costs on their own, with various counties extending additional help to some agencies. Typically, funding for the data collection by service providers is to be folded into the cost of doing business by including the cost in the unit rate for the services that are billed. Federal Block Grants are given to each state, and this money is expected to cover the cost of measuring the NOMs.

Staff education and training

Extensive guidelines exist that detail what administrators at state systems must do for reporting NOMs. For those states employing the NOMs perception of care measures, further guidance is given about how to administer these tools. All states use sampling for these measures, so there is limited need for extensive training.

Training has always been seen as a core activity affecting the success of Outcomes. At the outset of the initiative in Ohio, regional training was provided in a train-the-trainer mode. An Outcomes Implementation Toolkit was created and distributed that contained roles-based training modules for clinical staff, clinical supervisors, agency and programme administrative staff, adult consumers, family members of adult consumers, youth consumers and parents of youth consumers. These tools were also posted to the outcomes website. After several rounds of initial training, agencies assumed responsibility for training their staff. Periodically, ODMH provided training when new approaches or tools were developed.

Who completes what and when

Table 5.3 shows the instruments' contents, which are used for whom, and when they are administered. The actual instruments are available at http://www.mh.state.oh.us/what-we-do/protect-and-monitor/consumer-outcomes/instruments/index.shtml.

Ohio's completion levels

Reporting for adult and youth consumers went from 20% in September 2004 to 80% in June of 2008. The measure was the number of people with at least one outcome reported in the year, over the number of people who received any of the outcomes-qualifying services. The

Table 5.3 Ohio Mental Health Outcomes: who completes what and when

	Instrument				
	Adult Consumer Form	Adult Provider Form	Ohio Scales (Y-Form)	Ohio Scales (P-Form)	Ohio Scales (W-Form)
	(completed by consumer)	(completed by service provider)	(completed by youth ages 12–18)	(completed by parent/guardian for youth ages 5–18)	(completed by service provider for youth ages 5–18)
What is measured	Overall quality of life (12-item scale)	Functional status	Problem severity (20-item scale)	Problem severity (20-item scale)	Problem severity (20-item scale)
	Safety and health (7 independent items)	• Social (2 items)	Functioning (20-item scale)	Functioning (20-item scale)	Functioning (20-item scale)
	Symptom distress (15-item scale)	• Housing (2 items)	Hopefulness about life or overall well-being (4-item scale)	Hopefulness about caring for the identified youth (4-item scale)	Restrictiveness of living environment (ROLES) (computed score)
	Overall empowerment (28-item scale)	• Activities of daily living (8-item subscale)	Satisfaction with behavioural health services (4-item scale)	Satisfaction with behavioural health services (4-item scale)	
		• Meaningful activities (6-item subscale)			
		• Primary role (1 item)			
		• Problem behaviours (1 item)			
		Safety and health (9 independent items)			
When administered	Admission into one of the target services				
	Three months after admission (YOUTH INSTRUMENTS ONLY)				
	Six months after admission				
	Twelve months after admission				
	Annually thereafter				
	Termination: if Outcomes-qualifying services have occurred on three or more days since previous administration				

measurement of reporting rates is discussed in detail at http://b9962ed140049a571a710839f
1f71c989aaf09ce.gripelements.com/oper/outcomes/reports/rpt.missing.data.evolution.pdf

Resources available for providers/consumers/managers

A Procedural Manual and many other training and data use tools are available for consumers, family members, clinicians, support staff, IT staff, QI/PI staff and administrative staff.

See http://www.mh.state.oh.us/what-we-do/protect-and-monitor/consumer-outcomes/index.shtml.

IT support

ODMH has an Outcomes Support Team and IT staff (available by phone or e-mail) who provide support for three systems related to outcomes:

Agency Data Entry and Reports Generator: a Microsoft Access database that 50% of agencies have chosen to use (other agencies have the option to build or buy their own).

ODMH Production Database: outcomes data are sent in batch files to ODMH through the local boards and are scrubbed; status reports for each batch file are produced and the clean data uploaded to the production database. Support is provided for the testing process and to address data flow issues.

Outcomes Data Mart: described in the 'OM history in Ohio and the USA' section; users can get help with use or problem resolution.

Good or outstanding practices

Many features of Ohio's Outcomes System have been successful. Among the most successful have been:

Outcomes Support Team – having dedicated staff to serve as a help desk and consultancy for data use.

Creation of Agency Data Entry and Reports Generator for agencies – by absorbing the cost of development and working with clinicians and consumers, the creation of an application has enabled about 180 agencies to get up to speed in using outcomes data. It has been widely downloaded outside Ohio.

Creation of the Outcomes Data Mart – the Outcomes Data Mart was described in the 'OM history in Ohio and the USA' section. It has allowed many constituents access to the statewide database to look at any item or scale for their own agency, their own county or the whole state.

Development and use of the Ohio Scales for Youth – these scales share identically worded items for Parent, Worker, and Youth respondents that allow for direct comparison of viewpoints and have proven to be well-accepted as part of treatment planning and recognized in various youth-serving state agencies and around the country.

Development of the ARROW (Achieving Recovery and Resiliency the Outcomes Way) report – based on the Adult Consumer instrument, the report lists problematic items in ascending order on Maslow's hierarchy, and for each item lists a number of actions that the consumer can take to address the problem.

Consumer involvement in planning/implementation

Consumers have been involved at every major planning step. At least four adult consumers or parents of youth consumers were included on each of the workgroups, or 10% to 15% of the committee members. It has been difficult to retain input from parents of youth. ODMH covered expenses for consumers who do participate and offered a per diem stipend to ensure that financial issues are not a barrier to participation. The effect of consumers on the decision-making of the group is large. This reflects a commitment on the part of ODMH to include consumers in many aspects of planning. Consumers also provide Climbing into the Driver's Seat training, a programme that shows adult consumers how to use outcomes to promote their recovery.

What constituents think of Ohio's OM system

Ohio's Outcomes System has met with enthusiastic support all the way to enthusiastic opposition. In 2008, in the most comprehensive review of constituent opinion about outcomes, ODMH asked consumers, boards and agencies about the benefit and cost-effectiveness of the Outcomes System. Only one response was allowed from each responding board and agency, with mostly directors responding. Agencies reported only small to moderate benefits from Outcomes, and that costs outweigh benefits. Board opinion was somewhat better. Most adult and youth consumers and parents of youth consumers reported that Outcomes were just about the right length, done at the right frequency, and were somewhat to very useful. Presented with reasons Outcomes were helpful and not helpful, consumers' validated helpful reasons three times more often than not helpful reasons. The most common helpful and not-helpful reasons were that it helped people understand their problems, and that it was too long, respectively. The full survey result can be found at http://b9962ed140049a571a710839f1f71c9 89aaf09ce.gripelements.com/oper/outcomes/moe/survey-results-costs-benefits.pdf.

Obstacles

The five chief inter-related obstacles are 'bigger-than-outcomes', and are described fully in the final report of the OSQIG (2006) group discussed in the history section:

- *Financing and reimbursement* – agency finances are not systemically impacted by performance on Outcomes; funding is only contingent on Outcomes to the extent that Outcomes are required for continued certification of the agency, which is a three-year cycle in Ohio, and agencies are re-approved for certification so long as a plan of correction is in place. If Outcomes were seen as medically necessary (and therefore a Medicaid-required activity), everyone would use Outcomes.

- *Productivity and Quality* – as mentioned above, Medicaid set a ceiling on rates not changed since 1999. This caused agencies to focus on activities that are billable to Medicaid. Although using Outcomes in treatment is billable, clinicians completing Outcomes and clinician helping consumers complete Outcomes for non-mental-health related reasons are not billable, therefore do not contribute to 'productivity', so there is a strong motive to not attempt to use Outcomes.

- *Information technology* – one often overlooked IT problem is that agencies performing human services sometimes overlook that they are also technology management organizations, and therefore fail to invest resources in appropriate technical infrastructure and staffing. Acquisition of unrelated off-the-shelf applications can make integration of data difficult or impossible. Organizations that have installed 'best of breed' applications for given functions may not have access to the information needed for decision-making. Integrated behavioural health information systems answer many of the information system challenges agencies face. Vendors are not inclined to make changes without a state mandate for inclusion of specific functionality, especially around useful but optional outcomes reporting. Systems can be obsolete or outmoded by the time of implementation, leading to abandonment and/or resentment of users who know better technology is available. The nature and quantities of system demands on organizations require the use of technical and analytical tools (e.g. statistical software) which the organizations either lack or don't have appropriate people resources to utilize. There is little emphasis or outward valuing of data and its use for decision-making.

- *Workforce* – the success of initiatives is compromised by high levels of staff turnover, particularly of staff who have initiative-specific or technical skills, or are perceived as 'champions' for the initiative in question. Staff are being asked to do things for which they've never been trained. They lack the skills for approaching, asking questions of, analysing and understanding data. Agencies lack appropriate staff 'know-how' to use data to help achieve consumers' goals.

- *Organizational culture* – organizational culture is a major determinant of an organization's actions, decisions and performance as indicated by extensive literature in many fields. While the organizational culture operating in agencies and boards may, in many cases, be a direct function of the funding constraints they face, it does not necessarily follow that addressing the financing and reimbursement issues alone will change the culture for the positive. In fact, solving the financing problems may simply reinforce current decision-making methods that do not employ outcomes data. Bickman (2008) adeptly describes the benefits of NOT measuring outcomes for everyone but consumers.

Additionally, ODMH conducted a survey of barriers and facilitators that identify more specific operational barriers and methods to address them, available at http://b9962ed14004 9a571a710839f1f71c989aaf09ce.gripelements.com/oper/outcomes/planning_training/impl ementation.facilitators.barriers.pdf.

Advice for building OM systems

Ensure that the outcomes measures are reliable, valid and as short as possible.

Ensure constituents gets something from participating – consumers can benefit from better care; clinicians can get useful feedback; administrators can get useful feedback about programme data, and funders can get accountability information. Ask each what they want and build it into the system.

Build complete systems before going live – be sure enough features are operational at start-up that balance the cost and burden, especially for clinicians and consumers.

Integrate OM into clinical processes and documentation. As Lambert and his colleagues have shown (Slade et al., 2008), OM can be useful clinically (see Chapter 6 in this book by Michael Lambert). Outcomes measures and clinical assessment both tap the same constructs so an outcomes-centred approach to assessment can capitalize on outcomes data and thereby reduce burden.

Build programme/practice participation data into OM systems – outcomes data are more useful to everyone when they can be analysed for a specific programme or practice.

References

Attkisson, C. C. and Broskowski, A. (1978). Evaluation and the emerging human service concept. In C. C. Attkisson, W. A. Hargreaves, M. J. Horowitz and J. E. Sorenson, eds., *Evaluation of Human Service Programs*. New York: Academic Press.

Bellack, A. S., Green, M. F., Cook, J. A., et al. (2007). Assessment of community functioning in people with schizophrenia and other severe mental illnesses: a white paper based on an NIMH-sponsored workshop. *Schizophrenia Bulletin*, **33**, 805–22.

Bickman, L. (2008). A measurement feedback system (MFS) is necessary to improve mental health outcomes. *Journal of the American Academy of Child & Adolescent Psychiatry*, **47**, 1114–19.

Derogatis, L. R. (1983). *SCL-90-R Administration, Scoring, and Procedures Manual – II*. Towson, MD: Clinical Psychometric Research.

Hawkins, R. P., Almeida, M. C., Fabry, B. and Reitz, A. L. (1992). A scale to measure restrictiveness of living environments for troubled children and youths. *Hospital & Community Psychiatry*, **43**, 54–8.

Ohio Mental Health Outcomes Task Force (1998). *Vital Signs: A Statewide Approach to Measuring Consumer Outcomes in Ohio's Publicly Supported Community Mental Health System, (final report)*. Columbus, OH: Ohio Department of Mental Health, availabl;e at: http://b9962ed140049a571a71 0839f1f71c989aaf09ce.gripelements.com/ oper/outcomes/history/otf.vital.signs.pdf.

Rogers, E. S., Chamberlin, J., Langer Ellison, M. and Crean, T. (1997). A consumer-constructed scale to measure empowerment among users of mental health services. *Psychiatric Services*, **48**, 1042–7.

Slade, K., Lambert, M. J., Harmon, S. C., Smart, D. W. and Bailey, R. (2008). Improving psychotherapy outcome: the use of immediate electronic feedback and revised clinical support tools. *Clinical Psychology and Psychotherapy*, **15**, 287–303.

Section 1
Chapter

6

The *Outcome Questionnaire* system: a practical application for mental health care settings

Michael J. Lambert

The aim of the OQ system is to provide measures and methods to enhance treatment outcomes for psychological disorders, especially for patients whose progress and eventual positive outcome is in doubt, by providing progress information directly to practitioners. This system is owned and distributed by OQ Measures (www.OQMeasures.com), and consists of several adult and youth measures contained in a software application – OQ-Analyst. The central measure within the OQ-Analyst is the Outcome Questionnaire-45 (OQ-45), first developed and distributed in the United States in 1993. According to a survey conducted by Hatfield and Ogles (2004), it is the third most frequently used self-report instrument for measuring adult patient outcome in the USA in private practice. Unlike most psychological tests, it was developed specifically for use in monitoring patient well-being on a weekly basis during routine care. It was assumed that the measure would be taken prior to each treatment session, require about 5 minutes of patient time and be composed of items that would reflect the consequences of receiving care, while remaining stable in untreated controls.

The OQ-45 was originally developed for use in Managed Behavioural Care and applied in regional care settings that included intermountain states and a nation-wide private insurance company that served consumers from Alaska to Florida as a means of helping these companies engage in outcomes management, i.e. using patient treatment response data to improve care within their 6,000,000 population of potential consumers. Following development of this adult measure, OQ systems expanded to other patient populations, such as children and the severely mentally ill. A major development achieved by 2009 was the use of the OQ system in state-wide mental health in the states of Arkansas, Maine, Michigan and Utah.

Table 6.1 presents an overview of the OQ system measures and some of their characteristics. The major distinguishing feature of OQ Measures is their focus on managing the treatment response of individual patients by providing clinicians with graphs of patient progress, with alarm signals for predicted negative outcome that brings providers' attention to such cases. This is the most effective and certain way to maximize treatment effects for the patient. An important but secondary purpose of the measures is to document treatment effects for administrators and funding agencies. In addition to the outcome measures the reader will note the presence of a measure for adults and children (the Assessment for Signal Cases; ASC) which is a decision tool that guides problem-solving and interventions with cases at risk for treatment failure. The ASC is not taken by all clients, but is used with the approximately 25% of patients whose recovery is doubtful given their response to initial attempts to help.

The instrument manuals (e.g. Lambert et al., 2004) document excellent internal consistency: Cronbach's $\alpha \geq 0.90$, adequate test–retest reliability, and good to excellent validity with a wide variety of other standardized outcome measures that are frequently used in psychotherapy outcome research. These measures do a good job of distinguishing between patient and psychologically healthy samples. The instruments have been normed on patient and

Table 6.1 Outcomes Questionnaire instrument overview

Instrument	Number of items	Completed by	Subscales	Change metrics[a]	Treatment failure alerts[b]	Community normative score range	Clinical score range
OQ® 45.2 – Adult outcome measure (ages 18+)	45	Self	3	Yes	Yes	0 to 63	64 to 180
Y-OQ® 2.01 – Youth outcome measure (ages 4–17)	64	Parent	6	Yes	Yes	–16 to 46	47 to 240
Y-OQ® 2.0 SR – Youth outcome measure (ages 12–17)	64	Self	6	Yes		–16 to 46	47 to 240
OQ® 30.1 – Adult outcome measure (ages 18+)	30	Self	3	Yes	Yes	0 to 43	44 to 120
Y-OQ® 30.1 – Omni-form youth outcome measure (ages 12–18)	30	Parent	6	Yes	Yes	0 to 29	30 to 120
Y-OQ® 30.1 SR – Omni-form youth outcome measure (ages 12–18)	30	Self	6	Yes		0 to 30	31 to 120
S-OQ® 2.0 – Outcome measure for the severely and persistently mentally ill	45	Self or clinician	2	Yes		0 to 59	60 to 180
BPRS – Outcome measure for the severely and persistently mentally ill	24	Clinician	3	Yes		0 to 30	31 to 50 (outpatient) 51 to 129 (inpatient)
ASC (Assessment for Signal Clients) adult clinical support tool to help assess problems with therapeutic alliance, motivation, social supports and life events	40	Self	4		Yes	N/A	N/A

[a]Change metrics refers to an outcome measure's ability to use a Reliable Change Index (RCI) and cutoff score to define standards for clinically significant change achieved during mental health treatment (i.e. classifying patients as recovered, improved, no change, or deteriorated).
[b]Treatment failure alerts refers to an outcome measure's ability to use rational or empirically based algorithms to detect possible treatment failures and alert clinicians accordingly.

non-patient samples across the USA and throughout much of the world through translations into over 17 non-English languages. Normative comparisons have been employed to provide markers for individual patient progress based on Jacobson and Truax's (1991) formulas for reliable and clinically significant change, fulfilling a necessary use of the instrument to inform clinicians about the degree of success a patient they are treating is having.

The Severe Outcome Questionnaire (SOQ) is composed of the 30 items from the OQ-30 and an additional 15 items that capture symptoms and functioning of patients who have severe psychopathology such as bipolar, schizophrenia and other psychotic illness. It was created with the intention of being especially appropriate for use in settings where highly impaired patients seek treatment, such as community mental health centres. If patients are too disturbed to provide a valid self-report of their symptoms the Brief Psychiatric Rating Scale (BPRS, Ventura et al., 1993) is provided in the OQ-Analyst software so that an expert judge (the treating clinician) can rate mental health status. It is our belief that measuring outcomes is best accomplished by placing the burden on the client whenever possible, rather than placing the burden on clinicians who are already struggling with treating the patient.

We find patient acceptance of these procedures is very high, provided that the information they provide is actually used by clinicians during their treatment and the support staff are cooperative. Since the support staff in many clinics see themselves as advocates for the patient, it is important that they understand the measures are being given for the benefit of the patient, not simply for research purposes.

Deviations from a positive course of treatment

The central feature of the OQ system family of measures is not the measures themselves, although they were specifically made for the purpose of quantifying the impacts of treatment, but the creation of decision-making tools (laboratory tests) based on comparing an individual patient's progress with that of similar patients who have undergone treatment. From both research and practice perspectives, identifying 'signal' cases, or cases at risk for poor outcome, is a critical component of enhancing treatment outcome. Additionally, from a healthcare management perspective, with a focus on containing costs and providing quality assurance in mental health services, identifying signal cases is essential for efficient allocation of resources. Quality assurance is 'fundamentally a case-based issue' (Lueger et al., 2001, p. 150) that should enhance 'problem-patient-therapy-therapist matches' (p. 157). Patient-focused research (Howard et al., 1996) emphasizes case-based approaches for optimizing treatment for the individual patient, and a number of actuarial methods have been developed for predicting the course of treatment and identifying 'signal' cases, with the goal of preventing treatment failures (Finch et al., 2001, Lambert et al., 2002a, Lutz et al., 2006).

Traditionally, outcome prediction has utilized baseline characteristics of patients, therapists and the treatment context to predict treatment outcome. These variables are useful in creating models for casemix adjustment and can guide the placement of patients into services; however, we make use of ongoing treatment monitoring where patient progress (or lack thereof) is compared to data on the expected course of treatment from previously treated patients (Lambert et al., 2003). Ongoing treatment monitoring systems generally share a number of similar components. First, treatment monitoring requires routine assessment of patient functioning during the course of treatment. This assessment can be limited to pre–post measurement, though more commonly assessment occurs on a regular basis during the course of treatment, as frequently as every weekly session of therapy. Second, treatment monitoring requires the comparison of patient outcome to norms from similar patients. Third, treatment monitoring has the goal of feeding patient information back to the practice setting with the goal of informing treatment delivery in order to enhance outcomes. This feedback can range from reporting on the outcome of completed treatments, to management, and to ongoing feedback of session-by-session change to therapists and even patients.

While clinicians are confident in their ability to care adequately for patients in the absence of formal monitoring systems, as is pointed out shortly, therapists are highly reluctant to predict that an ongoing case is advancing in a manner consistent with final deterioration. In order to become more aware of pending treatment failure actuarial methods that take into account massive amounts of information about the treatment response of thousands of patients across thousands of therapists can be of considerable predictive benefit. For example, Finch et al. (2001) applied actuarial methods to a large data base consisting of 11,492 patients treated in a variety of settings including employee assistance programmes, university counselling centres, outpatient clinics and private practice settings and were able to identify 50 separate courses of recovery based on OQ-45 scores. Similar methods have been applied using the OQ-30, Y-OQ and Y-OQ-30.

We have found effective methods of predicting treatment (e.g. Lambert et al., 2002a, Spielmans et al., 2006) with accuracy varying from 85 to 100% identification of impending failure – compared to near zero accuracy by treating clinicians asked to make the same prediction (Hannan et al., 2005).

Collecting outcome data

The questionnaires are typically administered to patients by asking them to come 10 minutes early to their scheduled treatment session. The patient (or parent) is given a handheld computer, directed to a computer kiosk or provided with a hard copy of the scale. If treatment is provided in a patient's home, handheld administration and feedback can take place in that setting. Once the questionnaire is completed it is scored, algorithms are applied, the results are graphed and a report appears on the therapist's computer within seconds. Thus, before the patient even reaches the therapist's office the therapist can quickly see a progress graph since the inception of treatment. A sample of the clinician report is provided in Figure 6.1.

As can be seen the clinician is also able to view the patient's answers to several critical items such as substance use and suicide. We do not prescribe what the clinician does with the information provided, although a message at the bottom of the report makes some suggestions based on a comparison with answers given at the time the client entered treatment. In our minds, using information technology, instantaneous feedback of outcome information,and predictive methodologies is a significant advance in the way clinical services are offered. But does this help clinicians do a better job serving their clients?

Research on ongoing treatment monitoring

Comparisons of individual patient response to session-by-session normative data have been employed in five large randomized controlled studies to evaluate the impact of using the OQ system (OQ-45) to assess and modify ongoing treatment response (Lambert et al., 2001, 2002b, Whipple et al., 2003, Hawkins et al., 2004, Harmon et al., 2007). These studies each required about one year of data collection and included session-by-session measurement of over 4,185 patients. All five of the studies assessed the effectiveness of providing therapists with session-by-session progress data as measured by the OQ-45, with particular focus on identifying patients who were not responding well to treatment (signal-alarm cases). Progress data were

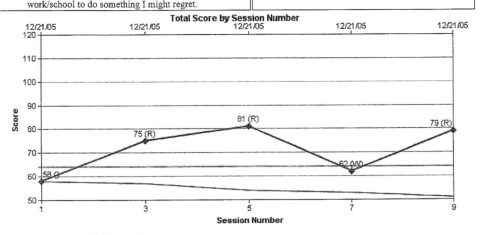

Name:	12, case	ID:	12
Session Date:	12/21/2005	Session: 9	
Clinician:	M , Mariana	Clinic:	Aigle
Diagnosis:	Unknown Diagnosis		
Algorithm:	Empirical		

Alert Status:	**Red**
Most Recent Score:	79
Initial Score:	58
Change From Initial:	Reliably Worse
Current Distress Level:	Moderate

Most Recent Critical Item Status:

8. **Suicide** - I have thoughts of ending my life. **Never**

11. **Substance Abuse** - After heavy drinking, I need a drink the next morning to get going. **Never**

26. **Substance Abuse** - I feel annoyed by people who criticize my drinking. **Never**

32. **Substance Abuse** - I have trouble at work/school because of drinking or drug use. **Never**

44. **Work Violence** - I feel angry enough at work/school to do something I might regret. **Rarely**

Subscales	Current	Outpat. Norm	Comm. Norm
Symptom Distress:	45	49	25
Interpersonal Relations:	18	20	10
Social Role:	16	14	10
Total:	**79**	**83**	**45**

Total Score by Session Number

81 (R)
75 (R)
79 (R)
58.0
62.0(W)

Session Number

Graph Label Legend:

(R) = **Red**: High chance of negative outcome (Y) = **Yellow**: Some chance of negative outcome

(G) = **Green**: Making expected progress (W) = **White**: Functioning in normal range

Feedback Message:

The patient is deviating from the expected response to treatment. They are not on track to realize substantial benefit from treatment. Chances are they may drop out of treatment prematurely or have a negative treatment outcome. Steps should be taken to carefully review this case and identify reasons for poor progress. It is recommended that you be alert to the possible need to improve the therapeutic alliance, reconsider the client's readiness for change and the need to renegotiate the therapeutic contract, intervene to strengthen social supports, or possibly alter your treatment plan by intensifying treatment, shifting intervention strategies, or decide upon a new course of action, such as referral for medication. Continuous monitoring of future progress is highly recommended.

REMINDER: THE USER IS SOLELY RESPONSIBLE FOR ANY AND ALL DECISIONS AFFECTING PATIENT CARE. THE OQ®-A IS NOT A DIAGNOSTIC TOOL AND SHOULD NOT BE USED AS SUCH. IT IS NOT A SUBSTITUTE FOR A MEDICAL OR PROFESSIONAL EVALUATION. RELIANCE ON THE OQ®-A IS AT USER'S SOLE RISK AND RESPONSIBILITY. (SEE LICENSE FOR FULL STATEMENT OF RIGHTS, RESPONSIBILITIES & DISCLAIMERS)

Figure 6.1 Example feedback report.

supplied in the form of a graph of OQ-45 scores detailing patient change over time and warning messages when improvement was not occurring or was not of the expected magnitude (see Figure 6.1 for example of a feedback report). Additionally, two of the studies assessed the impact of providing both therapists *and patients* with OQ-45 progress information, and two of the studies assessed the impact of providing therapists with additional feedback regarding the patient's assessment of the therapeutic relationship, readiness for change and degree of social support (termed Clinical Support Tools Feedback or CST Feedback). These latter three assessments were provided in concert with OQ-45 progress information when it was deemed that the patient was not progressing in treatment as well as expected and, in fact, predicted to leave treatment deteriorated.

The five studies summarized here include a number of commonalities. The most important of these are as follows. (1) Patients were randomly assigned into control (No Feedback) or experimental (Feedback) groups at intake (one study employed an archival control). (2) The same therapists who saw control-condition patients also saw experimental-condition patients, thus minimizing the possibility that measured differences are attributable to therapist effects. (3) The therapists represented a variety of treatment orientations, with the majority ascribing to cognitive behavioural or other eclectic orientations. (4) Professional therapists represented about 50% to 100% of the clinicians participating in each study, with the balance composed of graduate student or postdoctoral trainees.

Table 6.2 presents aggregated results for all patients in the five feedback studies who deviated significantly and negatively from their expected treatment course (i.e. Not-On-Track patients). Data are divided into three groups: Treatment as Usual (i.e. No Feedback); OQ-45 Feedback (Therapist Feedback and Therapist/Patient Feedback); and OQ-45 Feedback + Clinical Support Tools Feedback. Of particular note is the percentage of patients who deteriorated or ended treatment with negative change. As can be seen, OQ-45 feedback resulted in a decrease in the percentage of Not-On-Track patients who ended treatment with reliable negative change (20.1% to 14.9%). Deterioration rates were further reduced when Clinical Support Tools Feedback was provided in addition to the OQ-45 Feedback, with the percentage of deterioration falling to 7.8%. Additional benefits of feedback are seen in a comparison of Not-On-Track patients who meet criteria for Reliable Improvement and/or Clinically Significant Change, with percentages increasing from 22.0% for Treatment As Usual, to 32.5% for OQ-45 Feedback, and 44.8% for OQ-45 Feedback + CST Feedback. Taken together, results suggest that providing therapists with feedback on patient progress improves outcome for patients predicted to be treatment failures. Further, providing therapists with the patient's assessment of the therapeutic alliance, the patient's assessment of his or her own readiness for change and assessment of the strength of social support networks further improves treatment outcome.

In addition to changes in final treatment outcome, the results of the five studies indicate that session utilization may be affected by the provision of OQ-45 feedback. There were significant treatment-length differences between experimental and control participants in four out of the five studies (Lambert et al., 2001, 2002b, Whipple et al., 2003, Harmon et al., 2007), with Not-On-Track patients in the feedback conditions receiving significantly

Table 6.2 Final outcome categorizations of Not-On-Track patients by treatment group

Feedback:	TAU[a] n = 318 No		OQ-45 n = 582 Yes		OQ-45 + CST[b] n = 154 Yes	
Outcome classification	n	%	n	%	n	%
Deteriorated/reliable worsening	64	20.1	87	14.9	12	7.8
No reliable change	184	57.9	306	52.6	73	47.4
Reliable/clinically significant change	70	22.0	189	32.5	69	44.8

[a]TAU = Treatment as Usual; [b]CST = Clinical Support Tool.

more sessions than their Treatment As Usual counterparts. This result was not found in the study that was conducted at an outpatient hospital-based clinic where, in general, patients began treatment as more disturbed. This suggests that increases in treatment length may be just one mechanism of action by which feedback improves outcome. In two out of the five studies (Lambert et al., 2001, Whipple et al., 2003), patients who were On-Track for a positive outcome and in the experimental feedback condition received fewer sessions than On-Track controls. This suggests the possibility that the cost-effectiveness of psychotherapy can be positively impacted, with the most needy patients staying in treatment longer, and patients who recover quickly having fewer sessions when their therapist receives feedback on their progress.

Discussion of the OQ system in application to treatment monitoring

The studies summarized above clearly demonstrate the utility of the OQ-45 in assessing ongoing patient functioning during the course of treatment. Ongoing treatment monitoring shows great potential in improving the efficiency and effectiveness of psychotherapy. Additionally, monitoring treatment on a consistent basis has several advantages over more limited assessment (such as administering assessments at pre-treatment and post-treatment only). First, a central goal of quality assurance is the prevention of negative outcomes. Even under the best circumstances, such as in carefully crafted and controlled clinical trials research, roughly 10% of patients show negative outcome (deterioration), while another 25 to 40% will fail to improve and show no reliable change (Hansen et al., 2002). Consistent ongoing assessment is the only way to get 'real-time' measurement of patient functioning that can be fed back to therapists in a timely fashion to impact the treatment for that patient. Intermittent or pre–post assessment alone limits or makes impossible the provision of feedback to therapists that can inform their treatment decisions regarding the actual patients who are completing questionnaires. While such data are useful to inform treatment expectations for future patients, and to inform management about the utilization and effectiveness of clinical services, the application of such data to individual cases is limited.

Second, from a practical perspective, the logistics of maintaining an ongoing treatment monitoring system are easier to manage when assessment becomes a routine part of practice. A central question in such systems is 'who is responsible for data collection?', with the related questions of 'when are assessments administered?' and 'who keeps track of this?' Thus, if therapists administer questionnaires, do they do this before or after the session and, if assessment is intermittent, how does the therapist know to administer an assessment to patient A, but not to patient B? Is the therapist expected to keep track of this along with the patient case file, or is this handled on the management side and therapists are informed as needed? We have found that the most efficient system has been to simply make administration of assessments routine, with patients completing a questionnaire prior to each appointment in the clinic so there is no need to track who needs an assessment and who does not, and with assessments administered by clinic receptionists when patients check in for appointments. While there is a need for an employee who is responsible for gathering assessments, scoring them, managing the data and preparing feedback for clinicians, this process has become increasingly automated and can easily be handled as part of the routine tasks of administrative personnel using OQ-Analyst software. The National Registry of Evidence-based Programs and Practices (NREPP) has indicated that the OQ-Analyst is an evidence-based practice, and recently rated the OQ-Analyst a

3.9 (out of 4) as meeting their criteria for 'Readiness for Dissemination' based on user guides and step-by-step instructions for implementation (http://www.nrepp.samhsa.gov/).

Third, any treatment monitoring approach will be limited by patient dropout or premature termination of treatment. It is uncommon for therapists to know when treatment is going to end in such a way as to be ready with an assessment to obtain post-treatment data. Therefore data collection for post-treatment is frequently conducted at some point after termination and typically requires mailing the questionnaire to patients or contacting them by phone to administer the questionnaire. These methods have drawbacks, such as potentially violating confidentiality in contacting former patients, having biased data as a result of patients who are unwilling to complete forms or who cannot be located, and administrative time in delivering these assessments. With routine ongoing treatment monitoring, missing data is less of a drawback, as statistical methods are able to fill gaps from incomplete data, and session-by-session assessment data should be available up to the last session a patient attended. This provides a much more complete and accurate estimate of treatment outcome.

There are several barriers to the implementation of ongoing treatment monitoring, including clinician resistance to monitoring, the logistics of establishing routine and ongoing assessment of treatment, issues of scoring assessments and data management, and developing procedures to provide useful and timely feedback to clinicians and patients. Additionally, to make use of these treatment-monitoring methods, normative data from similar patients and treatments are required to compute treatment expectations. While data to develop such norms are available for many patient categories and treatment approaches (e.g. cognitive and interpersonal therapies for affective and anxiety disorders), such data are not available for many more specific treatment situations.

Of course, treatment monitoring is only as good as the measurement tool used. In the feedback studies just summarized, the OQ-45 was the instrument used. This measure was specifically developed to be brief and quickly administered, thus being acceptable for routine use. It has been shown to have stable scores across time in non-treatment settings, as well as being sensitive to change over the course of treatment. Additionally, a large amount of data has been accumulated on the clinical use of the OQ-45, such that normative data for treatment expectations are available across a large number of settings, treatments and patient categories. The utility of the OQ-45 in identifying patients who are expected to have negative outcomes has been established, as have procedures for informing clinicians (and patients) of treatment expectations. Clinical support tools have been developed which further augment the OQ system and serve to provide clinicians with a range of options to address patients who are not progressing as expected.

Given the large sample sizes of the individual studies in this summary, and a combined overall sample size of over 4,000 cases in our clinical trials, the current findings are compelling, though they are not without limitations. First, the majority of the data on ongoing treatment monitoring and therapist feedback were collected in a university outpatient clinic. Studies in other settings, and with different treatments and patient samples, are needed. For example, as our samples are composed of predominantly young adult patients with generally good prognosis, we have limited research data on the effects of feedback on chronic psychotic disorders, children and adolescents, and on older adults. Although a recent study of 30-day inpatient treatment in Switzerland (Berking et al., 2006) using similar methods has replicated the effects of treatment monitoring and feedback, many more studies will be needed before the limitations and generalizability of such interventions are known. We are currently conducting studies on substance abuse and inpatient eating-disorder samples.

Second, there were no evaluations or controls of how therapists made use of feedback or clinical support tools. While this methodological limitation increases the likelihood that the results reflect what will happen in other clinical settings, clinicians' actions with regard to looking at feedback, sharing it with clients, seeking supervision or consultation and modifying treatment remain largely unknown, with the exception of our two studies where we delivered feedback directly to patients (Hawkins et al., 2004, Harmon et al., 2007). This raises the issue of clinician acceptance of feedback, which is another potential limitation of this type of research and clinical management.

Generally speaking, clinicians do not see the value of frequent assessments based on standardized scales (Hatfield and Ogles, 2004); probably because they are confident in their ability to accurately respond to patients. Despite evidence which suggests psychotherapists are not alert to treatment failure (Yalom and Lieberman, 1971, Hannan et al., 2005), and strong evidence that clinical judgements are usually found to be inferior to actuarial methods across a wide variety of predictive tasks (Grove, 2005), therapist confidence in his/her own clinical judgement stands as a barrier to implementation of monitoring and feedback systems. In addition, clinicians are used to practising in private and with considerable autonomy. Monitoring patient treatment response makes the effects of practice somewhat public and transparent. Such 'transparency' inevitably raises evaluation anxiety and fears of losing control. Implementation requires the cooperation of therapists and takes time before it is apparent to clinicians that the feedback is helpful.

Finally, self-report and a single measure provide only one view of the impact of therapy on patients. The OQ system was designed to be a tool to aid clinical decision-making rather than to dictate or prescribe to clinicians. We are well aware of the fact that decisions regarding the continued provision of treatment, the modification of ongoing treatment, obtaining case consultation or supervision or the application of clinical support tools or other techniques cannot be made on the basis of a single questionnaire or independent from clinical judgement. Thus we envision the OQ system as analogous to a 'laboratory test' in medical treatment, which can supplement and inform clinical decision-making, rather than as a replacement for the clinician's judgement.

When one considers the many ways in which systems of care and clinicians attempt to improve patient outcomes, monitoring treatment response is an inexpensive alternative. Other methods such as continuing education to deliver evidence-based psychotherapy are quite costly and, of course, do not guarantee successful patient outcomes, nor provide accountability data. Monitoring treatment response through the means described costs just a few dollars per patient and is likely to improve outcomes for those whose improvement is most in doubt. By targeting non-responding clients, a specific solution to quality of care is being applied in real time on a case-by-case basis rather than relying on very general methods such as traditional studies of groups of patients.

While the focus of this chapter has been on a specific set of measures that were developed and applied as a means of improving outcomes, it is likely that improvements in patient outcome can be attained through the use of comparable measures provided that some basic guidelines are adhered to. These include: (a) a brief measure that is reliable and valid; (b) frequent assessments during the course of ongoing treatment; (c) valid cut-off scores for demarking reliable change and normal functioning; (d) application of actuarial prediction of impending treatment failure; (e) timely (computer-assisted) feedback of this information to therapists and perhaps clients; (f) clinical decision-making tools to prompt therapist actions with clients who are not responding positively; and (g) cooperation and support of clinical staff. I look forward to a time when formally tracking treatment response and the use of decision support tools become a part of routine practice. Certainly the research suggests that this is a feasible and effective evidence-based practice that maximizes positive patient outcomes while making treatment more cost-effective. In addition, these practices provide accountability data to administrators and policy makers, as well as impacting the scientific foundations of clinical practice.

References

Berking, M., Orth, U. and Lutz, W. (2006). How effective is systematic feedback of treatment progress to the therapist? An empirical study in a cognitive-behavioural-oriented inpatient setting. *Zeitchrift fur Klinishe Psychologie und Psychotherapie*, **35**, 21–9.

Finch, A. E., Lambert, M. J. and Schaalje, B. G. (2001). Psychotherapy quality control: the statistical generation of expected recovery curves for integration into an early warning system. *Clinical Psychology and Psychotherapy*, **8**, 231–42.

Grove, W. M. (2005). Clinical versus statistical prediction: the contribution of Paul E. Meehl. *Journal of Clinical Psychology in Medical Settings*, **61**, 1233–43.

Hannan, C., Lambert, M. J., Harmon, C., et al. (2005). A lab test and algorithms for identiying clients at risk for treatment failure. *Journal of Clinical Psychology*, **61**, 155–63.

Hansen, N. B., Lambert, M. J. and Forman, E. V. (2002). The psychotherapy dose-response effect and its implications for treatment delivery services. *Clinical Psychology: Science and Practice*, **9**, 329–43.

Harmon, S. C., Lambert, M. J., Smart, D. W., et al. (2007). Enhancing outcome for potential treatment failures: Therapist/client feedback and clinical support tools. *Psychotherapy Research*, **17**, 379–92.

Hatfield, D. R. and Ogles, B. M. (2004). The use of outcome measures by psychologists in clinical practice. *Professional Psychology: Research and Practice*, **35**, 485–91.

Hawkins, E. J., Lambert, M. J., Vermeersch, D. A., Slade, K. and Tuttle, K. (2004). The therapeutic effects of providing patient progress information to therapists and patients. *Psychotherapy Research*, **14**, 308–27.

Howard, K. I., Moras, K., Brill, P. L., Martinovich, Z. and Lutz, W. (1996). Efficacy, effectiveness, and patient progress. *American Psychologist*, **51**, 1059–64.

Jacobson, N. S. and Truax, P. (1991). Clinical significance: a statistical approach to defining meaningful change in psychotherapy research. *Journal of Consulting and Clinical Psychology*, **59**, 12–19.

Lambert, M. J., Whipple, J. L., Smart, D. W., et al. (2001). The effects of providing therapists with feedback on patient progress during psychotherapy: are outcomes enhanced? *Psychotherapy Research*, **11**, 49–68.

Lambert, M. J., Whipple, J. L., Bishop, M. J., et al. (2002a). Comparison of empirically derived and rationally derived methods for identifying clients at risk for treatment failure. *Clinical Psychology and Psychotherapy*, **9**, 149–64.

Lambert, M. J., Whipple, J. L., Vermeersch, D. A., et al. (2002b). Enhancing psychotherapy outcomes via providing feedback on client progress: A replication. *Clinical Psychology and Psychotherapy*, **9**, 91–103.

Lambert, M. J., Whipple, J. L., Hawkins, E. J., et al. (2003). Is it time for clinicians to routinely track patient outcome?: A meta-analysis. *Clinical Psychology: Science and Practice*, **10**, 288–301.

Lambert, M. J., Morton, J. J., Hatfield, D., et al. (2004). *Administration and Scoring Manual for the Outcome Questionnaire-45*. Salt Lake City: Utah, American Professional Credentialing Services.

Lueger, R. J., Howard, K. I., Martinovich, Z., et al. (2001). Assessing treatment progress of individual patients using expected treatment response models. *Journal of Consulting and Clinical Psychology*, **69**, 150–8.

Lutz, W., Lambert, M. J., Harmon, S. C., et al. (2006). The probability of treatment success, failure and duration – what can be learned from empirical data to support decision making in clinical practice? *Clinical Psychology and Psychotherapy*, **13**, 223–32.

Spielmans, G. I., Masters, K. S. and Lambert, M. J. (2006). A comparison of rational versus empirical methods in prediction of negative psychotherapy outcome. *Clinical Psychology and Psychotherapy*, **13**, 202–14.

Ventura, J., Green, M. F., Shaner, A. and Liberman, R. P. (1993). Training and quality assurance with the Brief Psychiatric Rating Scale: 'The drift busters'. *International Journal of Methods in Psychiatric Research*, **3**, 221–44.

Whipple, J. L., Lambert, M. J., Vermeersch, D. A., et al. (2003). Improving the effects of psychotherapy: The use of early identification of treatment failure and problem solving strategies in routine practice. *Journal of Counseling Psychology*, **58**, 59–68.

Yalom, I. D. and Lieberman, M. A. (1971). A study of encounter group casualties. *Archives of General Psychiatry*, **25**, 16–30.

Outcome measurement in Italy

Mirella Ruggeri

Introduction

This chapter provides an overview of outcome measurement initiatives conducted in Italian mental health services in Italy since the Reform that occurred 30 years ago, called 'Law 180', which radically changed the architecture of psychiatric care (De Girolamo et al., 2007).

Gaining in-depth knowledge of the outcomes of people with mental disorders who receive community care has been a great challenge for both researchers and clinicians in the last 20 years, due to the lack of an agreed conceptual and methodological framework to assess outcome. Several important achievements have been fulfilled in the last decade and an agreement on the various facets of this concept has been reached. It has first been made clear that outcome measurement is not independent of ethical principles and thus should provide a wider balance of information for health policy and clinical service decisions (Thornicroft and Tansella, 1999). Then, it has been stated that for outcome measurement to be valid, reliable and useful for both programme planning and evaluation of interventions, it should be based on the principle of *multiaxiality* (i.e. the assessment should consider the perspectives of all those involved in the care process, including clinicians, patients, caregivers, user representatives, third-party payers, etc.) and of *multidimensionality* (i.e. the assessment should consider an intervention's effect on various dimensions of the patients' life, including both clinical and social aspects) (Lasalvia and Ruggeri, 2007). In routine psychiatric settings, clinicians, patients and caregivers are all involved in the care process and all their perspectives should be considered when assessing mental health outcome. The fact that their views may markedly differ is a further confirmation that taking into account multiple perspectives and integrating these views is a necessary step when evaluating mental health outcomes.

Specifically, three types of studies concerning outcomes in routine services will be reviewed: (1) multicentre international studies involving one or more Italian centres; (2) multicentre studies conducted entirely in Italy; and (3) studies performed in defined Italian catchment areas which have focused on specific modalities of service functioning and may be useful to examine specific issues related to the implementation of community care. Data on the main outcome indicators will be systematically reported, including *clinical outcomes* such as psychopathology, disability and needs for care; and *self-perceived outcomes* such as quality of life and service satisfaction.

The psychiatric reform and its developments

Health care in Italy is provided, generally free of charge, to the whole population by the National Health Service (NHS) through 'Local Health Units' (LHU), each responsible for a geographically defined catchment area.

The 1978 psychiatric reform established four principal components: (1) a gradual phasing out of mental hospitals, with the cessation of all new admissions; (2) the establishment of general hospital psychiatric units for acute admissions, each having a maximum of 15 beds; (3) more restrictive criteria and administrative procedures for compulsory admissions (allowed only to meet the patient's needs of care, and no longer his/her dangerousness); and (4) the setting up of Community Mental Health Centres (CMHC) providing psychiatric care to geographically defined areas. Mental health services are at present organized through 211 Departments of Mental Health, covering the entire country, each responsible for a geographically defined area.

The law was basically a 'guideline' law ('legge quadro'), and Regions were entrusted with the specific tasks of drafting and implementing detailed norms, methods and timetables for the organizational translation of the law's general principles. Over time these conditions have led to an uneven national situation, with Regions adopting different standards in terms of service provision and different organizational frameworks (De Girolamo et al., 2007). This makes it sometimes difficult to grasp a comprehensive picture of mental health care at the national level.

In order to overcome this national lack of homogeneity, and to provide quantitative standards for services, the Ministry of Health launched a multi-year 'National Mental Health Plan' (NMHP) that spelled out, for the first time ever, a set of (mainly structural) standards to be achieved; however, standards of the NMHP are hardly considered as mandatory by Regions.

So far all 76 Italian mental hospitals have been closed. Most former long-stay, elderly patients have been transferred to different types of residential facilities (RF), nursing homes, etc. In the year 2000 throughout Italy there were 1,370 RFs with an average of 12.5 beds each.

According to a Ministry of Health survey in 2001, 707 Community Mental Health Centres were operating and they deliver the bulk of outpatient and non-residential care: they provide individual consultations and visits, organize a variety of daytime and domiciliary care activities for the most severely disabled patients, establish and maintain contacts with other health and social agencies and provide emergency interventions. In most Regions they operate 12 hours a day for 5 or 6 days a week; most CMHCs have a multidisciplinary staff, including psychiatrists, psychologists, social workers, nurses and educators. A more detailed account of the Italian mental health system can be found in Lora (2009).

Outcome measurement in Italian routine psychiatric services

Disappointingly few outcome studies have been carried out in Italy since 1978; they would have been invaluable for a systematic evaluation of the results of the radical change in mental health care, avoiding impressionistic or opinion-based statements. Most of these studies have been promoted in a few centres, such as Verona, Naples, L' Aquila and Milan.

The most systematic approach to outcome measurement in the 'real world' Italian mental health services – and one of the most comprehensive in the world – is the South Verona Outcome Project (SVOP). It is a naturalistic, longitudinal research project which aimed to assess the outcome of care provided by the South Verona CMHS. Its key features are that (a) data collection was conducted in the routine clinical practice setting of a well-established 'real world' psychiatric service, (b) professionals engaged in clinical work were systematically involved in the assessment process, (c) the assessment included a comprehensive set of both clinician-rated and patient-rated outcomes, and (d) regular checks of the reliability and quality of the data were conducted; more details can be found elsewhere (Lasalvia and Ruggeri, 2007). In brief, all patients on the caseloads of the South Verona CMHS were systematically assessed with a set of standardized instruments. Assessments took place twice a year, from April to June (wave A) and from October to December (wave B). During these periods all key workers (psychiatrist or psychologists) were asked to assess, at the first or, at the latest, the second visit in the period, both first-time patients and patients already in contact with the service. In wave A the assessment was done only by the key professional on the basis of the patient's condition in the previous month and included assessment of global functioning, psychopathology and disability in performing social roles. In wave B the assessment was made both by the key professionals (again the same assessments as in wave A, plus the assessment of needs for care) and by the patients, who were requested to assess their quality of life and satisfaction with mental health services in relation to their experience over the previous year.

All primary clinicians (psychiatrists and psychologists) were trained in the correct use of the standardized instruments. The psychometric characteristics of the instruments used by the SVOP had been assessed in the existing literature. These properties were also tested regularly within the SVOP (Lasalvia and Ruggeri, 2007).

The SVOP included assessment of a series of prevalence cohorts of patients attending the South Verona CMHS and a series of follow-up studies. Overall, SVOP data allowed examination of a series of research questions mainly focused on the issues of heterogeneity of outcomes, clinical course, characteristics and determinants of needs for care and quality of life that have a great relevance for clinical practice. The main SVOP results will be summarized next, together with contributions from other studies conducted in Italy.

(a) Continuity of care and drop out

Several studies conducted in Italian settings show a large variability in continuity of care and drop-out rates, depending on the local organization. Among 1,070 consecutively discharged patients from 21 inpatient departments in eight different Regions in Italy and recruited on a voluntary basis, only approximately half of the original cohort could be traced, indicating a widespread loss of contact after discharge, and large variability among sites (Barbato et al., 1992a, 1992b). In the entire Lombardy Region, among all first-time admitted patients in the year 2000, only 1 in 6 were in contact with public mental health services in the following year (Lora et al., 2002).

On the other hand, a study performed in a representative cohort of 495 patients seeking care in the South Verona CMHC has shown that only 17% of patients (and none with a diagnosis of schizophrenia) had dropped out after two years. Patients who were less satisfied with the professionals skill and behaviour of staff were more likely to drop out (Rossi et al., 2002). Another study conducted in the SVOP analysed the drop-out phenomenon with a six-year follow-up design, and confirmed that the main reason for dropping out is service dissatisfaction. The vast majority of the patients who interrupted their contacts with CMHS were affected by non-psychotic disorders; some of them at follow-up were shown to have long-term residual symptoms and disability and rarely sought help from other agencies (Ruggeri et al., 2007).

In conclusion, Italian community mental health services seem to have a variable capability to engage patients. A comprehensive model of community care might provide good continuity of mental health care to patients with psychosis, but it is likely that these services do not dedicate sufficient attention to patients with relatively less severe symptoms and less disability, even though they could potentially benefit from effective treatments. The consequent persistence of untreated psychopathology and disability is likely to cause high subjective distress and higher direct and indirect social costs. This should prompt a careful analysis of the objectives and priorities of mental health services organized according to a public health approach.

(b) Psychopathology and disability

The most extensive Italian longitudinal study on psychopathology and disability has been performed by the SVOP, in a representative cohort of 354 patients treated in the South Verona CMHS, followed-up over 6 years (with assessments made at baseline and at 2 and 6 years) by using a set of standardized measures exploring psychopathology with the Brief Psychiatric Rating Scale (BPRS, Ventura et al., 1993) and social disability with the Disability Assessment Schedule (DAS, World Health Organization, 1988) with the aims of (1) determining changes in symptoms and social disability, and (2) exploring predictors of clinical and social outcome in patients receiving community-based mental health care. Psychotic patients displayed a clinical and social outcome characterized by complex patterns of exacerbation and remission over time; however, a clear trend towards a deteriorating course was not found, thus challenging the notion that patients with psychosis are necessarily destined to a chronic course. Patients without psychosis reported a significant reduction in the core symptom of depression and in the observable physical and motor manifestations of tension and agitation, and a parallel increase of complaints about their physical health. Clinical and social dimensions of outcome are influenced by specific and different sets of predictors that depict a rather complex pattern (Lasalvia et al., 2007).

(c) Needs for care

Over the last decade a number of authors have questioned the traditional approach to mental health care provision based on symptoms and psychiatric diagnosis, proposing an alternative needs-led approach (Lasalvia and Ruggeri, 2007).

A growing body of evidence has consistently shown that mental health professionals and service users have different perceptions of needs and that there is not a single correct perspective according to which needs assessment should be performed. In this regard, a cross-sectional study conducted by the SVOP has shown that patients and staff disagree on both the presence of a need and on whether a need had been met or not; moreover, while staff tend to identify more needs in areas related to clinical aspects, patients tend to report more needs in social life and in domains related to everyday issues, with a strong correlation between clinical variables, such as symptomatology and disability, and staff-rated needs (Lasalvia et al., 2000).

These findings, together with other consistent evidence (Lasalvia and Ruggeri, 2007), suggest that clinicians assessing needs may have the tendency to use Camberwell Assessment of Need (CAN, Phelan et al., 1995) ratings as a proxy for patients' disability or illness severity, whereas patients may be more likely to include the social consequences of the disorder, thereby rating their own handicaps. This seems to confirm that patients and staff have different views on what constitutes their respective priorities and that both should be considered when planning and providing mental health care within a framework of a modern partnership model.

A study conducted by the SVOP aimed to investigate, in a 4-year prospective longitudinal design, the impact of meeting needs for care, as assessed by both patients and mental health professionals, to improve the subjective quality of life in a sample of patients receiving community-based psychiatric care. Improvement in patients' clinical conditions as well as the reduction in patient-rated unmet needs in the social domain predicted an increase in subjective quality of life over 4 years; changes in staff-rated needs did not show any association with changes in subjective quality of life. These data show that, if the main goal of mental health care is to improve the quality of life of users, a policy of actively addressing patient-rated needs should be implemented (Lasalvia et al., 2005). A subsequent study with the same follow-up design investigated whether a better staff–patient agreement on needs for care predicts more favourable outcome in patients receiving community-based psychiatric care. Controlling for the effect of sociodemographic variables, service utilization and changes in clinical status, better staff–patient agreement makes a significant additional contribution in predicting treatment outcomes not only on patient-rated but also on clinician-rated measures (Lasalvia et al., 2008).

Taken together, these findings clearly show that mental health care should be provided on the basis of a negotiation process involving both professionals and service users to ensure effective interventions; every effort should be made by services to implement strategies aiming to increase consensus between staff and patients.

(d) Quality of life

Several studies have investigated the quality of life (QOL) of patients treated in mental health services in Italy. Results obtained in the Epsilon Study of Schizophrenia involving five centres from five countries in Europe have shown that the average QOL in the Italian sample ($n = 104$) studied in South Verona was in the mid range of the samples studied in the other four sites (Gaite et al., 2002). Another study has compared psychopathology and QOL in patients suffering from schizophrenia in Boulder, Colorado, and in Bologna (Warner et al., 1998). Patients in Bologna reported several significant QOL objectively rated advantages over Boulder patients; patients in Bologna also scored lower on some dimensions of psychopathology. However, the QOL advantages, objectively rated by external assessors, rather than being the result of more effective or better organized mental health services, appeared to reflect at least in part the sociocultural differences between the two countries, especially in terms of family structure. As many as 74% of Bologna patients were living with their families, as compared to a much smaller percentage (17%) of Boulder patients: not surprisingly most advantages for Bologna patients were strictly dependent on their family ties and situation (housing situation, food, medical care, etc.).

QOL was measured by the WHOQOL-Bref (Division of Mental Health and Prevention of Substance Abuse, 1997) in 1,492 subjects living in 174 residential facilities randomly sampled in 15 Italian Regions and compared with those of healthy subjects and outpatients with schizophrenia. Mean WHOQOL scores of residents were similar to those of outpatients with schizophrenia, but substantially lower than those of healthy controls. Lower scores on WHOQOL domains were associated with schizophrenia and non-affective psychoses, unipolar depression, anxiety or somatoform disorders, shorter duration of illness, positive, negative or mood symptoms, lower levels of functioning, and no participation in internal activities. This suggests the need for well-designed rehabilitation plans, tailored to patients' needs, to foster the development of their independence and, ultimately, improve their QOL (Picardi et al., 2006).

Several studies conducted so far in South Verona using the Lancashire Quality of Life Profile (LQoLP, Oliver, 1991–92) have shown that subjective and objective QOL are distinct types of information. The most significant predictors of good objective QOL were higher education and being married. Predictors of good subjective QOL were: self-perceived psychopathology, and especially anxiety and depressive symptoms (Ruggeri et al., 2001), reduction in unmet needs (Lasalvia et al., 2005), service satisfaction with special regard to satisfaction with service efficacy and interventions provided, and self-esteem (Ruggeri et al, 2003). According to these findings, a patient's QOL is most likely to improve when the focus is on the subjective concerns of the patient, and not solely on the problems as defined by the clinician.

(e) Service satisfaction

In this area a major contribution has been made possible by the development of the Verona Expectations for Care Scale (VECS) and Verona Service Satisfaction Scale (VSSS), a tool for community mental health services that derives from the Service Satisfaction Scale (Ruggeri et al., 2006). These scales measure the expectations and satisfaction of patients, relatives and professionals with mental health services (Ruggeri and Dall'Agnola, 1993); the domain-specific measurement (Professionals' Behaviour and Manners, Access, Information, Efficacy, Type of Intervention, Relatives' Involvement) that they provide has been shown to have good psychometric properties and greater sensitivity than instruments that measure overall satisfaction (Ruggeri et al., 1993). Identification of the factorial structure of the VSSS has allowed the development of short versions – VSSS-54 and VSSS-32 (Ruggeri et al., 1996) – which retain good psychometric properties. The content validity of the VSSS has been demonstrated cross-nationally (Henderson et al., 2003). Within the broader framework of the Epsilon Study of Schizophrenia, a European version of the VSSS, the VSSS-EU, was developed for patients, with translations into English, Dutch, Danish and Spanish and adapted for use in these countries' psychiatric settings (Ruggeri et al., 2000). Translations and adaptations of the VSSS into English, French, German, Portuguese, Greek, Slovene, Norwegian, Polish, Japanese and Chinese are also available. The VSSS is currently used in the psychiatric services of many countries world-wide. Copies of the various versions for patients, relatives and staff are available on request. Several studies conducted in the Verona CMHS and in other settings have used the VSSS to explore the relationship between satisfaction and other indicators of outcome. These accomplishments have elicited sustained interest in Italy, from 1990 on, to the extent that in the National Mental Health Plan, Departments of Mental Health have been encouraged to promote regular assessments of service satisfaction.

Two studies have compared service satisfaction with an Italian community-based practice and traditional hospital-based care in London (Henderson et al., 2003, Ruggeri et al., 2006) and shown that patients' responses markedly favour the community service. Moreoever, service satisfaction in outpatients with schizophrenia has been compared across five different European sites; satisfaction with care provided in Amsterdam, Copenhagen and Verona has been shown to be higher than satisfaction in London and Santander, in the former case due to the difficulty of the local service in satisfying the demand for mental health care in a very deprived area, and in the latter due to lack of facilities and personnel. In all services the lowest satisfaction has been reported in the key areas relatives' involvement and information (Ruggeri et al., 2003).

Satisfaction studies conducted among outpatient samples in Verona (Ruggeri et al., 2001), among outpatients in Rome by Cozza et al. (1997) and by Gigantesco et al. (2002), in the suburbs of Milan (Lora et al., 2002) and in Bologna (Chiappelli and Berardi, 2000) have found fairly high levels of satisfaction among users and their relatives; satisfaction was much lower among inpatients, and in all studies the areas of information and relatives' involvement were considered the most critical.

Using the VSSS, a longitudinal study that aims to exemplify some applications of routine measurements of service satisfaction was conducted by the SVOP with the aims of (1) identifying strengths and weaknesses in the patients' perspectives of a 'real world' service; (2) monitoring whether this specific service provides satisfactory care over three years; and

(3) identifying whether there are any patient characteristics that might be associated with service dissatisfaction.

Good levels of overall satisfaction, and a good stability in service satisfaction, were maintained over time in the South Verona CMHS. Specifically, patients appreciated the behaviour and manners of professionals, the type of interventions provided and the overall aspects of service provision. The service model oriented towards comprehensive community care provision was considered satisfactory by most patients; however, a series of weaknesses that would require organizational changes, and that persisted over time, were identified: rapid staff turnover, which negatively affected continuity of care; poor physical layout of the facilities; insufficient involvement of relatives and carers; insufficient information provided on diagnosis, prognosis and the services available; need for closer attention to the interactions of the patients with some members of the staff; and more careful assessment of the social problems the patients must face. These two last aspects have been shown to be problematic areas in other European settings as well (Ruggeri et al., 2003).

After taking into account a comprehensive set of measures which included patients' socio-demographic, clinical and service use characteristics and the type of interventions provided, the main variable found to exert a significant effect in predicting service satisfaction was the length of the interaction with the service. Whether this reflects progressive lowering of efforts and enthusiasm by the service staff when providing care to patients with chronic and enduring disorders, or a more pessimistic view by long-term patients who perceive their own condition as substantially unchanged despite having undertaken a number of long-lasting treatments, is difficult to say.

The comprehensive set of measures taken into account explained only a modest percentage of the variance in satisfaction with community mental health services, possibly as the result of a large individual variability in the factors that determine patient satisfaction. These results might also suggest that the ability of mental health professionals in understanding the patients' requests and needs, and in adapting treatment provision accordingly, is the ultimate predictor of service satisfaction. Finally, the personal meaning to the patients of their mental health problems, and of mental health services, could also play a part.

Overall the data showed that satisfaction with psychiatric services can be considered as the result of both the ability of a service to provide a standard of care above a certain quality threshold, and the perception of each individual patient that the care received has been specifically tailored to his/her specific, individual needs (Ruggeri et al., 2003).

(f) Heterogeneity of clinician-rated and self-rated outcomes

A three-year follow-up study addressed the issue of heterogeneity of outcomes in a prevalence cohort of 107 patients with schizophrenia attending the South Verona CMHS (Ruggeri et al., 2004), by measuring several outcomes simultaneously (psychopathology, functioning, needs and quality of life) and identifying discrepancies in the results obtained in each domain. Mean symptom severity was stable in 74% of patients, worsened in 18% and improved in 8%. Patients had 4.8 and 4.6 needs as assessed by their key workers at baseline and follow-up respectively out of the 22 problem areas assessed by the scale. Social and functioning needs for care worsened, while basic needs improved. The majority of subjects rated their quality of life as medium–high and on average showed no change over time. In three years, functioning worsened in 47% and improved in 30% of subjects. Depending on the inclusion of objective or subjective variables in the definition of 'good' and 'poor' outcome, the percentage of patients with a bad outcome ranged from 3% to 31%, and percentages of 'good' outcome ranged from 0% to 24%, showing that only a minority of subjects affected by schizophrenia can be placed at the extremes of the range of possible outcomes, and that care should be taken in extrapolating the results of studies based on single indicators of outcome. These results convey an important piece of information for clinical practice, i.e. that additional treatments targeted to problem areas beyond symptoms become especially important as they may offer more opportunities to reduce disability and to increase quality of life and subjective well-being.

The road ahead

In Italy, psychiatric reform has been applied unevenly when considering the most comprehensive set of facilities and requirements but it is clear that changes that have occurred in the last 30 years have placed community treatments at the very centre of psychiatric care. As was noted more than two decades ago: 'monitoring and evaluation are important aspects of change: planning and evaluation should go hand in hand and evaluation should, wherever possible, have an epidemiological basis' (Tansella and Williams, 1987). Unfortunately, in Italy this has not happened on a large scale and no governmental decision has promoted the fulfilment of such requirements. However, some Italian centres of excellence, with a long tradition in the area of psychiatric epidemiology, have conducted studies that compare favourably with the international standards and proved that outcome assessment in Italian routine practice is not only sustainable, but advantageous in the medium and long term (Lasalvia and Ruggeri, 2007, Ruggeri et al., 2007). The methodology successfully tested by several Italian mental health services should thus be more extensively used in multicentre studies and in evaluating the effectiveness of psychosocial interventions. The groundwork has been laid for these changes, and can benefit from the contribution of recent developments in psychiatric epidemiology. Some actions are to be prioritized:

(a) encouraging mental health services' participation in evaluation activities – and rewarding staff members for participating in them; in fact, this type of assessment is typically conducted on a voluntary basis, with no proper methodological support, no staff incentives and, quite frequently, no dedicated funding;

(b) allocating resources for intervention studies based on the mandatory criteria of (i) an evidence base for any intervention proposed, (ii) rigorous assessment of treatment fidelity to the original model and careful documentation of all reasons for adapting treatment to routine practice or to a specific local condition, (iii) a proper assessment of the intervention's effectiveness, (iv) implementation and testing of the intervention on a larger scale, (v) an assessment of implementation results and (vi) dissemination of findings;

(c) promoting decision-making processes that rely more strictly on evidence and on epidemiological assessment; not only is such an attitude currently lacking in Italy (and abroad; Goldberg, 2008), but the field's capacity for coordinating its existing body of knowledge is as poor as the data on routine practices are scarce.

Implementation of these three actions can lead to a cultural change among Italian mental health service staff members, which in turn will facilitate the establishment of a revision-of-practice process, greater acceptance of the importance of evidence and a predisposition to put it into practice, a better understanding by researchers of the limitations of academic studies and, consequently, an increase in the number and quality of studies conducted in routine, real-world services.

References

Barbato, A., Terzian, E., Saraceno, B., Barquero, F. M. and Tognoni, G. (1992a). Patterns of aftercare for psychiatric patients discharged after short inpatient treatment. An Italian collaborative study. *Social Psychiatry and Psychiatric Epidemiology*, 27, 46–52.

Barbato, A., Terzian, E., Saraceno, B., De Luca, L. and Tognoni, G. (1992b). Outcome of discharged psychiatric patients after short inpatient treatment: an Italian collaborative study. *Social Psychiatry and Psychiatric Epidemiology*, 27, 192–7.

Chiappelli, M. and Berardi, S. (2000). [Pattern of intervention and patients' satisfaction with community mental health services in Bologna]. *Epidemiologia e Psichiatria Sociale*, 9, 272–81.

Cozza, M., Amara, M., Butera, N., et al. (1997). [The patient and family satisfaction with the department of mental health in Rome]. *Epidemiologia e Psichiatria Sociale*, 6, 173–83.

De Girolamo, G., Bassi, M., Neri, G., Ruggeri, M., Santone, G. and Picardi, A. (2007). The current state of mental health care in Italy: problems, perspectives, and lessons to learn. *European Archives of Clinical Neurosciences*, 257, 83–91.

Division of Mental Health and Prevention of Substance Abuse (1997). *WHOQOL – Measuring quality of life*. Geneva.

Gaite, L., Vazquez-Barquero, J. L., Borra, C., et al. and the EPSILON study group (2002). Quality of life in patients with schizophrenia in five European countries: the Epsilon Study. *Acta Psychiatrica Scandinavica*, 105, 283–92.

Gigantesco, A., Picardi, A., Chiaia, E., Balbi, A. and Morosini, P. (2002). Patients' and relatives' satisfaction with psychiatric services in a large catchment area in Rome. *European Psychiatry*, 17, 139–47.

Goldberg, D. (2008). Improved investment in mental health services: value for money? *British Journal of Psychiatry*, 192, 88–91.

Henderson, C., Hales, H. and Ruggeri, M. (2003). Cross-cultural differences in the conceptualisation of patient's satisfaction with psychiatric services: content validity of the English version of the Verona Service Satisfaction Scale. *Social Psychiatry and Psychiatric Epidemiology*, 38, 142–8.

Lasalvia, A. and Ruggeri, M. (2007). Assessing the outcome of community-based psychiatric care: building a feedback loop from 'real world' health services research into clinical practice. *Acta Psychiatrica Scandinavica Supplementum*, 437, 6–15.

Lasalvia, A., Ruggeri, M., Mazzi, M. A. and Dall'Agnola, R. B. (2000). The perception of needs for care in staff and patients in community-based mental health services. The South-Verona Outcome Project 3. *Acta Psychiatrica Scandinavica*, 102, 366–75.

Lasalvia, A., Bonetto, C., Malchiodi, F., et al. (2005). Listening to patients' needs to improve their subjective quality of life. *Psychological Medicine*, 35, 1655–65.

Lasalvia, A., Bonetto, C., Salvi, G., et al. (2007). Predictors of changes in needs for care in patients receiving community psychiatric treatment: a 4-year follow-up study. *Acta Psychiatrica Scandinavica Supplementum*, 437, 31–41.

Lasalvia, A., Bonetto, C., Tansella, M., Stefani, B. and Ruggeri, M. (2008). Does staff-patient agreement on needs for care predict a better mental health outcome? A 4-year follow-up in a community service. *Psychological Medicine*, 38, 123–33.

Lora, A. (2009). An overview of the mental health system in Italy. *Annali Dell Istituto Superiore Di Sanita*, 45, 5–16.

Lora, A., Bezzi, R., Di Vietri, R., et al. (2002). I pacchetti di cura nei Dipartimenti di Salute Mentale della Regione Lombardia [Packages of care in the departments of mental health in Lombardy]. *Epidemiologia e Psichiatria Sociale*, 11, 100–15.

Oliver, J. P. J. (1991–92). The social care directive: development of a quality of life profile for use in community services for the mentally ill. *Social Work & Social Sciences Review*, 3, 5–45.

Phelan, M., Slade, M., Thornicroft, G., et al. (1995). The Camberwell Assessment of Need: the validity and reliability of an instrument to assess the needs of people with severe mental illness. *British Journal of Psychiatry*, **167**, 589–95.

Picardi, A., Rucci, P., de Girolamo, G., et al. (2006). The quality of life of the mentally ill living in residential facilities: findings from a national survey in Italy. *European Archives of Psychiatry and Clinical Neuroscience*, **256**, 372–81.

Progetto Obiettivo 'Tutela Salute Mentale 1998–2000'; (1999). Decreto del Presidente della Repubblica (Gazzetta Ufficiale n. 274 del 22.11.1999).

Rossi, A., Amaddeo, F., Bisoffi, G., et al. (2002). Dropping out of care: inappropriate terminations of contact with community-based psychiatric services. *British Journal of Psychiatry*, **181**, 331–8.

Ruggeri, M. and Dall'Agnola, R. (1993). The development and use of the Verona Expectations for Care Scale (VECS) and the Verona Service Satisfaction Scale (VSSS) for measuring expectations and satisfaction with community-based psychiatric services in patients, relatives and professionals. *Psychological Medicine*, **23**, 511–23.

Ruggeri, M., Dall'Agnola, R., Bisoffi, G. and Greenfield, T. (1996). Factor analysis of the Verona Service Satisfaction Scale – 82 and development of reduced versions. *International Journal of Methods in Psychiatric Research*, **6**, 23–38.

Ruggeri, M., Lasalvia, A., Dall'Agnola, R., et al. and the EPSILON study group (2000). Development, internal consistency and reliability of the European version of the Verona Service Satisfaction Scale – EU Version (VSSS-EU). *British Journal of Psychiatry*, **177**, S41–8.

Ruggeri, M., Warner, R., Bisoffi, G. and Fontecedro, L. (2001). Subjective and objective dimensions of quality of life in psychiatric patients: a factor-analytic approach. The South Verona Outcome Project 4. *British Journal of Psychiatry*, **178**, 268–75.

Ruggeri, M., Lasalvia, A., Bisoffi, G., et al. (2003). Satisfaction with mental health services among people with schizophrenia in five European sites: results from the Epsilon Study. *Schizophrenia Bulletin*, **29**, 229–45.

Ruggeri, M., Lasalvia, A., Tansella, M., et al. (2004). Heterogeneity in multi-dimensional outcomes of schizophrenia: 3 year follow-up for treated prevalent cases. *British Journal of Psychiatry*, **184**, 48–57.

Ruggeri, M., Greenfield, T. and Dall'Agnola, R. (2006). The VSSS-EU Scale. In G. Thornicroft, T. Becker, M. Knapp et al., eds., *International Outcome Measures in Mental Health. Quality of Life, Needs, Service Satisfaction, Costs and Impact on Carers. Scales to Measure Mental Health Outcomes*. London: Gaskell.

Ruggeri, M., Salvi, G., Bonetto, C., et al. (2007). Outcome of patients dropping out from community-based mental health care: a 6-year multiwave follow-up study. *Acta Psychiatrica Scandinavica Supplementum*, **437**, 42–52.

Tansella, M. and Williams, P. (1987). The Italian experience and its implications. *Psychological Medicine*, **17**, 283–9.

Thornicroft, G. and Tansella, M. (1999). Translating ethical principles into outcome measures for mental health service research. *Psychological Medicine*, **29**, 761–7.

Ventura, J., Green, M. F., Shaner, A. and Liberman, R. P. (1993). Training and quality assurance with the Brief Psychiatric Rating Scale: 'The drift busters'. *International Journal of Methods in Psychiatric Research*, **3**, 221–44.

Warner, R., de Girolamo, G., Belelli, G., et al. (1998). Quality of life and psychopathology in Boulder, Colorado, and Bologna, Italy. *Schizophrenia Bulletin*, **24**, 559–68.

World Health Organization (1988). *Disability Assessment Schedule (DAS-II)*. Geneva.

Outcome measurement in Germany

Sylke Andreas, Thomas Becker, Holger Schulz and Bernd Puschner

Organization of mental health service provision in Germany

Unlike many other Western countries, the organization of the German health care system is 'multi-centre', i.e. there is no central organization with overall responsibility, let alone power, for planning of service provision. The German government can only provide a legal framework and define overarching goals. Specific responsibilities are shared between federal authorities, the 16 states, local authorities and semi-statutory organizations. 'Free doctor choice' is one of the central principles of the German system, and – in contrast to most other countries – there is so far little restriction of access to specialist care.

By international standards, the Federal Republic of Germany system has a particularly densely developed provision of mental health care (Salize et al., 2007). Settings include inpatient or day care in psychiatric or psychosomatic hospitals, psychiatric and psychosomatic units at general hospitals and outpatient treatment by psychiatrists and psychotherapists of various theoretical backgrounds, e.g. CBT or psychodynamic and GPs; see Puschner et al. (2006). While in most Western countries, inpatient care of patients with mental disorders takes place in psychiatric wards of general hospitals or psychiatric clinics, in Germany a comprehensive inpatient health care system has been established within the medical rehabilitation sector (see Figure 1, Schulz et al., 2008). This development was influenced by a neglect of psychotherapeutic approaches in the postwar period and a strong neurological-biological focus, while there was an emphasis on psychotherapeutic treatment of mental disorders within the framework of medical rehabilitation (Koch and Potreck-Rose, 1994). Since the 1990s the psychiatric-psychotherapeutic health care system has identified the shortcomings of psychotherapeutic services, and substantial progress has been made to incorporate psychotherapeutic interventions as a routine part of care.

As seen in Table 8.1, in Germany inpatient psychiatric-psychotherapeutic and psychosomatic-psychotherapeutic health care takes place both within the framework of hospital treatment and in the rehabilitation sector. The former is provided in wards (in general hospitals) and in psychiatric and psychotherapeutic hospitals as well as in hospitals and wards for psychosomatic medicine and psychotherapy. Health care is mainly provided to patients with statutory health insurance and also to a limited number of private patients and self-paying patients. A further part of health care takes place within the field of rehabilitation of patients with mental disorders. This service is mainly provided to patients with statutory pension insurance within the framework of medical rehabilitation and to a limited number of patients within the statutory health insurance. Finally inpatient psychiatric-psychotherapeutic health care is also provided within the framework of consultation and liaison psychiatry in general hospitals. German outpatient psychiatric-psychotherapeutic health care is provided primarily through medical specialists in psychiatry and psychotherapy (and neurologists) in private practice and through psychological and medical psychotherapists and child & youth

Outcome Measurement in Mental Health: Theory and Practice, ed. Tom Trauer. Published by Cambridge University Press.

Table 8.1 The mental health care system of Germany

Service provision			Financing[a]
Inpatient	Psychiatry	(53,021 beds)	SHI / PHI
	Psychosomatic	(4,412 beds)	
	Medical rehabilitation	(12,477 beds)	SHI / SPI / PHI
Partial inpatient	Day clinics		SHI / SPI / PHI
Outpatient	Private practice		SHI / PHI
	Private practice		
	Outpatients		

[a]SHI, statutory health insurance; PHI, private health insurance; SPI, statutory pension insurance.

psychotherapists. This outpatient care is mainly financed by statutory health insurance (Schulz et al., 2008).

Quality assurance in Germany

In Germany the legal basis for quality assurance lies in the health care reform passed in 1989 and the Social Code Book amendments, which came into effect in January 2000. By law health service providers are liable for the assurance and advancement of the services they provide. These have to adhere to the current state of scientific knowledge and have to be provided to a professionally adequate standard. Thus all mental health providers have to participate in external quality assurance comprising multiple professions and institutions (including certified hospitals, SHI (Statutory Health Insurance)-authorized physicians and providers of preventive and rehabilitation services). The German Social Code Book also stipulates that certified hospitals, inpatient preventive clinics and inpatient rehabilitation clinics must introduce a quality management system within their institution (Kawski et al., 2005).

The first approaches towards an introduction of quality assurance measures in the field of psychotherapeutic and psychosomatic health care services into routine care only started in the mid-1990s (Kawski and Koch, 2004). Compared to other countries, this is a young and still evolving branch of quality assurance in health care.

Outcome measurement in Germany

In general, assessment of the quality of health services can be described under the headings of inputs, processes and outcomes. Direct and indirect information on each of these can in principle be obtained from the perspective of any stakeholer, including payors. However, the means for the direct assessment of illness severity as the pivotal component of outcome of mental health services are ratings by the patient or the clinician.

Self-evaluation measures have several advantages and are therefore more frequently used in clinical practice and research than rating measures performed by clinicians. A large amount of clinically relevant information can only be collected by means of information provided directly by the patient (e.g. patient mood or perception of his or her overall mental state). Furthermore, self-evaluation measures are less time-consuming for personnel and can thus be carried out more frequently. On the other hand, clinician ratings are advantageous when the patient is unable to provide information due to such factors as compliance and cognitive capacity (Andreas et al., 2007).

Efforts to measure outcome and to actively use outcome data in Germany have been restricted to specific settings or occur at a local level. We will describe some of the relevant initiatives.

Documentation of basic features of routine care in different service settings

(a) Inpatient psychiatric-psychotherapeutic services

Basic concepts and principles of quality assurance in mental health care have been described in detail by Gaebel (2001), who recommended the introduction of a feasible documentation system and the establishment of structures for internal and external quality assurance.

A major effort in this direction began 15 years ago when a team at Regensburg University developed a basic documentation system (BADO) which has been recommended for use in psychiatric hospitals in Germany by the German Association for Psychiatry and Psychotherapy (DGPPN, Cording et al., 1995) and is now in use in many German psychiatric hospitals.

The BADO has about 70 items and focuses on the assessment of patient sociodemographic (e.g. age, living situation) and illness characteristics (e.g. illness onet, diagnosis), as well as on elements of treatment (e.g. medication and psychotherapy). Aspects of treatment outcome include suicidality, use of compulsory measures and discharge against clinician advice. Furthermore, clinicians are asked to complete the Global Assessment of Functioning Scale (GAF, Endicott et al., 1976) and Clinical Global Impressions (CGI, Guy, 1976). Motivated to evaluate the effects of routine care, the team at Regensburg University used BADO data to study questions such as the validity of diagnoses, suicidality and pathways of care (Spiessl, 2009).

The main drawback of the BADO is the limited focus on standardized assessment of outcome using rather crude measures with questionable psychometric properties. Also, the quality of data is rather poor (Frick et al., 2003), and clinicians receive no formal training in using these instruments. Furthermore active use of routine data generated this way is far from optimal, i.e. it is generally restricted to the team of original developers.

While this version was intended to be used in inpatient psychiatric care, several offshoots have been developed for other service settings, e.g. the BADO-K for complementary psychiatric community care (Schützwohl and Kallert, 2009) which has been widely implemented in Saxony and also includes the Health of the Nation Outcome Scales (HoNOS, see below) (Wing et al., 1998, Andreas et al., 2007), the AmBADO for psychiatric outpatient clinics (Spengler, 2009), and Psy-BADO for Psychosomatics and Psychotherapy (see below). Some initiatives extended the BADO in order to carry out external quality assurance including comparisons between inpatient service providers and benchmarking. First, during 1998 to 2000, a quality assurance programme for diagnosis and treatment of depression was implemented in the federal state of Baden-Wuerttemberg (Härter et al., 2004). The quality of in-patient care of over 3,000 patients with depressive disorders has been documented at 24 psychiatric/psychotherapeutic hospitals. Outcome measures included the staff-rated Hamilton Depression Rating Scale (HAM-D, Hamilton, 1960), Clinical Global Impression Scale (CGI, Guy, 1976) and the user-rated instruments the Beck Depression Inventory (BDI, Beck et al., 1961) and a patient satisfaction questionnaire (ZUF-8, Schmidt et al., 1989). The hospitals received an evaluation which included a detailed comparison of performance and quality indicators.

Second, in 1997/1998, with the goal of developing and implementing a feedback system for quality comparison, comprehensive data were collected for 1,042 inpatients with a diagnosis of schizophrenia in four psychiatric hospitals in the state of Northrhine-Westphalia (Janssen et al., 2000). Instruments used included Brief Psychiatric Rating Scale (Overall and Gorham, 1962), Social and Occupational Functioning Assessment Scale (SOFAS, Goldman et al., 1992), CGI (Guy, 1976) and ZUF-8 (Schmidt et al., 1989). Quality profiles including selected information of structural, process and outcome indicators were considered useful in order to quickly compare clinic performance. However, use of outcome profiles was limited due to lack of systematic control of casemix.

(b) Inpatient psychosomatic-psychotherapeutic services

The first intensive efforts for external quality assurance measures in Germany started in the inpatient hospital care sector and they were pioneered both in the medical rehabilitation sector within the statutory pension insurance and in some inpatient mental health services. In 1994 a quality assurance programme also including the field of 'psychosomatic-psychotherapeutic rehabilitation' was begun. The core features of this programme comprised structural investigations, assessment of process quality via peer reviews and interviewing of patients (Cording et al., 1995).

Since the year 2000 this quality assurance programme has been further developed within the framework of rehabilitation of the statutory health insurance (including the indications of psychosomatic rehabilitation). This advance mainly includes a stronger focus on the aspect of outcome quality (multiple time-point measurements at the level of patients and consultants).

In the mid-1990s a psychotherapy documentation system was developed for the psychotherapeutic care sector by a number of different psychotherapeutic associations (Basisdokumentation in der Psychotherapie) (Heuft and Senf, 1998). This Psy-BaDo system incoporates all therapeutic and health care approaches; however, it has not been implemented into health care as much as was originally intended. A parallel and advanced version was developed for the inpatient and psychosomatic health care sector, the Psy-BaDo-PTM (Schulz et al., 2008), which by now has been implemented in 17 institutions. Data management is carried out by the Institute for Quality Assurance in Psychotherapy and Psychosomatics (Institut für Qualitätssicherung in der Psychotherapie und Psychosomatik, IQP). Of the 17 participating clinics eight are rehabilitation clinics, four are hospitals and five include both rehabilitation and hospital care. In total, hospital care includes 479 beds while rehabilitation comprises 1,431 beds. Still limited in size, this cannot be regarded as an external quality assurance programme reflecting the typical health care structure in the psychotherapeutic hospital care sector.

Use of outcome measures in routine care: examples of good practice

(a) The Stuttgart Heidelberg model

The Stuttgart Heidelberg model (Kordy and Bauer, 2003) was initially designed as an 'active-internal' quality assurance model. It is primarily based on a documentation system as well as on measures for the assessment of outcome quality (therapist and patient perspectives). This model calculates differences between the actual and expected values in the course of treatment. When a calculated difference exceeds a certain threshold an 'attention signal' is reported to the therapist. The system has been implemented in a large number of clinics, and a first external clinic comparison is now available at Heidelberg University's Center for Psychotherapy Research (Schulz et al., 2008).

(b) The TRANS-OP study

The 'Transparency and Outcome Orientation in Outpatient Psychotherapy' (TRANS-OP) study undertook comprehensive repeated tracking of treatment outcome for outpatient psychotherapy. Between September 1998 and February 2000, 787 insurees of a major German health insurance company who received outpatient psychotherapy gave informed consent to participate in this study. Participants applied for the following treatments eligible for reimbursement in the German health insurance system: psychodynamically oriented psychotherapy (52%), cognitive behavioural therapy (31%) and psychoanalytic psychotherapy (17%). During a two-year period, participants' health status was comprehensively assessed on five occasions using standardized instruments. Hierarchical linear modelling was used to estimate courses of improvement in and transitions between the phases before, during and after treatment.

Figure 8.1 shows that – with some variation – psychological impairment improved substantially in all three forms of treatment.

Such an approach could be used as the basis for comprehensive quality management in outpatient psychotherapy. Currently, this is being tried in a model project of a public health insurance company ('Techniker Krankenkasse') (Fydrich et al., 2003). In several regions in Central and Southern Germany, a quality-monitoring system, including collection of standardized outcome data at intake, during treatment and at termination, is being tested as an alternative to the traditional peer review which is still necessary for the approval of reimbursement of the costs of psychotherapy by health insurers.

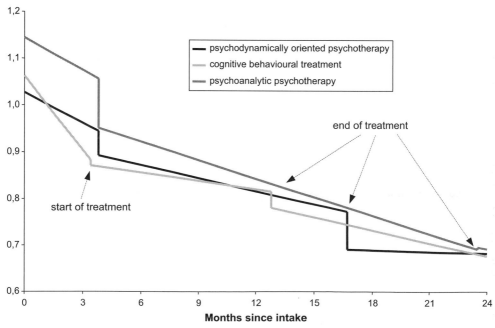

Figure 8.1 Symptom severity (SCL-90-R Global Severity Index) before, during and after outpatient psychotherapy (adapted from Puschner et al., 2007).

(c) Outcome management in inpatient psychiatric care: the EMM study

Recently, a cluster-randomized trial entitled 'Outcome monitoring and outcome management in inpatient psychiatric care' (EMM) investigated the efficacy of weekly feedback of treatment outcome management to users and staff at a large psychiatric hospital in rural Bavaria (Puschner et al., 2009). All 294 patients who participated filled in the *Ergebnisbogen EB-45* (Lambert et al., 2002), the German version of the *Outcome Questionnaire 45.2* (OQ-45.2, (Lambert et al., 1996), a scale widely used for outcome assessment in mental health services (see Chapter 6 by Michael Lambert in this book). Shortly after having completed the EB-45, patient and clinician received a summary of the information provided. Feedback was given in paper on a single page with the following information: (a) a graph showing the EB-45 total scores over time; (b) a written summary consisting of illness course, illness status and a treatment recommendation; (c) a sentence in red text on suicidality in case the relevant EB-45 item had been rated higher than 0 ('alarm item'); (d) a disclaimer saying that this information is based on the patient's view only, which might differ from the clinician's appraisal, and encouraging patient and clinician to talk about this feedback. Clinicians received additional information: (a) a coloured dot (red, yellow, green or white) corresponding to type of change; (b) a table with all EB-45 total scores at admission, subsequent and current assessment, including a summary of change and status. Drawing upon Hawkins et al. (2004), patient and clinician versions of short text messages were formulated for each feedback type in plain language. As a rule, feedback was optimistic, i.e. even in the case of repeated unfavourable outcomes (no change or deterioration), the recommendation was to continue the treatment. The summary statements and treatment recommendations were formulated in a positive, non-threatening way.

Table 8.2 Use and appraisal of outcome management (of last feedback received)

		n	%
Clinician			
Agree	Supplemented my view	296	37.5%
	Confirmed my view	308	39.0%
	Changed my view	14	1.8%
Disagree	Underestimated impairment	99	12.4%
	Overestimated impairment	52	6.5%
	Neglected other important areas	48	6.0%
Talked about with someone	Yes	666	83.3%
Talked about with patient	Yes	559	69.9%
Use for treatment planning	Not at all	96	12.0%
	Hardly	272	34.0%
	Yes, a little	302	37.8%
	Yes, a lot	96	12.0%
Time spent	min., M (SD)/N	6.2 (5.9)/792	
Patient			
Talked about with someone	Yes	306	44.6%
Talked about with therapist	Yes	123	22.3%

After each feedback received, patients and clinicians were invited to answer a few questions on feasibility of feedback. Of the 1,339 feedbacks received from the intervention group, 126 patients answered the feasibility questionnaire 686 times (51.2%) and 20 clinicians 800 times (59.7%).

As shown in Table 8.2, clinicians spent 6 minutes with a given feedback on average. Most clinicians agreed with the outcome information given, and those who did mostly reported that feedback supplemented or confirmed their clinical judgement. If clinicians disagreed, this was mostly because in their view the patient tended to underreport symptoms. Self-reported use of outcome feedback for treatment planning by clinicians was mixed.

Most striking is the finding that, according to patients, their clinicians talked to them in only about one-fifth of feedbacks received, yet according to clinicians this was the case three times as often. Furthermore, only half the clinicians reported that they used feedback for treatment planning.

(d) Clinician perspective: feedback on the Health of the Nation Outcome Scales (HoNOS)

Since 2004 an internationally widely used outcome instrument, The Health of the Nation Outcome Scales (HoNOS) (Wing et al., 1998, Andreas et al., 2007, 2010), has been available in Germany as a clinician-rating of severity, and is used routinely as a feedback of outcome quality in the quality assurance programme of national health insurance schemes in the rehabilitation sector. In the following an example of the HoNOS is presented to illustrate the feedback of outcome quality to the clinics.

In Germany the national health insurance schemes are responsible for approximately 70 million people. The national confederations of regional associations of health insurance developed a procedure for external quality assurance, on the basis of the legal framework and requirements, measuring the dimensions of structure, process and outcome quality and patient satisfaction: the QS-Reha®-Verfahren (QS-Rehab System). Subsequent to the instrument development the derived procedures for the indication of mental disorders and substance-related disorders were tested in 11 inpatient clinics within a pilot phase. Following the analysis of the results of the pilot phase, instruments and measures were customized and modified. The routine phase started in autumn 2004 and by 2009 included 22 further clinics.

The reports to the clinics include risk-adjusted analyses in different areas of outcome quality (e.g. drop-out analyses and therapy goals).[1] Following the feedback of the sample distribution in the index clinic compared to all other clinics taking part in the QS-Rehab System, the following parameters are now also reported to the clinic: employment status, absence due to incapacity to work and sick leave during the last 6 months, application for pension due to reduced earning capacity, prior treatments, diagnoses, chronicity of main illness, therapy motivation and treatment duration. Due to difficulties in the assessment of treatment success by therapists, who thereby also indirectly assesses their own work, patient assessments are the most important measure of outcome quality in clinic comparisons.

For the risk adjustment of the QS-Rehab System a regression analysis approach was chosen (Iezzoni, 1997). In order to avoid data loss due to missing values, these were replaced with interval scaled variables by means of the Expectation Maximization Method

---

[1] Rabung, S., Andreas, S., Bleich, C., et al. (2009). Comparing outcomes across mental health care providers – necessity and limitations of risk adjustment. Unpublished manuscript.

(Little and Rubin, 2002). Categorical variables were recoded into dummy-coded variables, which enabled monitoring for possible systemic effects of missing values and also allowed the use of the complete data set for the assessment of regression weights and expected values.

By means of this analysis individual outcome values within outcome areas were predicted for each patient, controlling for values of the theoretically supported or empirically identified confounding variables, from which mean expected values were calculated across all patients of one clinic. In order to account for the inaccuracy of psychometric measurements, a 95% confidence interval was calculated for the difference between the expected and observed mean values (see note 1, this chapter).

A wide range of sociodemographic and diagnostic variables were included as outcome predictors, as well as impairment at the beginning of treatment measured across the different psychometric measures. Thereby the regression analyses allow for a prediction of symptom burden and severity of impairment, as expected from the size of the confounding variables in the patient population, and a comparison of this predicted value with the achieved value. The ratio between risk-adjusted expected values and achieved values at the end of treatment in the respective test procedure represents a central parameter of outcome quality. For all tests and their subscales high values indicate a high degree of symptoms and problem impairment. In Figure 8.2 the expected values are represented by a dashed line, while the achieved values are represented by solid symbols. The upper and lower limits of the 95% confidence intervals for the difference between achieved and expected mean values are shown as vertical error bars in the figure. In cases where the achieved value of a clinic lies below the confidence interval of the expected value this generally indicates a significantly better treatment outcome than expected from the presented patient characteristics in the clinic and accounted for by the risk adjustment (marked as a diamond; see Figure 8.2). In cases where the achieved value of a clinic lies above the confidence interval of the expected value, this indicates a poorer treatment

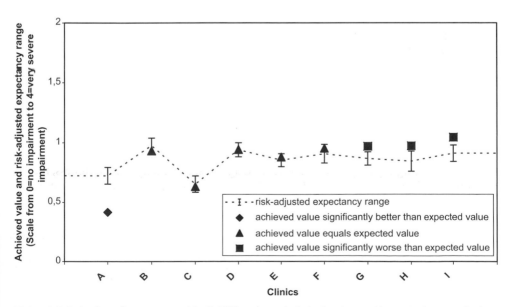

Figure 8.2 Risk-adjusted comparison of the HoNOS total severity index (mean score) between the example clinic (F) and the reference clinics (see note 1, this chapter); mean score of the HoNOS = total score divided by 10.

outcome than expected from the presented patient characteristics in the clinic (marked as a square) (see note 1, this chapter).

With regard to the degree of impairment at the time of discharge, patients of the example clinic 'F' do not show significantly different impairment, with a mean HoNOS-D total score of 0.95 (SD = 0.47, in comparison with the expected value from the distribution of the risk factors within the sample of 0.91) as depicted in Figure 8.2 (see note 1, this chapter).

Empirical studies supported the practicality of the HoNOS, as demonstrated by the small number of missing values and the average administration time (Andreas et al., 2007). Despite the existence of some evidence that HoNOS training does not necessarily improve inter-rater reliability (Rock and Preston, 2001), our own study showed that HoNOS training is necessary and meaningful (Andreas et al., 2009). Moreover, with regard to reliability and validity the HoNOS shows satisfactory values in routine mental health care (Andreas et al., 2007, 2010).

Conclusions

Even though numerous instruments with good psychometric properties and feasibility are available to assess treatment outcome in people with mental illness, use of these measures in routine care is rather arbitrary and is mostly restricted to research settings. Use of outcome measurement in Germany could be considered a patchwork. There are initiatives at a local level or in certain service settings that stand out as examples of best practice.

Also many clinicians, especially in large inpatient institutions, complain about being over-burdened with clinical duties and paperwork and are hard to convince to spend extra time using standardized instruments. This is especially difficult when the information obtained is not actively used, as often happens with BADO data, which in some clinics end up in 'data cemeteries' (Spiessl, 2009). On the other hand, as shown by the example of the EMM study, patients in general are able and willing to fill in outcome data on a regular basis.

Thus, acceptance of outcome data largely depends upon implementing adequate strategies in an effort to convince patients and clinicians of the necessity of standardized assessment of treatment outcome. One of the most promising strategies to actively use outcome data is to directly feed back the information obtained to stakeholders. This can be done at an institutional level, e.g. by benchmarking among different comparable service providers, or at an individual level by reporting back information obtained in a meaningful way to service users and their clinicians. Best practice examples for these two approaches have been described above (the QS-Rehab project and the EMM study). However, such approaches consume considerable resources, and need experienced research staff in order to support feedback, e.g. via quality circles.

Further research in this vein should extend the findings of a recent meta-analysis (Knaup et al., 2009) which has shown that feedback of standardized treatment outcome was more effective if it was given to both patients and clinicians (versus clinicians only), was reported at least twice (versus only once), and comprised information on patient progress (versus on status only), and should be continued after the change of service provider (e.g. hospital discharge).

The main reason for the lack of a common strategy for outcome measurement in mental health care in Germany is the fragmentation of the service system, with the lack of a central body responsible for coordinating the different initiatives. The road towards achieving the goal of stakeholders acting more in concert than against one another could be made less rocky by researchers identifying ingredients of best practice in close collaboration with clinicians.

The main task is to find strategies of outcome assessment which are deemed meaningful by clinicians for use in their daily practice – and not, as it is often the case now, as just another part of tedious paperwork.

Outcome measurement in mental health care is often viewed as having a value in itself, or even an 'ethical obligation for the health professions in the modern healthcare systems' (Mainz, 2008). Obviously, informed improvement of mental health services can only take place based upon a solid empirical foundation. However, there is a great need for cost-effectiveness showing how much improvement in mental health at a population or individual level is achieved by the implementation of often complex outcome measurement applications (staff, equipment, space and other resource costs). Thus, future research could produce convincing arguments against sceptics, especially among busy clinicans, arguing that much of outcome measurement is just an end in itself.

References

Andreas, S., Harfst, T., Dirmaier, J., et al. (2007). A psychometric evaluation of the German version of the 'Health of the Nation Outcome Scales, HoNOS-D': on the feasibility and reliability of clinician-performed measurements of severity in patients with mental disorders. *Psychopathology*, **40**, 116–25.

Andreas, S., Rabung, S., Horstmann, D., et al. (2009). Ist eine Schulung von Ratern zur differenzierten Beurteilung des Schweregrades bei Patienten mit psychischen Störungen in der Routineversorgung notwendig? [Training of mental health care professionals in routine outcome assessment – necessary or dispensable?]. *Psychologische Medizin*, **20**, 117.

Andreas, S., Harfst, T., Rabung, S., et al. (2010). The validity of the German version of the Health of the Nation Outcome Scales (HoNOS-D): an expert-rating for the differential assessment of the severity of mental disorders. *International Journal of Methods in Psychiatric Research*, **19**, 50–62.

Beck, A. T., Ward, C. H., Mendelson, M., Mock, J. E. and Erbaugh, J. T. (1961). An inventory for measuring depression. *Archives of General Psychiatry*, **4**, 561–71.

Cording, C., Gaebel, W. and Sengler, A. (1995). Die neue psychiatrische Basisdokumentation. Eine Empfehlung der DGPPN zur Qualitätssicherung im (teil-) stationären Bereich [An innovative basic documentation system. Recommended by the DGPPN for quality assurance in inpatient services]. *Spectrum*, **24**, 3–38.

Endicott, J., Spitzer, R. L., Fleiss, J. L. and Cohen, J. (1976). The Global Assessment Scale: a procedure for measuring overall severity of psychiatric disturbance. *Archives of General Psychiatry*, **33**, 766–71.

Frick, U., Krischker, S. and Cording, C. (2003). *Freiwillige Krankenhausvergleiche zur externen Qualitätssicherung in der Psychiatrie [Voluntary Hospital Comparisons for External Quality Assurance in Psychiatry]*, Bonn: Bericht an das Bundesministerium für Gesundheit und Soziale Sicherung.

Fydrich, T., Nagel, A., Lutz, W. and Richter, R. (2003). Qualitätsmonitoring in der ambulanten Psychotherapie: Modellprojekt der Techniker Krankenkasse [Monitoring of quality assurance in outpatient psychotherapy: A pilot project of the statutory health insurance Techniker Krankenkasse]. *Verhaltenstherapie*, **13**, 291–5.

Gaebel, W. (2001). *Quality assurance in psychiatry*. In F. H. H. Helmchen, H. Lauter and N. Sartorius, eds., *Contemporary Psychiatry*, vol. 2. Berlin: Springer.

Goldman, H. H., Skodol, A. E. and Lave, T. R. (1992). Revising Axis V for DSM-IV: a review of measures of social functioning. *American Journal of Psychiatry*, **149**, 1148–56.

Guy, W. (1976). *ECDEU Assessment Manual for Psychopharmacology – Revised*. Rockville, MD: U.S. Department of Health,

Education, and Welfare, Public Health Service, Alcohol, Drug Abuse, and Mental Health Administration, NIMH Psychopharmacology Research Branch, Division of Extramural Research Programs.

Hamilton, M. (1960). A rating scale for depression. *Journal of Neurology, Neurosurgery and Psychiatry*, **23**, 56–62.

Härter, M., Sitta, P., Keller, F., et al. (2004). Externe Qualitätssicherung bei stationärer Depressionsbehandlung: Modellprojekt der Landesärztekammer Baden-Württemberg [External quality assurance program for in-patient treatment of depression]. *Nervenarzt*, **75**, 1083–91.

Hawkins, E. J., Lambert, M. J., Vermeersch, D. A., Slade, K. and Tuttle, K. (2004). The therapeutic effects of providing patient progress information to therapists and patients. *Psychotherapy Research*, **14**, 308–27.

Heuft, G. and Senf, W. (1998). Praxis der Qualitätssicherung in der Psychotherapie. Das Manual der Psy-BaDo [Practical Issues of Quality Assurance in Psychotherapy. The Manual of the Basis Documentation System in Psychotherapy], Stuttgart: Thieme.

Iezzoni, L. I. (1997). The risks of risk adjustment. *JAMA*, **278**, 1600–7.

Janssen, B., Burgmann, C., Held, T., et al. (2000). Externe Qualitätssicherung der stationären Behandlung schizophrener Patienten: Ergebnisse einer multizentrischen Studie [External quality assurance of inpatient treatment in schizophrenia – results of a multicenter study]. *Der Nervenarzt*, **71**, 364–72.

Kawski, S. and Koch, U. (2004). Qualitätssicherung in der medizinischen Rehabilitation in Deutschland. Entwicklungsstand und Perspektiven [Quality assurance in the field of medical rehabilitation in Germany. State of the art and perspectives]. *Bundesgesundheitsblatt Gesundheitsforschung Gesundheitsschutz*, **47**, 111–17.

Kawski, S., Koch, U., Lubecki, P. and Schulz, H. (2005). Qualitätssicherung der Psychotherapie [Quality assurance in psychotherapy]. In W. Senf and M. Broda,

eds., *Praxis der Psychotherapie – Ein integratives Lehrbuch [Practical Issues of Psychotherapy – An Integrative Educational Book]*. Stuttgart: Thieme.

Knaup, C., Koesters, M., Schoefer, D., Becker, T. and Puschner, B. (2009). Effect of feedback of treatment outcome in specialist mental healthcare: meta-analysis. *British Journal of Psychiatry*, **195**, 15–22.

Koch, U. and Potreck-Rose, F. (1994). Stationäre psychosomatische Rehabilitation – ein Versorgungssystem in der Diskussion. In B. Strauß and A. E. Meyer, eds., *Psychoanalytische Psychosomatik – Theorie, Forschung und Praxis*. Stuttgart: Schattauer.

Kordy, H. and Bauer, S. (2003). The Stuttgart-Heidelberg model of active feedback driven quality management: means for the optimization of psychotherapy provision. *International Journal of Clinical and Health Psychology*, **3**, 615–31.

Lambert, M. J., Burlingame, G. M., Umphress, V. J., et al. (1996). The reliability and validity of the Outcome Questionnaire. *Clinical Psychology and Psychotherapy*, **3**, 106–16.

Lambert, M. J., Hannöver, W., Nisslmüller, K., Richard, M. and Kordy, H. (2002). Fragebogen zum Ergebnis von Psychotherapie: Zur Reliabilität und Validität der deutschen Übersetzung des Outcome Questionnaire 45.2 (OQ-45.2) [Questionnaire on the results of psychotherapy: reliability and validity of the German translation of the Outcome Questionnaire 45.2 (OQ-45.2)]. *Zeitschrift für Klinische Psychologie und Psychotherapie*, **1**, 40–7.

Little, R. and Rubin, D. (2002). *Statistical Analysis with Missing Data*. New York: John Wiley.

Mainz, J. (2008). Quality measurement can improve the quality of care – when supervised by health professionals. *Acta Psychiatrica Scandinavica*, **117**, 321–2.

Overall, J. E. and Gorham, D. R. (1962). The Brief Psychiatric Rating Scale. *Psychological Reports*, **10**, 799–82.

Puschner, B., Kunze, H. and Becker, T. (2006). Influencing policy in Germany. In M. S. S. Priebe, ed., *Choosing Methods in Mental*

Health Research: Mental Health Research from Theory to Practice. London: Routledge.

Puschner, B., Kraft, S., Kächele, H. and Kordy, H. (2007). Course of improvement during two years in psychoanalytic and psychodynamic outpatient psychotherapy. *Psychology and Psychotherapy: Theory, Research and Practice*, **80**, 51–68.

Puschner, B., Schöfer, D., Knaup, C. and Becker, T. (2009). Outcome management in inpatient psychiatric care. *Acta Psychiatrica Scandinavica*, **120**, 308–19.

Rock, D. and Preston, N. (2001). HoNOS: is there any point in training clinicians? *Journal of Psychiatric and Mental Health Nursing*, **8**, 405–9.

Salize, H.-J., Roessler, W. and Becker, T. (2007). Mental health care in Germany: Current state and trends. *European Archives of Psychiatry and Clinical Neuroscience*, **257**, 92–103.

Schmidt, J., Lamprecht, F. and Wittmann, W. W. (1989). Zufriedenheit mit der stationären Versorgung: Entwicklung eines Fragebogens und erste Validitätsuntersuchungen [Satisfaction with inpatient management. Development of a questionnaire and initial validity studies]. *Psychotherapie, Psychosomatik, Medizinische Psychologie*, **39**, 248–55.

Schulz, H., Barghaan, D., Harfst, T. and Koch, U. (2008). *Gesundheitsberichterstattung des Bundes – Psychotherapeutische Versorgung [Health related reporting in Germany – Mental health care]*. Robert Koch Institut.

Schützwohl, M. and Kallert, T. W. (2009). Routine-Daten im komplementären Bereich [Routine data in the complementary sector]. In H. S. W.Gaebel and T . Becker, eds., *Routinedaten in der Psychiatry: Sektorenübergreifende Versorgungsforschung und Qualitätssicherung [Routine Data in Psychiatry: Trans-sectoral Service Research and Quality Assurance]*. Heidelberg: Steinkopf.

Spengler, A. (2009). Routine-Daten in der PIA [Routine data in psychiatric outpatient clinics]. In H. S. W.Gaebel and T . Becker, eds., *Routinedaten in der Psychiatry: Sektorenübergreifende Versorgungsforschung und Qualitätssicherung [Routine Data in Psychiatry: Trans-sectoral Service Research and Quality Assurance]*. Heidelberg: Steinkopf.

Spiessl, H. (2009). Von der BADO zum sektorübergreifenden Daten-Set [From the basic documentation toward trans-sectoral data]. In H. S. W.Gaebel and T . Becker, eds., *Routinedaten in der Psychiatry: Sektorenübergreifende Versorgungsforschung und Qualitätssicherung [Routine Data in Psychiatry: Trans-sectoral Service Research and Quality Assurance]*. Heidelberg: Steinkopf.

Wing, J. K., Beevor, A. S., Curtis, R. H., et al. (1998). Health of the Nation Outcome Scales (HoNOS). Research and development. *British Journal of Psychiatry*, **172**, 11–18.

Outcome measurement in mental health services in Norway

Torleif Ruud

This chapter gives an overview of the use of outcome measures in clinical work in mental health services in Norway. As there is no previous publication on this topic, the presentation is based on a combination of the author's knowledge from mental health services research, discussions with some other researchers, and a few publications giving information on some aspects. The use of outcome measures in research is only partly covered, and is referred to mainly in relation to how the use of outcome measures in studies influences the use of outcome measures in clinical practice.

Mental health services in Norway

Specialized mental health services in Norway are organized together with general hospital services in 20 health authorities, run by four regional health authorities on behalf of the Ministry of Health and Care Services (Norwegian Ministry of Health and Care Services, 2005). Within a health authority the mental health services are organized as a division with inpatient and outpatient services for children and adolescents, adults, the elderly and persons with substance abuse. Almost two-thirds of the inpatient services for adults are in psychiatric wards in hospitals and the rest are in community mental health centres that also have outpatient clinics, mobile teams and day treatment units (Ruud and Hauff, 2003, Johnsen, 2006, Olson, 2006). Psychiatrists and clinical psychologists with their own practices are also part of the mental health services. Almost all the mental health services are public. There are only a few private hospitals and community mental health centres, and these and the psychiatrists and clinical psychologists running their own practices are also mostly funded by the state through agreements with the regional health authority. The child and adolescent mental health services (CAMHS) are also run by the health authorities and consist mainly of outpatient clinics and some inpatient services. The substance abuse and addiction services, with a mixture of outpatient and inpatient services, were included in the health authorities by a reform in 2004. Municipalities are responsible for primary care, including general practitioners (GPs) and social and health services, which often include mental health teams. Most referrals to the mental health services come from the GPs, yet the GPs refer fewer than one in five patients with mental health problems. Norway has 4.8 million inhabitants.

Professional guidelines and instructions on the professional aspects of the health services are mostly given by the Norwegian Directorate of Health, a subdivision of the Ministry of Health and Care Services. There has been a major increase in resources and funding of mental health services in primary care and community mental health centres as part of a National Plan for Mental Health 1999–2008 agreed upon in 1998 by all political parties in Norway on the basis of a parliamentary white paper on mental health. The use of outcome measures was not a specific focus in this plan.

The use of outcome measures in mental health services

Thirty years ago outcome measures were rarely used in the mental health services in Norway, except in research studies. During the last two decades the use of outcome measures has increased in clinical work, but usually more selectively and not in a systematic way that involves all patients. The clinics that have tried to use outcome measures routinely have found this to be difficult to implement consistently, especially in the phase of ending the treatment. The clinicians are more motivated to use systematic measurements to plan treatment in the assessment phase, than to repeat the use of such measures in the last phase of the treatment to measure outcome.

Most of the psychiatrists and psychologists with their own practices use the same software for management of their practice, and this includes a few outcome measures. The proportion of these specialists who use one or more of these measures is not known, but there are probably very few who use such measures routinely with all their patients.

(a) Initiatives from national health authorities

The Directorate of Health and Social Affairs has developed a national strategy for quality in social and health services where effective services are defined as one of the domains for quality (Directorate of Health and Social Affairs, 2005). However, there is no legislative framework or specific demands for use of outcome measures in health services in Norway except what is mentioned below.

In 1999 the Norwegian health authorities decided that a national minimum data set should be used by all mental health services from 2000. This national data set includes rating a split version of the Global Assessment of Functioning Scale (GAF, American Psychiatric Association, 1994) with separate scales for symptom severity and impaired functioning as a routine measure at the beginning and end of each treatment episode. This split version of GAF was developed in Norway (Loevdahl and Friis, 1996) parallel to a similar version published by Goldman et al. (1992), and it has become the version of GAF used in Norway.

GPs receive a fee for using the Montgomery and Åsberg Depression Rating Scale (MADRS, Montgomery and Åsberg, 1979) for assessment and rating of depression. This has been used mostly for assessment, but also to measure outcome in order to monitor improvement in therapy.

The Norwegian Board of Health Supervision has published clinical guidelines for assessment and treatment of anxiety disorders (Norwegian Board of Health Supervision, 1999), eating disorders (Norwegian Board of Health Supervision, 2000a), schizophrenia (Norwegian Board of Health Supervision, 2000b) and mood disorders (Norwegian Board of Health Supervision, 2000c). These guidelines recommend the use of outcome measurement and list instruments that could be used for assessment and outcome measurement, but they give few specific recommendations. The guidelines have contributed to selective use of such instruments for assessment, but they have not led to a general use of outcome measures. There is no systematic study on the implementation of these guidelines, and no mental health authority is known to have implemented any of them on a regular basis.

In recent years the National Knowledge Centre for the Health Services has established the website The Health Library (www.helsebiblioteket.no) for information for health professionals and for the public. The mental health section of the Health Library has included a subsection on measures, including outcome measures. By June 2009 most of the outcome measures mentioned in this chapter were available on this website with copies of the instruments and instructions.

There were efforts in one regional health authority to agree on a set of instruments for the mental health services, but this had not been implemented by the time this regional health authority was merged with another, and there is as yet no decision in the new and expanded regional health authority on the use of outcome measures.

(b) Initiatives from professional organizations

There have been a few publications recommending instruments including outcome measures. An overview of scales and questionnaires used in Norway and the other Nordic countries at that time was published in 1993 (Bech et al., 1993). A Test Battery for Group Psychotherapy (TBG) recommended outcome and process measures (Ruud and Lorentzen, 1999), and the use of this test battery has been taught as a part of a five-year training programme at the Institute of Group Analysis in Norway. A software version of the TBG for use in clinical practice has had limited dissemination and has only been used by a few group therapists.

Professional organizations and user organizations have promoted various aspects of treatment in mental health services and primary care, but a report from the Norwegian Medical Association on the needs for improvement of the health services for mental disorders (Fryjordet et al., 2004) did not contain specific recommendations regarding regular use of outcome measures in clinical practice, and the largest user organization, Mental Health Norway, has not given any specific written statements on outcome measurements.

Outcome measures most widely used

All outcome measures that are used in Norway have been imported from other countries. Symptom Checklist 90-R (SCL-90R, Derogatis, 1983) is the most widely used outcome measure, covering a broader range of symptoms. It has been used in many research studies and in clinical work in many parts of the mental health services. The Inventory of Interpersonal Problems (IIP, Horowitz et al., 1988) was developed to measure interpersonal problems in a similar way as SCL-90R measures symptoms. These two instruments or shorter versions of them have increasingly been used together to give information on both psychiatric symptoms and problems in interpersonal relationships.

There is a growing interest in using Outcome Questionnaire 45 (OQ-45, Lambert et al., 1994) in outpatient clinics, and a pilot project has been prepared where patients fill in OQ-45 on a handheld computer in the waiting room, so that the therapist may have the result in the session as a part of monitoring the treatment process. There is also some interest in the Clinical Outcomes in Routine Evaluation – Outcome Measure questionnaire (CORE-OM, Evans et al., 2002). Among many psychologists in adult mental health services and among parts of the CAMHS there has also been an increasing interest in the brief measure Outcome Rating Scale (ORS, Miller et al., 2003). A survey has shown that clinicians in half of the child and adolescent outpatient clinics in the largest health region used or were interested in using ORS (Tuseth et al., 2006).

The Health of the Nation Outcome Scales (HoNOS, Wing et al., 1998) was the main outcome measure in a Multicentre study of Acute Psychiatry carried out by a network involving most of the acute mental health services in Norway in 2005–2006 (Ruud et al., 2006). This and some other larger projects have exposed clinicians in many parts of the mental health services to HoNOS. Many clinicians have commented that they find HoNOS more useful than GAF, as HoNOS ratings give more specific and useful clinical information.

In addition to the broader outcome measures mentioned above, there are some fairly widespread measures covering specific types of symptoms or problems. Among these the

Beck Depression Inventory (BDI, Beck et al., 1996) and the Montgomery and Åsberg Depression Rating Scale (MADRS, Montgomery and Åsberg, 1979) are the most widely used for measuring depression. The Positive and Negative Syndrome Scale (PANSS, Kay et al., 1987) has become a major rating scale in research projects on schizophrenia, and it seems to be increasingly used in clinical practice. Two of the most used outcome measures for anxiety disorders are the Hospital Anxiety Depression Scale (HADS, Snaith and Zigmond, 1983), also covering depression, and the Beck Anxiety Inventory (BAI, Beck et al., 1988). Instruments targeted at other specific patient groups are also in use.

In the substance abuse services the Alcohol Use Disorder Identification Test (AUDIT, Babor et al., 2001) and Drug Use Disorders Identification Test (DUDIT, Berman et al., 2005) are increasingly used to measure abuse of alcohol and drugs, and these now seem to be to the best candidates for outcome measures of substance abuse in clinical practice.

In the CAMHS the four main outcome instruments in use are Health of the Nation Outcome Scales for Children and Adolescents (HoNOSCA, Gowers et al., 1999), Children's Global Assessment Scale (CGAS, Schaffer et al., 1983), Strength and Difficulties Questionnaire (SDQ, Goodman, 1997) and ORS. These have been used in research studies, but are also used to some extent in clinical practice. One child and adolescent outpatient clinic that took part in a research study has continued to use the first three of these instruments to measure outcome with repeated measurements for all patients.

Rating of target complaints defined by the patient is a type of individualized scale that may be used as an outcome measure and that may be very meaningful in clinical practice. This seems to be used fairly seldom compared to the standard instruments mentioned above.

In the last few years the use of remission as an outcome measure has been proposed in scientific journals, and criteria for remission have been developed for some of the major mental disorders. While rating scales and questionnaires usually measure improvement on a continuous scale, remission requires that criteria for a diagnosis present at the start of treatment are no longer present at the end of the treatment. Assessment of remission should be a natural part of clinical practice, but this is not yet practised with systematic outcome measures. The Symptom Checklist 90 Revised (SCL-90R) may be the only outcome measure that has been standardized on the Norwegian population with identification of cut-off points between illness and health (Vassend and Skrondal, 2003), which is useful for identification of remission.

Major projects and implementations

Information about outcome measures and their use has been disseminated from several larger research projects, and some of these are mentioned below. There are also many national and regional centres of competence in relation to assessment and treatment of specific patient groups. These centres seem to have had a varying degree of influence on clinical practice and on use of outcome measurements.

(a) Research networks involving clinicians

Research studies involving many sites in a multicentre study have recommended sets of instruments for use in specific settings or for specific patient groups, contributing to dissemination of outcome measurement.

The Day Treatment Network has been a success since it was established in 1994 (Karterud et al., 2003). Fifteen day units in the south-eastern region of Norway have taken part in the network on a regular basis over several years. The network has succeeded in keeping clinicians interested and engaged by involving them in training and in the use of outcome measures, by giving regular feedback to each site on their outcome compared with other sites, and by involving them in regular professional meetings and the research process. The day units in the network use outcome measures on a daily basis for all patients.

The Multicentre study on Acute Psychiatry (Ruud et al., 2006) was developed as a joint undertaking by a network for evaluation and research on acute psychiatric services involving most acute units in Norway. While the inclusion period and data collection in this study and network were limited in time to a few months, a few of the acute wards have continued to use parts of the registration forms used in the study, including HoNOS.

As mentioned above, parts of the CAMHS and many psychologists in the adult mental health services are involved in a network of people interested in the use of ORS in clinical practice. Another example is a research network on bipolar disorders.

(b) Large research studies

Large and successful research studies also contribute to the use of outcome measures even if they are not a part of a formal network with clinicians. Some clinicians may be involved in data collection using outcome measures, and they may be trained in the use of such measures by researchers who have had time and opportunity to be well trained and gain much experience in using the instruments.

A research project on outcome measures in CAMHS is a good example of such studies. Several child and adolescent outpatient clinics in the country were involved in the study, and many clinicians were trained in using HoNOSCA and other outcome measures achieving adequate levels of inter-rater reliability (Hanssen-Bauer et al., 2007).

There are also several large studies that have contributed to dissemination of outcome measures even if the instruments were not used as outcome measures in these studies. One of the largest and most recent examples is the research programme for the Thematic Area Psychoses (TOP) selected as one of the strategic research priorities by the Faculty of Medicine at the University of Oslo. In this project the same core instruments are used in many sub-studies (doctoral theses) to assist in the building of a large data base on severe mental disorders. With many research fellows having been trained in the same instruments in order to secure a good enough inter-rater reliability across studies in the TOP project, this has led to well-organized training and to training for many researchers who later may train clinicians. The TIPS study of early identification of and intervention in first psychosis (Johannessen et al. 2000) is another example of a large study having impact on the use of outcome measures for psychotic disorders.

Current issues and concerns
(a) Low levels of completion and compliance

The use of GAF as a part of the national data set on treatment episodes in the mental health services for adults has been the only outcome measure required by the national health authorities. Analysis of data reported to the National Patient Register for 2007 based on the national data set for treatment episodes in mental health services shows that split GAF scores for symptoms and functioning had been registered for 66% patients at admission and for 55% at discharge (personal communication, Per Bernhard Pedersen, SINTEF, 5 June 2009).

In the Multicentre study on Acute Psychiatry the acute units were asked to report the use of instruments in the assessments at admission, and the average proportion of patients across sites assessed with any rating scale was 8% in acute inpatient wards and 6% in crisis resolution teams (Ruud et al., 2006). There was no requirement to report the use of measures at discharge in order to assess outcome, but this was probably even less frequent. In a recent survey of group therapy in mental health services for adults more than half of the 426 groups reporting data used a questionnaire as an outcome measure, and one in six used rating scales (Lorentzen, personal communication, June 2009).

(b) Low quality of the outcome measurements

The quality of the routine GAF ratings as a part of the national data set for the adult mental health services is unknown, but it has been questioned as there is great variation in whether the services have procedures to ensure the quality of these (Loevdahl and Friis, 1996, Fallmyr and Repål, 2002). In a study of the GAF scores of symptoms and functioning of 82 consecutive admissions, the ratings done by clinicians according to department procedures had low inter-rater reliability (ICC coefficients of 0.39 and 0.59) when compared to GAF ratings by two trained researchers, while it was high (ICC coefficients of 0.81 and 0.85) between the two researchers (Vatnaland et al., 2007).

Due to incomplete data and questionable reliability, the GAF scores are not routinely reported in national statistics, and the data are not published or used locally in a systematic way. The Directorate of Health is considering removing GAF from the national data set, since it is not used as intended and probably has low data quality.

(c) Limited systematic training of staff

There are no national programmes or instructions for training of staff in use of outcome measures, but research studies have established such training programmes, and these are sometimes adopted by clinical services. Such training is often based on models from those that developed the instruments. On a few occasions the inter-rater reliability is tested, but most often this is not the case, and often outcome measures are used in clinical practice without adequate training and with unknown quality.

As the split GAF scale is the only rating scale that has been mandatory in the mental health services, there has been some activity in running training for this. Such half-day trainings have been arranged in several health authorities. One recent doctoral thesis on the use of the psychometric properties of GAF and some other instruments has shown that the most cost-effective quality assurance of GAF ratings is done by having two clinicians rate GAF together (Pedersen et al., 2007). Further improvement in quality may be obtained by including more raters, but not to the extent that it can justify the additional use of resources.

The psychologist who wrote the dissertation mentioned above also established a website for training in GAF rating (Pedersen, 2008) as a part of the work with the Day Treatment Network. At this website clinicians can improve their GAF rating by rating 20 case vignettes and getting individual feedback on their own rating compared with a 'gold standard' set by 25 experts rating the same case vignettes. Many clinicians have found this to be a useful way to get feedback on their skills in rating GAF.

(d) Time pressure and lack of motivation

In acute wards with much to accomplish during short stays and in outpatient clinics with a high number of patients per clinician the reluctance to systematically use outcome measures may be especially strong. Use of outcome measures is more likely to be implemented in settings with lower time pressure and no obligation to give emergency assessments or treatments; but also in such settings large-scale implementation of outcome measurement is difficult.

(e) Lack of adequate IT support

Outcome measures need to be easily available in the information system with patient records in order to be used consistently on a routine basis. No outcome measure except GAF is made available for all the mental health services in this way. Some outcome measures are made available in some of the services, but this requires that the specific services have paid for such options. There is a growing interest among mental health services leaders to include outcome measures as a standard, and this may change the situation over the next few years.

Thoughts for the future

In Norway the most successful attempts at implementing outcome measurement have been done in the context of research networks involving clinicians in the mental health services, and often with a multicentre research study as a major component in the network. The Day Treatment Network is the best example, being the largest and most longstanding network. Having a centre with resources and motivation for creating and maintaining the infrastructure and coordination makes it easier for the clinical units to take part. The experience of being a part of a larger project that contributes to knowledge and clinical practice makes the effort meaningful, and feedback on their own results in relation to results in other clinics keeps the clinics engaged in the network. Collecting the data as a part of a network and research study also contributes to better data quality from training in the use of instruments, from testing of inter-rater reliability, and from the fact that the outcome data are actually used.

Thus, based on these experiences in Norway, network of clinics with focus on clinical practice and research may be one of the best ways to implement the use of outcome measures on a larger scale with adequate quality of the measurements.

The implementation of GAF as a part of a national data set for all treatment episodes in the mental health services has not been successful. The alternative choices seem to be to remove GAF from the national data set, or to 'take it seriously' and require adequate training, regular repetition and testing of rating skills to obtain quality data, and to use these data locally.

An alternative way to implement outcome measures in routine practice may be to define as a standard that mental health services should use outcome measurement with all patients, but that the choice of instrument should be based on the target group of patients, the treatment setting and the time frame for the treatment episodes.

Any large-scale implementation of outcome measurement needs to be supported by health authorities, managers, clinicians and user organizations in order to be successful. Other important prerequisites are choice of measures that are relevant to patient groups and clinical setting, acknowledgement of the time and resources necessary for training and use of outcome measurements, adequate IT support, active use of measurements in monitoring outcome, including joint decision-making with the patient, use of the data as feedback in improvement of the services, and an equal or greater emphasis on outcome in relation to productivity.

Acknowledgements

The following researchers have contributed to the content of the chapter by sharing their knowledge and views regarding the use of outcome measurements in mental health services in Norway: Rolf W. Gråwe, Ketil Hanssen-Bauer, Per Høglænd, Siv Kvernmo, Anne Landheim, Egil W. Martinsen and Lars Tanum.

References

American Psychiatric Association (1994). *Diagnostic and Statistical Manual of Mental Disorders – Fourth Edition.* Washington DC: American Psychiatric Association.

Babor, T. F., Higgins-Biddle, J. C., Saunders, J. B. and Monteiro, M. G. (2001). *AUDIT. The Alcohol Use Disorders Identification Test. Guidelines for Use in Primary Care.* Geneva: World Health Organization.

Bech, P., Malt, U. F., Dencker, S. J., et al. (1993). Scales for assessment of diagnosis and severity of mental disorders. *Acta Psychiatrica Scandinavica Supplementum,* **87**, suppl 372.

Beck, A. T., Epstein, N., Brown, G. K. and Steer, R. A. (1988). An inventory for measuring clinical anxiety: psychometric properties. *Journal of Consulting and Clinical Psychology,* **56**, 893–7.

Beck, A. T., Steer, R. A. and Brown, G. K. (1996). *Beck Depression inventory – II Manual.* San Antonio: Psychological Corporation.

Berman, A. H., Bergman, H., Palmstierna, T. and Schlyter, F. (2005). Evaluation of the Drug Use Disorders Identification Test (DUDIT) in Criminal Justice and Detoxification Settings and in a Swedish Population Sample. *European Addiction Research,* **11**, 22–31.

Derogatis, L. R. (1983). *SCL-90-R Administration, Scoring, and Procedures Manual – II.* Towson, MD: Clinical Psychometric Research.

Directorate of Health and Social Affairs (2005). *And it's going to get better. . . National Strategy for Quality Improvement in Health and Social Services (2005–2015).* Oslo: Directorate of Health and Social Affairs.

Evans, C., Connell, J., Barkham, M., et al. (2002). Towards a standardised brief outcome measure: psychometric properties and utility. *British Journal of Psychiatry,* **180**, 51–60.

Fallmyr, Ø. and Repål, A. (2002). Evaluering av GAF-skåring som del av Minste Basis Datasett [Evaluation of GAF-rating as part of the Minimum Data Set.] *Tidsskrift for Norsk Psykologforening,* **180**, 51–60.

Fryjordet, J., Kveldstad, M., Ruud, T., Stubhaug, B. and Walstad, M. (2004). *Statusrapport: Psykiske lidelser – Faglighet og verdighet. Rett til utredning, diagnostisk vurdering og målrettet behandling. [Status report: Mental disorders – Professionality and dignity. The right to assessment, diagnostic assessment and targeted treatment].* Oslo: The Norwegian Medical Association.

Goldman, H. H., Skodol, A. E. and Lave, T. R. (1992). Revising Axis V for DSM-IV: a review of measures of social functioning. *American Journal of Psychiatry,* **149**, 1148–56.

Goodman, R. (1997). The Strengths and Difficulties Questionnaire: a research note. *Journal of Child Psychology and Psychiatry,* **38**, 581–6.

Gowers, S. G., Harrington, R. C., Whitton, A., et al. (1999). Brief scale for measuring the outcomes of emotional and behavioural disorders in children. Health of the Nation Outcome Scales for Children and Adolescents (HoNOSCA). *British Journal of Psychiatry,* **174**, 413–16.

Hanssen-Bauer, K., Aalen, O. O., Ruud, T. and Heyerdahl, S. (2007). Inter-rater reliability of clinician-rated measures in child and adolescent mental health services. *Administration and Policy in Mental Health,* **34**, 504–12.

Horowitz, L. M., Rosenberg, S. E., Baer, B. A., Ureno, G. and Villasenor, V. S. (1988). Inventory of Interpersonal Problems: psychometric properties and clinical applications. *Journal for Consulting and Clinical Psychology,* **56**, 885–92.

Johannessenn, J. O., Larsen, T. K., McGlashan, T. and Vaglum, P. (2000). Early intervention in psychosis: The TIPS project, a multi-centre study in Scandinavia. eds. B. Martindale, A. Bateman and F. Margison *Psychosis: Psychological approaches and their effectiveness.* London: Gaskell/Royal College of Psychiatrists.

Johnsen, J. R. (2006). *Health Systems in Transition: Norway.* Copenhagen: WHO Regional Office for Europe on behalf of the European Observatory on Health Systems and Policies.

Karterud, S., Pedersen, G., Bjordal, E., et al. (2003). Day treatment of patients with personality disorders: experiences from a Norwegian treatment research network. *Journal of Personality Disorders*, **17**, 243–62.

Kay, S. R., Fiszbein, A. and Opler, L. A. (1987). The positive and negative syndrome scale (PANSS) for schizophrenia. *Schizophrenia Bulletin*, **13**, 261–76.

Lambert, M. J., Lunnen, K. M., Umphress, V., Hansen, N. B. and Burlingame, G. (1994). *Administration and scoring manual for the Outcome Questionnaire (OQ 45.1)*. Salt Lake City.

Loevdahl, H. and Friis, S. (1996). Routine evaluation of mental health: reliable information or worthless 'guesstimates'? *Acta Psychiatrica Scandinavica*, **93**, 125–8.

Miller, S. D., Duncan, B. L., Brown, J., Sparks, J. and Claud, D. A. (2003). The Outcome Rating Scale: a preliminary study of the reliability, validity, and feasibility of a brief visual analog measure. *Journal of Brief Therapy*, **2**, 91–100.

Montgomery, S. A. and Åsberg, M. (1979). A new depression scale designed to be sensitive to change. *British Journal of Psychiatry*, **134**, 382–9.

Norwegian Board of Health Supervision (1999). Angstlidelser – kliniske retningslinjer for utredning og behandling [Anxiety disorders – clinical guidelines for assessment and treatment]. Statens helsetilsyns utredningsserie 4–99., IK 2694.

Norwegian Board of Health Supervision (2000a). Alvorlige spiseforstyrrelser – retningslinjer for behandling i spesialisthelsetjenesten [Severe eating disorders – guidelines for treatment in specialized health services]. Statens helsetilsyns utredningsserie 7–2000, IK 2714.

Norwegian Board of Health Supervision (2000b). Schizofreni – kliniske retningslinjer for utredning og behandling [Schizophrenia – clinical guidelines for assessment and treatment]. Statens helsetilsyns utredningsserie 9–2000, IK 2726.

Norwegian Board of Health Supervision (2000c). Stemningslidelser – kliniske retningslidelser for utredning og behandling [Affective disorders – clinical guidelines for assessment and treatment]. Statens helsetilsyns utredningsserie 3–2000, IK 2695.

Norwegian Ministry of Health and Care Services (2005). *Mental health services in Norway. Prevention – treatment – care.* Oslo: Norwegian Ministry of Health and Care Services.

Olson, R. P. (ed.) (2006). *Mental Health Systems Compared: Great Britain, Norway, Canada and the United States.* Springfield: Charles C Thomas.

Pedersen, G. (2008). *Global Assessment of Functioning – Splittet versjon [Split version]*, available at: http://www.personlig hetsprosjekt.com/gaf/, retrieved 27 August 2009.

Pedersen, G., Hagtvet, K. A. and Karterud, S. (2007). Generalizability studies of the Global Assessment of Functioning – Split version. *Comprehensive Psychiatry*, **48**, 88–94.

Ruud, T. and Hauff, E. (2003). Community Mental Health Services in Norway. *International Journal of Mental Health*, **31**, 3–14.

Ruud, T. and Lorentzen, S. (1999). Testbatteri i gruppepsykoterapi [Test Battery in Group Psychotherapy]. The Research Committee in the Norwegian Group Psychotherapy Association (NGPF), 1992 (1st edn) and 1999 (2nd edn].

Ruud, T., Gråwe, R. W. and Hatling, T. (2006). *Akuttpsykiatrisk behandling i Norge – resultater fra en multisenterstudie. SINTEF-rapport A310. SINTEF Helse [Acute Psychiatric Treatment in Norway – Results from a multicentre study. SINTEF Report A310]*. Trondheim/Oslo: SINTEF Health Research.

Schaffer, D., Gould, M. S., Brasic, J., et al. (1983). A children's global assessment scale (CGAS). *Archives of General Psychiatry*, **40**, 1228–31.

Snaith, R. P. and Zigmond, A. S. (1983). Hospital Anxiety and Depression Scale. *Acta Psychiatrica Scandinavica*, **67**, 361–70.

Tuseth, A. G., Sverdrup, S., Hjort, H. and Friestad, C. (2006). *Å spørre den det gjelder. Rapport. Regionsenter for barn o gunges psykiske helse [To ask whom it concerns. Report. Regional Centre for Mental Health of children and adolescents].* Oslo: Helseregion øst og sør [Health Region East and South].

Vassend, O. and Skrondal, A. (2003). *Interpretation of the SCL-90-R. A psychometric study based on a Norwegian national sample.* Norwegian Psychological Association.

Vatnaland, T., Vatnaland, J., Friis, S. and Opjordsmoen, S. (2007). Are GAF scores reliable in routine clinical use? *Acta Psychiatrica Scandinavica*, **115**, 326–30.

Wing, J. K., Beevor, A. S., Curtis, R. H., et al. (1998). Health of the Nation Outcome Scales (HoNOS). Research and development. *British Journal of Psychiatry*, **172**, 11–18.

Outcome measurement in Canada: one province's experience with implementation in community mental health

David Smith

Introduction

Like many parts of the world, mental health outcome measurement in Canada has a long history of development (Adair et al., 2003). Canada has a complex system of healthcare planning and outcome measurement as a result of its localized planning structures. There is no consistent 'pan-Canadian' approach any more than there is a single world approach. Most importantly though in examining approaches to outcome measurement is the benefit of the lessons that every attempt should offer to the next. The lesson from this chapter will be an understanding of the importance of a good implementation methodology in producing valid and reliable outcome data. The experience of introducing a common assessment in the Canadian province of Ontario will be the project from which these lessons are drawn.

For those outside Canada, some context on the Canadian health system is necessary. To begin, the Canadian healthcare system is not actually a national system. Healthcare planning and spending is not the responsibility of the Canadian government but rather the governments of the ten provinces, two territories and numerous First Nations which make up the country. Each of these governments plans and manages its health system somewhat independently although within the context of various national policies or strategies. The most important Canada-wide condition is that all healthcare is free at the point of delivery. The first national mental health strategy was in the process of being developed in 2009.

Depending on the province, territory or First Nation, there may also be further devolution of planning responsibilities down to local districts. Ontario is the largest of the provinces, with a population of over 12 million. In the province, there are 14 local districts and these are further divided into delivery agencies, of which community mental health has several hundred. In the context of outcome measurement there are therefore many levels at which outcomes can be measured. This has led to dozens and possibly hundreds of assessment and outcome measurement tools being used across the country.

Some notable attempts have been made at national outcomes measurements, beginning with a historical mental health database that is held with the Canadian Institute of Health Informatics. This database has been collecting limited information on mental health since the 1920s. Other programmes have begun to collect more extensive data, including the Canada Health Infoways project with Vancouver Island Health Authority, the Ontario Mental Health Reporting System for inpatient services and the Common Data Set for Community Mental Health. These have been very helpful in providing quality data for mental health. In Ontario, though, there was still a need for further development of client-level outcome data for community mental health.

Outcome Measurement in Mental Health: Theory and Practice, ed. Tom Trauer. Published by Cambridge University Press.
© Cambridge University Press 2010.

The Ontario Community Mental Health Common Assessment Project

The Ontario Community Mental Health Common Assessment Project began in the autumn of 2006. The purpose of the project was to lead the provincial community mental health providers of the province through a process of choosing and implementing a common tool or tools for use at a clinical level. The tool(s) would ultimately also provide information for planning and decision-making at various levels of governance.

The project had three phases. The first was the selection of an appropriate tool for the sector. All phases were led by a partnership of consumer leaders, sector leaders and planning leadership from both the province and the local planning areas (in Ontario these planning bodies are called Local Health Integration Networks (LHINs)). Envisioning debate about the outcome of this process, the project employed procurement expertise to ensure that the process of choosing was fair and appropriately involved all stakeholders. The selection process took over 8 months and more than 70 criteria were identified for an appropriate tool. There was a review of over 80 tools and a full evaluation of 26 finalist tools, including presentations by advocates, and a final paper on eight leading options and combinations, for piloting. In the end, the provincial Steering Committee chose the Camberwell Assessment of Need (CAN, Phelan et al., 1995) with the condition that further development work be undertaken to add data elements or training to cover criteria that the tool did not meet.

The CAN is a 22-item tool that looks at various domains of an individual's life and has the assessor rate them according to whether they is no need, a met need or an unmet need, and then rate the level of support provided by formal and informal help and finally indicate whether additional supports are necessary. Complementary to the CAN is the CAN-P (Trauer et al., 2008), which is a consumer self-assessment which asks service users to rate need as met, unmet or 'no need' for the same 22 domains. The key strengths of the tool in the opinion of the provincial Steering Committee were the ease of use by practitioners of various backgrounds, its recovery focus and its complementary consumer and staff versions. The complementary versions were especially important as the provincial Steering Committee had committed itself to a consumer-led approach to assessment.

The second phase of the project began by setting up sector-led working groups to oversee the development of the additional data elements and training requirements. Pilot organizations were selected to test the tool and associated processes. The information collected from the pilots informed the Steering Committee recommendations on the usefulness and implementation details for the tool. The recommendations also incorporated a revision of the assessment that included all the lessons from the pilot study. The final tool is now known as the Ontario Common Assessment of Need or OCAN.

At the time of writing the final recommendations had been submitted to the Ontario Ministry of Health and Long Term Care for consideration, and piloting was continuing. The last phase of the project is expected to be a province-wide implementation as recommended by the Steering Committee.

Traditional challenges to implementation of outcome measures

The team charged with implementing a community mental health common assessment in Ontario was facing a significant barrier in that previous performance measurement efforts fell short of stated aspirations. The generally agreed goal of an outcome measurement tool is high-quality data to inform planning and a desire to track consumer progress. However, the expectation of consistent high-quality data is rarely met.

Sector experience of poor data quality appeared to have several underlying causes. First, it appeared that buy-in at a direct service level was low. In early interviews for the OCAN, stakeholders who had experience in several earlier attempts complained that outcome measurement was an administrative exercise, tying up considerable resources for little or no benefit to consumers and direct service staff. Staff and managers indicated that often they did not receive reports back for many months and these were often difficult to understand, did not appear to represent their services and had little relevance to improving local services. Managers also spoke of the resistance of their staff to the new measures and a lack of appropriate resources to support the implementation.

Interestingly though, the other consistent message from stakeholders was that they felt there was clearly a need for measuring outcomes and conducting assessments. Planners felt they needed better information to allocate resources more effectively. Managers who were leading services felt they needed more information to make arguments for the usefulness of their services and to identify areas for improvement. Direct service and clinical staff indicated they wanted more feedback on how well their service was doing and to help quantify the 'gaps' in services. They also talked about needing consistent approaches across organizations and the sector. Consumers wanted some consistency to the information gathered so that they could expect the same level of service wherever they accessed the system. They also wanted to reduce the repetitive telling of their story to each new service provider.

With the knowledge of these historical implementation problems it was important to look at similar prior projects that had gone well. There was some work already under way in Ontario healthcare on a new approach. Thoughtful leadership of other recent assessment projects (beyond mental health) had begun to form a consistent approach to implementation of a common assessment. The first, and probably most important, shift in approach was in defining the goal of data collection. Experience with implementations in healthcare had made it clear that in order to get good data, support was needed from the people producing the data, namely direct service staff and consumers. Clearly the focus of the implementation had to shift in order to get their support. The primary goals of any common assessment or measurement process should therefore be those of the direct service staff and consumers. By focusing foremost on the clinical outcomes and care planning needs valued by clinicians and consumers, the overall reliability and validity of the data were expected to increase.

As a result of this shift in focus, many of the previous challenges could be minimized. If an assessment tool was implemented that met the needs of the direct service providers and consumers then they would work hard to produce better data quality and display much more enthusiasm for implementation of the OCAN. The dual purposes of clinical improvement and planning data had always been there; they had just been emphasized in the wrong order.

Emphasis on data collection for clinical outcomes and care planning was an important breakthrough and fortunately the learning did not stop there. A portion of the previously experienced resistance also came from a lack of support and available expertise to successfully implement. Staff resisted when they were worried that they would not be able to do the job correctly. The OCAN project had to ensure they were given a maximum level of support and the resources necessary to do the job correctly. A level of oversight was also necessary to determine when the support was not sufficient and when to make adjustments.

This lesson from stakeholder interviews and earlier implementations led to the approach that was used for choosing and introducing a common assessment tool in Ontario – the OCAN.

A new approach to implementation

The case was then made to move away from historical approaches and to develop a new outcome measurement implementation methodology. The implementation methodology that was used successfully to introduce the OCAN in Ontario was based on learning from two parallel projects in other healthcare sectors. The first was in Community Care Access Centres, where a common assessment was introduced to support case managers in allocating community resources (eHealthOntario.ca, no date-a). The second project was a similar assessment implementation in the long-term care sector (eHealthOntario.ca, no date-c). All three projects also benefited from the contracting in of leadership with considerable prior experience in change management and the support of strong leadership already based in the Ontario Ministry of Health and Long Term Care. Since these original projects, several new projects have begun to further support the sector in using and collecting information to support clients and planning (eHealthOntario.ca, no date-b).

The new approach focused more intensely on the management of change and transferred the ownership for the process of implementation to those who ultimately need to make it work, the direct service providers and the service consumers. This shift required a considerable degree of trust and foresight from decision-makers. They needed the confidence to provide key necessary resources at the front end of implementation to reduce the false starts, resistance, compliance and data-quality problems before they began.

The methodology that was used focuses on nine key areas, namely (a) focusing on delivering benefits for key stakeholders; (b) involving key stakeholders in leading the project; (c) using subject-matter experts; (d) maximizing supports; (e) implementing ongoing monitoring; (f) piloting; (g) delivering meaningful reporting early; (h) conducting formal evaluation, and (i) undertaking continual improvement.

(a) Focus on benefits

First and most important was to concentrate on defining, communicating and delivering tangible benefits. The focus was on the self-identified benefits of all the key stakeholders, beginning with those most relevant to the consumer. In the OCAN implementation, identifying benefits that helped consumers and staff to 'buy-in' to the process and begin to trust in the implementation was crucial to its success. Benefits also needed to be found for system planners and management. The focus for these needed to be tailored to the unique needs of each group.

In the Ontario process, the identification of benefits began with the initial fact-finding engagement with the sector and continued throughout the project. The process used for identifying benefits was lengthy, but employing resources that helped to find the correct mix of benefits and messages was very important to the methodology. These messages were then communicated to stakeholders using a variety of media. Sector associations (Ontario Peer Development Initiative, no date), direct presentations, email newsletters, community consultations (Community Mental Health Common Assessment Project, no date-a), conferences, ministry and LHIN meetings as well as the use of sector champions were all employed to get key messages to the sector. The communication of these benefits during the OCAN project was central to the messaging to the sector and generated considerable goodwill.

(b) Involve stakeholders

A critical feature of the methodology was involvement of stakeholders in all levels of project governance to understand their viewpoints. Often this engagement step is left to later in the outcome measurement process, once many of the decisions have already been made. With the development of the OCAN tool, representatives of consumers, staff, sector leadership and planning bodies were all involved from the beginning. They set down the processes, chose the tool, led the change, piloted the tool and communicated their decisions and the benefits to their peers.

Choosing and recruiting the right stakeholders is often a very difficult process. The need to bring in sector champions that can truly represent their peers is essential. This can lead to intense and challenging debate early on in the project but paid off during the OCAN implementation as these leaders became champions of a process that they truly owned. The involvement of key stakeholders needs to be considered carefully from the outset of any outcomes project.

(c) Use subject-matter experts

The process for setting up such an extensive stakeholder involvement required specific skills and experience. The third key element of the methodology involved using subject-matter experts. Many public-sector implementations suffer from a reliance on the resources that are available rather than seeking out those that are most needed.

In the implementation of OCAN, subject-matter experts were employed from a wide variety of disciplines. First among these were the people experienced in the management of large, long-term implementations and well-skilled in change management. They were instrumental in building a successful implementation plan. Following the recruitment of the leadership, experts were engaged to help understand the current state of services and outcome measurement in the sector. This included the recruitment of clinical and business analysis expertise. These resources led the selection of the tool, supported by procurement and project management expertise. They were further assisted by a strong communications team to create and disseminate the benefits messages and to build support in the sector.

Consumer expertise was also brought to the project in several forms. First, consumers were included in all of the Steering Committees and Working Groups. These consumer representatives were selected from provincial bodies at first. In later stages of the project, consumers also came from organizations that had implemented and also recruited at presentations or consultation events. As the project moved to implementation, consumers were also recruited to support educational events and to help problem-solve within the project team.

As the project progressed, additional technical expertise was required to automate the OCAN. This was followed by developers, systems analysts and privacy and security expertise. Then, to lead the piloting of the OCAN, a strong education team staffed with professional adult educators was assembled to build the education materials and deliver the training.

(d) Maximize support

Once the subject matter expertise was in place, channels were established so the sector could access it in a timely and helpful manner. Live user support, web access to documents, frequent communications (e.g. education opportunities, networking opportunities, process changes, etc.) and education were some of the more successful support mechanisms used on the OCAN project.

The other key support needed was the ability to process the OCAN electronically and send the resulting data to a central data store from which reports could be drawn. The selection and testing of an appropriate strategy for automation was a large stream of supporting work. In order to minimize the scope of change required for staff, the OCAN was built into existing case management systems in mental health organizations. In the 16 pilot organizations, there were six different vendors supplying the organization's principal case management system. The technical subject matter experts supported organizations in working with their software vendors to get the OCAN successfully built into all six software programs.

(e) Ongoing monitoring

Support and expertise needs differ from project to project. The OCAN project monitored a number of indicators, including the use of supports, understanding of the tool, effectiveness of education materials and overall satisfaction. To do this well, consideration was given to ongoing monitoring of results at a very early stage. Critical to this process was consideration of what needed monitoring from the onset.

Monitoring plays several roles. Most importantly, it provides feedback to determine whether something is not working well. Ongoing monitoring makes it possible to change direction quickly and show responsiveness to the needs of the sector, often before any major problems arise. Monitoring also permits communication of what is going well. Success stories, facts about implementation efforts and communication of the use of supports all help to build the project's profile with its stakeholders.

Monitoring can also support any key adjustments or corrections that are necessary throughout the course of the implementation. Such corrections are often the hardest to predict but are made easier by early warning and by having a broad range of expertise and supports available.

(f) Piloting

Piloting is crucial to a successful implementation, allowing for many of the 'bugs' to be worked out prior to a larger rollout. Those organizations that are most likely to be successful are most likely to volunteer and will help problem-solve many of the inevitable challenges that arise. The project sought to include a range of programme types from a variety of locations in the pilot phase. A total of 16 agencies joined in the process in the original pilots. Later, a system-level pilot was added as all (23) organizations in the North East LHIN participated in a second pilot. In addition to understanding the inter-agency issues associated with implementation, there was additional learning around the use of the OCAN with First Nations and French populations (North East Local Health Integration Network (LHIN), no date).

Lessons from the pilots were important to support decisions, make the case for change and give the leadership team the confidence to continue implementation. They also supported the case for stopping and rethinking approaches when that was necessary. Most important, the pilots became the 'champions' to the rest of the sector and allowed for the building of case studies and testing of secondary processes that continued to ease the way for the sector even after the formal end of the pilot stages.

(g) Delivering meaningful reporting at an early stage

Developing meaningful reporting was one of the most difficult parts of the project. Various audiences wanted different feedback from the assessment as it was implemented. Consumers indicated they would like to see their progress over time and staff members wanted similar feedback as well as tools to help organize the resulting information for care planning. Managers wanted to understand how programmes were meeting people's needs and planners wanted to better understand system-level impacts of interventions and services.

In keeping with the project philosophy of making assessment meaningful at the service level, the greatest initial effort was in response to the needs of consumers and staff members. Reports were developed to give live feedback from the assessment on needs and capabilities for prioritizing those with accompanying actions and comments. Printouts were also developed for the consumers and staff members to have take-away versions.

Work on development of reports for managers and planners continues but several early reports show promise and the continued involvement of stakeholders from these groups is leading to more and more meaningful reports.

(h) Formal evaluation

The pilot phase of the project was subjected to a formal evaluation by an external consultant. The intention was to obtain objective information to support or refute the lessons being identified by the internal monitoring mechanisms.

The evaluation study examined the impact of the common assessment process on people seeking services and on community mental health staff, gathered feedback on the assessment process and identified emerging best practices on use of the tool. The consultants used both online surveys as well as on-site focus groups to obtain feedback from consumers and staff.

The evaluation findings were reviewed by the project Steering Committee and informed decisions on various processes, including support for consumers, programme-by-programme effectiveness reviews and service level views of the various supports provided. Most importantly, the independently gathered success stories helped to communicate to other organizations the many benefits of the project.

(i) Continuous improvement

Piloting was a critical part of the Ontario methodology and allowed improvements to occur with selected early adopters prior to implementation across the whole sector. This continuous improvement approach was the final element of the Ontario approach (Community Mental Health Common Assessment Project, no date-b). By offering strong support and good monitoring, there were more opportunities to catch problems early. The development of a good pool of expertise and dynamic pilots then ensured that there were strong resources to use in problem-solving.

In any change implementation, ignoring problems or leaving them to someone else seldom works. Many of the problems that arise are very complex and require considerable time and effort to solve. Starting early is critical. Setting up a clear process and appropriate stakeholder groups is required to fully consider issues. On the OCAN project, significant goodwill with the sector was earned because problem identification was encouraged and solution development processes were built into the project.

Benefits of the methodology

The Ontario experience identified many benefits to approaching the implementation of outcome measurement in the manner that was used in the OCAN project. The first and greatest of these was the very real difference in the manner in which service was provided to community mental health consumers. Additionally there was more initial uptake, more engaged staff and consumers, champions for further implementation and an unexpected benefit of reducing the mistrust of measurement.

In the OCAN project there were several very important findings regarding how services were provided as a direct result of the common assessment tool. The findings of the evaluation of the pilot project showed that 84% of consumers felt that the assessment helped their workers understand them better and 74% said it was useful for assessing their needs (Caislyn Consulting Inc., 2008a, 2008b). Many consumers noted through focus groups that the pilot assessment represented the first time they were asked directly about their needs and they were impressed with the range of life domains covered by the instrument. Among workers, 81% felt that OCAN provided an accurate assessment of consumers' needs. Most importantly to changing practice, 56% of staff found that OCAN helped identify needs earlier than their previous processes and another 56% found it helped identify a greater number of needs. In other words, there was a clear clinical benefit to both consumers and workers in using the OCAN in a more inclusive assessment process.

As organizations become aware of the support offered using this methodology, they are more willing to attempt early adoption. Over 50 organizations (out of roughly 300 eligible) volunteered to be pilots for the OCAN project. Of the 16 organizations that were selected as pilots the engagement with the team was considerable. They attended over 50 in-person training sessions and dozens of teleconferences and logged over 1600 contacts with the support centre. They additionally logged over 100 weekly hits on the pilot-only web portal.

The enthusiasm of the pilot sites further came into play as they began to take on roles as champions of the project. Pilot sites participated in conferences, engaged in speaking events, arranged conversations with local planners and convinced their peers through word of mouth. Many of the pilot sites have volunteered as mentors for a further piloting to 32 organizations. They have also volunteered to support the project in further lessons around reassessment, reporting, mentoring and the testing of improved versions of the OCAN.

An unexpected benefit arising out of the methodology in the OCAN project was the reduction of mistrust around outcome measurement and assessment. As workers are supported to understand the clinical value of the tool, they seem to worry less about the use of the information, possibly because they know it accurately reflects their core work. In the OCAN project there was a discernible shift in people's trust, overtly noticeable through acceptance of previously resisted data collection for items such as the provincial health number and personal health information. There was also an enthusiasm among consumer-run organizations to engage in the formal collection of individual outcome data that had not previously been noted.

Conclusion

The implementation of outcome measurement tools in mental health is a difficult process. The process often encounters unforeseen difficulties and results in poor-quality data. The most important lesson from the recent piloting of OCAN in Ontario was that the generation of good-quality data was substantially increased by supporting a strong implementation methodology focused on support and change management. By delivering tangible benefits to consumers and staff, it was possible to shift the focus of outcome measurement efforts away from the data and towards clinical utility. The effect of this approach was magnified when supported by strong stakeholder engagement, the use of subject-matter experts, maximizing support mechanisms, using monitoring to reassess progress, learning through piloting and continually improving according to the information from monitoring and evaluation. Ultimately, the methodology employed produced very high levels of engagement and data quality and is expected to continue to produce similar results.

References

Adair, C. E., Simpson, L., Birdsell, J. M., et al. (2003). *Performance Measurement Systems in Health and Mental Health Services: Models, Practices and Effectiveness. A State of the Science Review.* Calgary, Alberta: The Alberta Heritage Foundation for Medical Research, available at: http://www.ahfmr.ab.ca/grants/docs/state_of_science_reviews/Adair_Review.pdf, retrieved 18 August 2009.

Caislyn Consulting Inc. (2008a). Caislyn Pilot Report. Executive Summary, available at: www.ontario.cmha.ca/docs/ehealth/CaislynPilotReport_ExecutiveSummary.pdf, retrieved 18 August 2009.

Caislyn Consulting Inc. (2008b). *Common Assessment Project.* Final report. Toronto, Ontario: Community Mental Health Common Assessment Project.

Community Mental Health Common Assessment Project (no date-a). Consultation Questions and Answers, available at: www.ontario.cmha.ca/docs/ehealth/CMHCAP_consultation_QA_20070925.pdf, retrieved 18 August 2009.

Community Mental Health Common Assessment Project (no date-b). Lessons Learned Summary, available at: www.ontario.cmha.ca/docs/ehealth/CMHCAP_lessons_learned_summary_200812.pdf, retrieved 18 August 2009.

eHealthOntario.ca (no date-a). Community Care Access Centres, available at: www.ehealthontario.ca/portal/server.pt?open=512&;objID=2201&mode=2&in_hi_userid=11862&cached=true, retrieved 18 August 2009.

eHealthOntario.ca (no date-b). Community Care Information Management (CCIM), available at: www.ehealthontario.ca/portal/server.pt?open=512&;objID=220&PageID=0&cached=true&mode=2&userID=11862, retrieved 18 August 2009.

eHealthOntario. ca (no date-c). Long Term Care (LTC), available at: www.ehealthontario.ca/portal/server.pt?open=512&;objID=2199&mode=2&in_hi_userid=11862&cached=true, retrieved 18 August 2009.

North East Local Health Integration Network (LHIN) (no date). Community Mental Health Common Assessment Pilot Information Workshop, available at: www.nelhin.on.ca/workarea/linkit.aspx?ItemID=3504, retrieved 18 August 2009.

Ontario Peer Development Initiative (no date). available at: http://opdi.org/newstogo/ opdi_newstogo_issue_224_-_june_26_2009/, retrieved 18 August 2009.

Phelan, M., Slade, M., Thornicroft, G., et al. (1995). The Camberwell Assessment of Need: the validity and reliability of an instrument to assess the needs of people with severe mental illness. *British Journal of Psychiatry*, **167**, 589–95.

Trauer, T., Tobias, G. and Slade, M. (2008). Development and evaluation of a patient-rated version of the Camberwell Assessment of Need Short Appraisal Schedule (CANSAS-P). *Community Mental Health Journal*, **44**, 113–24.

Outcome Measurement in Specific Groups and Settings

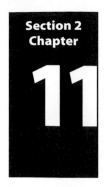

Section 2
Chapter

11

Routine outcome measurement in child and adolescent mental health

Peter Brann

Introduction

Routine outcome measurement (ROM) in child and adolescent mental health has its own particular set of challenges in addition to those outlined in other chapters of this volume. This chapter will focus on ROM in child and adolescent mental health services (CAMHS) with particular emphasis on the Australian situation. The aim of this chapter is to illustrate progress, and hopefully inspire the reader to consider potential areas for development in their own area of influence. Unless otherwise stated, the term children includes adolescents.

Mental health difficulties are not uncommon in children and adolescents, with estimates of prevalence ranging between 9% and 20%, and an Australian survey finding a rate of 14% (Sawyer et al., 2000, Rutter and Stevenson, 2008). Prevalence rates usually exceed the rates of treatment (Rutter and Stevenson, 2008). Of the children who scored in the clinical range of a screening questionnaire, and whose parents reported needing help, fewer than 20% had attended a psychiatrist, CAMHS or hospital-based Department of Psychiatry (Sawyer et al., 2000). In the USA, Weisz and Jensen (1999) estimated only 20–33% of children with a disorder received help. With limited resources, questions of value will be entwined with questions of effectiveness (Hunter et al., 1996).

Meta-analyses have indicated the effectiveness of child psychotherapy over no treatment (Kazdin, 1997, Weisz et al., 2005) although the relative lack of effective treatments implemented in clinical practice has been noted (McLennan et al., 2006). While knowledge of efficacious treatments has increased, there has been less examination of treatment effectiveness: 'Although the evidence for efficacy of preventive, psychopharmacological and psychosocial interventions is ample, and covers many child and adolescent mental health problems, studies testing the effectiveness of treatments in real-world settings and the cost-effectiveness of interventions to diffuse efficacious approaches to child mental health problems were not found.' (Graeff-Martins et al., 2008, p. 347).

What is particular about children and ROM?

(a) Children grow

Children are located in a developmental pathway and assessments must be informed by their developmental stage. The meaning of any behaviour or experience is informed by a child's developmental status. Instruments suitable for ROM need to account for development through specifying expectations or using the developmental knowledge of the informant. The success of an intervention must be judged by reference to both the available developmental pathways as well as relative to their baseline functioning (Hoagwood et al., 1996). The problem status of symptomatology in children differs from that of adults in that it is more obviously dynamic. Instruments that build on clinical judgements may be better able to capture developmental changes than instruments with fixed reference points.

(b) Children are connected

The seminal question of Leginski et al., 'Who receives what services from whom, at what cost, and with what effect?', highlights another major issue (Leginski et al., 1989). With adults, 'who' can be readily understood as the client whereas with children there are usually other significant figures, typically including parents, siblings, other family members, teachers and other health, welfare and education staff. Child assessments in particular require multiple informants and ROM should reflect this.

The absence of multiple informants in ROM may reveal biases. For example, only including clinicians' perspectives tends to privilege symptoms (Dickey and Wagenaar, 1996). Parents' views are more likely to be biased towards family burden and externalizing symptoms, while children are likely to be more aware of internalizing symptoms (American Academy Child and Adolescent Psychiatry, 1997). Parent reports are also correlated with their own mental health difficulties (Kazdin and Weisz, 1998). In some symptom areas, adolescents report greater severity than their clinicians (Gowers et al., 2002). Different informants produce at best low to moderate agreement when rating child psychopathology (Lambert et al., 1998). Even the same informant may differ across domains (Brookman-Frazee et al., 2006). Hunter et al. (1996) concluded that parents' and children's reports are simply not interchangeable and neither are clinicians' reports.

The development of ROM in Australian CAMHS

The Bickman et al. (1998) report was a major milestone for ROM. It proposed ROM needed to cover 15 domains: functional impairment; symptom severity; symptom acuity; parent–child relationship; quality of life; satisfaction with services; environmental safety; stressful events; family resources; maltreatment; treatment goals; treatment modality, strategy, tactics, timing and dosage; therapeutic alliance; motivation to change; and treatment adherence. This extensive list was modified by consideration of several criteria.

Feasibility is the most demanding criterion and refers to the applicability, acceptability and practicality of a system. Repetition of even the briefest task reduces the time available for other activities. Many clinicians consider face-to-face clinical work to be the 'real' work and resent intrusions into that activity. Parents are typically busy juggling multiple demands.

> In our clinic, we have observed that increasing more rigorous monitoring, assessment, and alternative treatment and control conditions reduces the likelihood that children and families will comply with the treatment program. (Chorpita et al., 1998, p. 9)

Comprehensiveness refers to an instrument's coverage of important domains. Surveys in the USA and Australia have indicated that symptom reduction and family and child functioning are the most important domains (Bickman et al., 1998, Garland et al., 2004).

Flexibility refers to the capacity of an outcome measurement system to be adapted according to the resources and focus of different services. Services will differ in their capacity to implement outcome systems.

In order to *improve clinical services*, Bickman et al. (1998) proposed that outcome data be accompanied by information about modifiable structures or processes.

Psychometric soundness refers to validity and reliability. The question of meaningful change is important and must reflect more than instrument imprecision (Ogles et al., 1996).

Developmental sensitivity is critical if an instrument is to be useful for children.

Cultural sensitivity is also critical in understanding the meaning of symptoms and burden.

Following the reports by Bickman et al. for children and Andrews et al. (1994) for adults, Australian state and territory governments agreed to implement a national routine outcome system for mental health. The minimum dataset for CAMHS has two clinician instruments, one parent and one adolescent self-report measure. These instruments are collected at assessment, reviews and discharge (Department of Health and Ageing, 2003). The majority of mental health care for severe presentations is provided by the public sector in outpatient settings.

The key clinician instruments are the Health of the Nation Outcome Scales for Children and Adolescents (HoNOSCA, Gowers et al., 1999) and the Children's Global Assessment Scale (CGAS, Schaffer et al., 1983). HoNOSCA comprises 15 scales assessing different domains of symptoms and functioning. Each scale is rated from No Problems to Very Severe Problems and the first 13 scales are summed to produce a total score (Gowers et al., 1999). HoNOSCA has been found to have moderate to good inter-rater reliability and has had its validity demonstrated in a number of studies (Garralda et al., 2000, Brann et al., 2001, Bilenberg, 2003, Manderson and McCune, 2003, Hanssen-Bauer et al., 2007b). The total score has been found to function as a measure of symptom severity, and the brief time taken to complete it is consistent with that required for routine use (Brann et al., 2001). The Children's Global Assessment Scale (CGAS) is a single-score clinician estimate on a 1–100 point scale summarizing the child's level of functioning. CGAS has been extensively studied and found to have fair to substantial inter-rater reliability and good validity (Schorre and Vandvik, 2004, Pirkis et al., 2005b).

The Strength and Difficulties Questionnaire (SDQ, Goodman, 2001) covers a range of symptoms and functioning and their impact on the child's life. It is available in parent, teacher and adolescent self-report versions. The SDQ has become widely used for epidemiological, clinical and research purposes (Vostanis, 2006). It has five subscales tapping four areas of difficulty (emotional, conduct, hyperactivity-inattention, peer problems) and one of strength (prosocial behaviour). The SDQ has been found to have good internal consistency, test–retest reliability and concurrent validity (Pirkis et al., 2005b). It has been found to predict the level of psychopathology at 3-year follow up, to discriminate between clinical and community samples, and is associated with mental health service use (Bourdon et al., 2005, Goodman and Goodman, 2009).

Where are we up to?

Significant progress has been made since the seminal reports of Bickman et al. (1998) and Hunter et al. (1996). In addition to Australia, routine collection in CAMHS has occurred in Denmark (Bilenberg, personal communication, August 2005) and New Zealand (Chipps et al., 2006). Other states (e.g. Ohio, Nova Scotia) and clusters of services (e.g. Norway, United Kingdom, California) around the world have implemented routine outcome measurement as part of clinical practice (Young et al., 2000, Johnston and Gowers, 2005, Pirkis et al., 2005a, Hanssen-Bauer et al., 2007a, Kisely et al., 2007). A comprehensive approach in Hawaii has seen the system-wide integration of client outcome measures with population measures and evidence-based interventions (Daleiden et al., 2006).

Of the key instruments used in Australia, the SDQ continues to be utilized at consumer and population levels. It has appeared in both examinations of cross-cultural differences (Heiervang et al., 2008) and prediction of change (Ford et al., 2007). Service provision has been examined in family support services and CAMHS (Mathai et al., 2003, Anderson et al., 2005). The SDQ continues to have its psychometric properties examined (Goodman and Goodman, 2009, Warnick et al., 2009). Intriguingly, the internal reliability of the SDQ for 8–11 year olds has been found to be similar to adolescents (Mellor, 2004).

HoNOSCA has been used in different contexts, including the impact of government policies on eating disorder outcomes (Ayton et al., 2009), and as part of a quality improvement framework in an in-patient setting (Lesinskiene et al., 2007). It has also been used to evaluate change in secure residential units (Yates et al., 2006), family support services (Vostanis et al., 2006), adolescent inpatient units (Harnett et al., 2005), a combined educational and mental health programme (McShane et al., 2007) and in research around diagnostic groups such as depression (Vitiello et al., 2006) and eating disorders (Ayton et al., 2009).

By July 2007 in ambulatory settings, valid records of over 130,000 HoNOSCA, 30,000 parent SDQs and 19,000 youth self-report SDQs had been collected across Australia (http://reports.mhnocc.org/cgi-bin/menu.cgi?menu=child-collection-occasion-summaries, last accessed 29 April 2009).

What do people think of ROM?

Few studies examine the attitudes of CAMHS clinicians to any outcome measure in routine clinical settings (Garland et al., 2003). The oft-quoted study 'Psychiatrists in the UK do not use outcome measures' did not survey any child psychiatrists (Gilbody et al., 2002). With child-focused clinicians, Hatfield and Ogles (2004) note an increase from Bickman et al.'s (2000) finding of outcome measures being used by 23% of clinicians to the 54% of psychologists in their survey. Outcome measures were used more by younger therapists and those working in public settings. Those who spent more time providing therapy were more likely to engage in outcome measurement. Common reasons for engaging in ROM were reported to have included 'tracking client progress' and determining if a 'change in the treatment plan' was required.

Surveys in the USA and the UK found difficulties arising from resource constraints. Feasibility was a major concern in the USA, where the core clinician instrument took from 10 to 60 minutes to rate. Many clinicians reported using intuition and clinical observation as their prime technique for evaluating therapy. The majority did not use these outcome data to inform practice, although 60% acknowledged the useful contribution the instruments made to the clinical process (Garland et al., 2003).

In the UK, 29% of services surveyed were using routine outcome measures, while 87% reported some form of quantitative evaluation. HoNOSCA was used by 39% (Johnston and Gowers, 2005). Over a 7-month period and without any active follow up, clinicians' completion rate of HoNOSCA at Eastern Health CAMHS was 84% (Brann et al., 2001) and 76% over 18 months (Brann, 2006). While the perceived subjectivity of HoNOSCA has concerned some (Jaffa, 2000) its emphasis on privileging perceptions of clinical significance may actually be a strength. Unlike many instruments, HoNOSCA does not ask clinicians to overlook their judgement.

A phone survey of CAMHS clinicians in New Zealand found approximately 20% used outcome measures (Merry et al., 2004). The majority supported introducing ROM to assist both clinical work and service delivery. Most were supportive of HoNOSCA as the clinician measure while acknowledging that no single measure should be seen as sufficient for all purposes.

While the SDQ has been used extensively, there are few published studies examining its acceptability. A sample of mothers of low-risk children found that they preferred the SDQ over the well-researched but longer Child Behaviour Checklist (Goodman and Scott, 1999). Young people and families themselves have been found to prefer the SDQ over the instrument clinicians recommended for them (Merry et al., 2004). The young children wanted their own self-report measure, like the SDQ. A major issue for these participants was that they should be involved in implementation, results should be accessible, privacy respected, and ROM viewed in the context of a trusting clinical relationship. Importantly, it was stressed that ROM should be accompanied by routine outcome discussion between children, clinicians and families.

Lawton and Marland (2008) reported a survey of 110 families; while unfamiliar with the term 'outcome measures', respondents found the SDQ easy to complete and believed it helped the clinician better understand their situation. Clinicians were described as rarely discussing the clinician measures (HoNOSCA and CGAS) with them, although families reported this as very helpful when it did occur.

Does it help with anything?

Unlike wilderness, ROM cannot exist for its own sake; it needs to be used to justify its existence. The following sections present examples of uses that have occurred in a number of services, including the author's.

(a) Individually

Outcome data have been used graphically to present the progress of individual clients at clinical reviews. This has been used to supplement clinical discussions, promote case reflection and facilitate dialogue with clients and their family. As an example, a five-step team review process, focusing on HoNOSCA, has been described by Stewart (2008). First, does the outcome measure suggest this is the right service? Second, the concordance over the ratings between the rater, other clinicians, the client and parents is discussed. While this may relate to inter-rater reliability, it became apparent to the Australian raters during a cross-national reliability study (Hanssen-Bauer et al., 2007b) that different views also reflected differing assumptions and knowledge. Third, the team discuss areas that have changed since the last rating. The team fourthly focus on remaining concerns with the necessity for treatment plans guided by the ratings for each scale, and finally the team review identifies one or two areas where change is most necessary.

A survey of clinicians' use of feedback about individual client outcomes produced a return rate of 87% (Brann, 2006). No directions about use were provided. Over 70% reported using feedback for reviewing case progress, 58% for decisions about discharge, and 66% to reflect on their own strengths and weaknesses.

> [It is] another tool that helps you reflect on what is happening for clients – which is useful because it is a different way of thinking about it. This can then have an impact on the way you work. (p. 305)

A second theme was collaborative uses. Approximately 31% took the feedback to peer reviews, while 25% discussed it in reviews with children and family members. The process of sharing perceptions of outcome can be threatening to clinicians; it draws attention to areas that may have been expected to alter with treatment. It may threaten engagement. This demands some clarity from the CAMHS field about expected change and when a lack of change would be considered a failure of this therapeutic encounter. Clinicians understandably may have some trepidation about this and facilitate processes that support engagement and bypass disagreements about the child's progress.

(b) Service improvement

While aggregated data may appear less interesting to clinicians and consumers, they have a large impact on service provision. In the author's service, HoNOSCA scores from admission to discharge were examined by diagnostic groups. One diagnosis with little change was targeted for increased training. Recommendations for a treatment pathway were developed; however, this revealed a substantial split in opinion about optimal treatment. Unfortunately, the paucity of outcome data from other services and the literature at the time made it difficult to determine the optimal approach. In another example, outcomes were examined by referral source and the results were used to improve consultation and referral pathways. Once again we were reminded of the value of local evidence of effectiveness.

Across Victorian CAMHS, a consultation group has formed to improve the quality of the state-wide outcomes system, share training approaches, develop resources and clarify processes and instrument-related questions. A recent training programme had clinicians present cases incorporating HoNOSCA and SDQ ratings. Participants were shown how to use the Australian Mental Health Outcomes and Classification Network (AMHOCN) Decision Support Tool to compare initial ratings with national comparative data (http://wdst.mhnocc. org/, last accessed 29 April 2009), which shows the national distribution of HoNOSCA total scores obtained at the start of any community episodes, with a given child's score superimposed (Figure 11.1). For this child's score, the accompanying text reads: '90.0% of assessments for consumers at Admission to Ambulatory care score 22 or less on the HoNOSCA Total Score; 10.0% of assessments for consumers like this score more than 22 on the HoNOSCA Total Score'. Clinicians were shown the Youth in Mind website and entered the parent or adolescent's SDQ online (http://www.youthinmind.net/Aus/index.html, last accessed 29 April 2009). The resulting report was incorporated into a role play where clinicians, parents and adolescents discussed the results

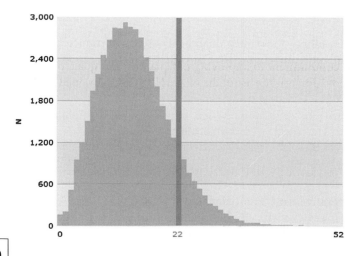

Figure 11.1 AMHOCN Web Decision Support Tool comparing a child's HoNOSCA total score against the national distribution.

together and used the fidelity checklist developed by AMHOCN to assess the quality of the interaction (Coombs, 2006).

(c) Research programmes

Adolescent day programmes (ADP) are intensive compared with outpatient treatment. Eighty-four adolescents participating in a non-residential ADP were compared with an out-patient-only group matched for age, gender, diagnosis and initial severity. Analysis revealed not only significant improvements for both ADP and outpatient participants, but showed significantly greater improvement for the ADP group (Kennair et al., in press). These results focused the programme's attention on outcomes and contributed to increases in funding.

A comparison of self-harming and non-self-harming young people admitted to hospital was found to be coherent in terms of the outcome profiles (Jones and Tardif, 2008). The results highlighted a potential lead for clinical intervention from this research. Of those who had been admitted, the sizable proportion discharged without community follow-up had higher HoNOSCA scores for substance use problems. ROM may indicate the intensity of required follow-up as well as symptom status at discharge.

(d) Service reform

Within the author's service, a clinical data group is addressing the prioritizing of complex cases for review through identifying children who have been in treatment for 6 months and either deteriorated or not changed. While this approach is limited in statistical sophistication, it is preferable to use outcomes to provide some guidance in the absence of sufficient resources to intensively review all cases.

Across Australia, national outcomes advisory groups have been established. The CAMHS outcomes expert group advises governments on opportunities and barriers relating to ROM. It has ensured inclusion of a parent and adolescent measure, trialled training packages and disseminated new approaches. It has argued for feedback and reference material such as the AMHOCN Decision Support Tool and is considering the issues around measuring outcomes with infants, and self-reporting by young children.

With a considerable degree of synergy with ROM, six Australian CAMHS engaged in a national benchmarking project. A number of key performance indicators, including ROM participation rates and outcome scores, were examined. The purported different models of care were clarified by HoNOSCA data. Services targeting more severe presentations did in fact have more severe ratings, and variation within those services in outcomes appeared related to length of treatment episode. While acknowledging the tentative nature of the findings, the process increased services' commitment to improving the quantity and quality of their collections. One interesting innovation was the use of the intake HoNOSCA by one CAMHS to ensure that clinicians maintained a caseload balanced for severity. (http://www.mhnocc. org/Benchmarking/BenchmarkingProject/, last accessed 29 April 2009).

Conclusion

There are substantial barriers in any system-wide reform of mental health and ROM is no different in that respect. Significant progress has been made, although increasing the use of the obtained outcomes remains an ongoing task. This increased use will occur through case discussions, treatment planning, service reviews and evaluation projects. The question of the connection between outcomes and interventions will be explored both through investigations of elements common to interventions and through evaluating distinct interventions. However, it is also clear that the inherent system complexity around children will challenge us to understand the multiple perspectives on outcomes without succumbing to either the paralysis of information overload or the temptation to simplify by privileging only one informant or domain.

It is clear that effectively helping children requires knowledge of their outcomes. This chapter has shown the progress some services have made in using ROM to improve the quality of mental health services to children.

References

American Academy Child and Adolescent Psychiatry (1997). Practice parameters for the psychiatric assessment of children and adolescents. *Journal of the American Academy of Child and Adolescent Psychiatry*, **36**, 4s–20s.

Anderson, L., Vostanis, P. and O'Reilly, M. (2005). Three-year follow-up of a family support service cohort of children with behavioural problems and their parents. *Child Care, Health & Development*, **31**, 469–77.

Andrews, G., Peters, L. and Teesson, M. (1994). *The Measurement of Consumer Outcome in Mental Health: a Report to the National Mental Health Information Strategy Committee*. Sydney: Clinical Research Unit for Anxiety Disorders.

Ayton, A., Keen, C. and Lask, B. (2009). Pros and cons of using the Mental Health Act for severe eating disorders in adolescents. *European Eating Disorders Review*, **17**, 14–23.

Bickman, L., Nurcombe, B., Townsend, C., et al. (1998). *Consumer Measurement Systems in Child and Adolescent Mental Health*. Canberra: Department of Health and Family Services.

Bickman, L., Rosof-Williams, J., Salzer, M. S., et al. (2000). What information do clinicians value for monitoring adolescent client progress and outcomes? *Professional Psychology: Research and Practice*, **31**, 70–4.

Bilenberg, N. (2003). Health of the Nation Outcome Scales for Children and Adolescents (HoNOSCA). Results of a Danish field trial. *European Child & Adolescent Psychiatry*, **12**, 298–302.

Bourdon, K. H., Goodman, R., Rae, D. S., Simpson, G. and Koretz, D. S. (2005). The Strengths and Difficulties Questionnaire: U.S. normative data and psychometric properties. *Journal of the American Academy of Child & Adolescent Psychiatry*, **44**, 557–64.

Brann, P. (2006). *Routine outcome measurement in child adolescent mental health services: HoNOSCA: reliable enough, valid enough and feasible enough?* Unpublished doctoral dissertation, Monash University, Clayton, Victoria, Australia.

Brann, P., Coleman, G. and Luk, E. (2001). Routine outcome measurement in a child and adolescent mental health service: an evaluation of HoNOSCA. *Australian and New Zealand Journal of Psychiatry*, **35**, 370–6.

Brookman-Frazee, L., Haine, R. A. and Garland, A. F. (2006). Innovations: child and adolescent psychiatry: measuring outcomes of real-world youth psychotherapy: whom to ask and what to ask? *Psychiatric Services*, **57**, 1373–5.

Chipps, J., Stewart, M. and Humberstone, V. (2006). *NZ Mental Health standard measures of assessment and recovery (MH-SMART) initiative. Information collection protocol.*1.0 edn. Auckland: The National Centre of Mental Health Research and Workforce Development. Te Pou o Te Whakaaro Nui.

Chorpita, B. F., Barlow, D. H., Albano, A. M. and Daleiden, E. L. (1998). Methodological strategies in child clinical trials: advancing the efficacy and effectiveness of psychosocial treatments. *Journal of Abnormal Child Psychology*, **26**, 7–16.

Coombs, T. (2006). Rater and Clinical Utility Training Manual: Child and Adolescent. In *Australian Mental Health Outcomes and Classification Network*, 1st edn. Sydney: NSW Institute of Psychiatry.

Daleiden, E., Chorpita, B., Donkervoet, C., Arensdorf, A. and Brogan, M. (2006). Getting better at getting them better: health outcomes and evidence-based practice within a system of care. *Journal of the American Academy of Child & Adolescent Psychiatry*, **45**, 749–56.

Department of Health and Ageing (2003). *Mental Health National Outcomes and Casemix Collection: Technical Specification of State and Territory Reporting Requirements for the Outcomes and Casemix components of 'Agreed Data' (Version 1.50)*. Canberra.

Dickey, B. and Wagenaar, H. (1996). Evaluating health status. In L. I. Sederer and B. Dickey, eds., *Outcomes Assessment in Clinical Practice*. Baltimore: Williams & Wilkins.

Ford, T., Collishaw, S., Meltzer, H. and Goodman, R. (2007). A prospective study of childhood psychopathology: independent predictors of change over three years. *Social Psychiatry & Psychiatric Epidemiology*, **42**, 953–61.

Garland, A. F., Kruse, M. and Aarons, G. A. (2003). Clinicians and outcome measurement: what's the use? *Journal of Behavioral Health Services & Research*, **30**, 393–405.

Garland, A. F., Lewczyk-Boxmeyer, C. M., Gabayan, E. N. and Hawley, K. M. (2004). Multiple stakeholder agreement on desired outcomes for adolescents' mental health services. *Psychiatric Services*, **55**, 671–6.

Garralda, M. E., Yates, P. and Higginson, I. (2000). Child and adolescent mental health service use – HoNOSCA as an outcome measure. *British Journal of Psychiatry*, **177**, 52–8.

Gilbody, S. M., House, A. O. and Sheldon, T. A. (2002). Psychiatrists in the UK do not use outcome measures. *British Journal of Psychiatry*, **180**, 101–3.

Goodman, A. and Goodman, R. (2009). Strengths and Difficulties Questionnaire as a dimensional measure of child mental health. *Journal of the American Academy of Child and Adolescnt Psychiatry*, **48**, 400–3.

Goodman, R. (2001). Psychometric properties of the Strengths and Difficulties Questionnaire. *Journal of the American Academy of Child and Adolescent Psychiatry*, **40**, 1337–45.

Goodman, R. and Scott, S. (1999). Comparing the Strengths and Difficulties Questionnaire and the Child Behavior Checklist: is small beautiful? *Journal of Abnormal Child Psychology*, **27**, 17–24.

Gowers, S., Levine, W., Bailey-Rogers, S., Shore, A. and Burhouse, E. (2002). Use of a routine, self-report outcome measure (HoNOSCA-SR) in two adolescent mental health services. *British Journal of Psychiatry*, **180**, 266–9.

Gowers, S. G., Harrington, R. C., Whitton, A., et al. (1999). Brief scale for measuring the outcomes of emotional and behavioural disorders in children. Health of the Nation Outcome Scales for Children and Adolescents (HoNOSCA). *British Journal of Psychiatry*, **174**, 413–16.

Graeff-Martins, A. S., Flament, M. F., Fayyad, J., et al. (2008). Diffusion of efficacious interventions for children and adolescents with mental health problems. *Journal of Child Psychology & Psychiatry*, **49**, 335–52.

Hanssen-Bauer, K., Aalen, O. O., Ruud, T. and Heyerdahl, S. (2007a). Inter-rater reliability of clinician-rated measures in child and adolescent mental health services. *Administration and Policy in Mental Health*, **34**, 504–12.

Hanssen-Bauer, K., Gowers, S., Aalen, O. O., et al. (2007b). Cross-national reliability of clinician-rated outcome measures in child and adolescent mental health services. *Administration & Policy in Mental Health*, **34**, 513–8.

Harnett, P. H., Loxton, N. J., Sadler, T., Hides, L. and Baldwin, A. (2005). The Health of the Nation Outcome Scales for Children and Adolescents in an adolescent in-patient sample. *Australian and New Zealand Journal of Psychiatry*, **39**, 129–35.

Hatfield, D. R. and Ogles, B. M. (2004). The use of outcome measures by psychologists in clinical practice. *Professional Psychology: Research and Practice*, **35**, 485–91.

Heiervang, E., Goodman, A. and Goodman, R. (2008). The Nordic advantage in child mental health: separating health differences from reporting style in a cross-cultural comparison of psychopathology. *Journal of Child Psychology & Psychiatry & Allied Disciplines*, **49**, 678–85.

Hoagwood, K., Jensen, P. S., Petti, T. and Burns, B. J. (1996). Outcomes of mental health care for children and adolescents: I. A comprehensive conceptual model. *Journal of the American Academy of Child and Adolescent Psychiatry*, **35**, 1055–63.

Hunter, J., Higginson, I. and Garralda, E. (1996). Systematic literature review: outcomes measures for child and adolescent mental health services. *Journal of Public Health Medicine*, **18**, 197–206.

Jaffa, T. (2000). HoNOSCA: is the enthusiasm justified? *Child Psychology and Psychiatry Review*, **5**, 130.

Johnston, C. and Gowers, S. (2005). Routine outcome measurement: a survey of UK child and adolescent mental health child and services. *Child and Adolescent Mental Health*, **10**, 133–9.

Jones, M. and Tardif, H. (2008). Self harm presentations to hospitals in West Australian 0–18 year olds: what can outcome measure profiles add to the understanding of trajectory? *Australian and New Zealand Journal of Psychiatry*, **42**, A7.

Kazdin, A. E. (1997). A model for developing effective treatments: progression and interplay of theory, research and practice. *Journal of Clinical Child Psychology*, **26**, 114–29.

Kazdin, A. E. and Weisz, J. R. (1998). Identifying and developing empirically supported child and adolescent treatments. *Journal of Consulting and Clinical Psychology*, **66**, 19–36.

Kennair, N., Mellor, D. and Brann, P. (in press). Evaluating the outcomes of adolescent day programs in an Australian child and adolescent mental health service. *Clinical Child Psychology & Psychiatry*.

Kisely, S., Campbell, L. A., Crossman, D., Gleich, S. and Campbell, J. (2007). Are the Health of the Nation Outcome Scales a valid and practical instrument to measure outcomes in North America? A three-site evaluation across Nova Scotia. *Community Mental Health Journal*, **43**, 91–107.

Lambert, W., Salzer, M. S. and Bickman, L. (1998). Clinical outcome, consumer satisfaction, and ad hoc ratings of improvement in children's mental health. *Journal of Consulting and Clinical Psychology*, **66**, 270–9.

Lawton, R. and Marland, P. (2008). Consumer experience of outcome measures in a CAMHS context. *Australian and New Zealand Journal of Psychiatry*, **42**, A8.

Leginski, W. A., Croze, C., Driggers, J., et al. (1989). *Data Standards for Mental Health Decision Support Systems. A Report of the Task Force to Revise the Data Content and System Guidelines of the Mental Health Statistics Improvement Program.* Washington DC.

Lesinskiene, S., Senina, J. and Ranceva, N. (2007). Use of the HoNOSCA scale in the teamwork of inpatient child psychiatry unit. *Journal of Psychiatric and Mental Health Nursing*, **14**, 727–33.

Manderson, J. and McCune, N. (2003). The use of HoNOSCA in a child and adolescent mental health service. *Irish Journal of Psychological Medicine*, **20**, 52–5.

Mathai, J., Anderson, P. and Bourne, A. (2003). Use of the Strengths and Difficulties Questionnaire as an outcome measure in a child and adolescent mental health service. *Australasian Psychiatry*, **11**, 334–7.

McLennan, J. D., Wathen, C. N., MacMillan, H. L. and Lavis, J. N. (2006). Research-practice gaps in child mental health. *Journal of the American Academy of Child & Adolescent Psychiatry*, **45**, 658–65.

McShane, G., Bazzano, C., Walter, G. and Barton, G. (2007). Outcome of patients attending a specialist educational and mental health service for social anxiety disorders. *Clinical Child Psychology & Psychiatry*, **12**, 117–24.

Mellor, D. (2004). Furthering the use of the Strength and Difficulties Questionnaire: reliability with younger respondents. *Psychological Assessment*, **16**, 396–401.

Merry, S., Stasiak, K., Parkin, A., et al. (2004). *Child and youth outcome measures: Examining current use and acceptability of measures in mental health services and recommending future directions.* Auckland, available at: http://www.hrc.govt.nz.

Ogles, B. M., Lambert, M. J. and Masters, K. S. (1996). *Assessing Outcome in Clinical Practice.* Boston, MA: Allyn & Bacon.

Pirkis, J., Burgess, P., Coombs, T., et al. (2005a). Routine measurement of outcomes in Australia's public sector mental health services. *Australia and New Zealand Health Policy*, **2**, 8.

Pirkis, J., Burgess, P., Kirk, P., Dodson, S. and Coombs, T. (2005b). *Review of standardised measures used in the national outcomes and casemix collection (NOCC). Version 1.2*, Sydney: Australian Mental Health Outcomes and Classification Network.

Rutter, M. and Stevenson, J. (2008). Using epidemiology to plan services: a conceptual approach. In M. Rutter, D. Bishop, D. Pine et al., eds., *Rutter's Child and Adolescent Psychiatry*, 5th edn. Oxford: Blackwell Publishing.

Sawyer, M. G., Arney, F. M., Baghurst, P. A., et al. (2000). *The Mental Health of Young People in Australia: Child And Adolescent Component of the National Survey of Mental Health and Wellbeing.* Canberra: Australian Government Publishing Service.

Schaffer, D., Gould, M. S., Brasic, J., et al. (1983). A children's global assessment scale (CGAS). *Archives of General Psychiatry*, **40**, 1228–31.

Schorre, B. and Vandvik, I. (2004). Global assessment of psychosocial functioning in child and adolescent psychiatry. A review

of three unidimensional scales (CGAS, GAF, GAPD). *European Child & Adolescent Psychiatry*, **13**, 273–86.

Stewart, M. (2008). Making the HoNOS(CA) clinically useful: a strategy for making HonOS, HoNOSCA, and HoNOS65+ useful to the clinical team. *Australian and New Zealand Journal of Psychiatry*, **42**, A5.

Vitiello, B., Rohde, P., Silva, S., et al. (2006). Functioning and quality of life in the Treatment for Adolescents with Depression Study (TADS). *Journal of the American Academy of Child & Adolescent Psychiatry*, **45**, 1419–26.

Vostanis, P. (2006). Strengths and Difficulties Questionnaire: research and clinical applications. *Current Opinion in Psychiatry*, **19**, 367–72.

Vostanis, P., Anderson, L. and Window, S. (2006). Evaluation of a family support service: short-term outcome. *Clinical Child Psychology & Psychiatry*, **11**, 513–28.

Warnick, E., Weersing, V., Scahill, L. and Woolston, J. (2009). Selecting measures for use in child mental health services: a scorecard approach. *Administration & Policy in Mental Health*, **36**, 112–22.

Weisz, J. R. and Jensen, P. S. (1999). Efficacy and effectiveness of child and adolescent psychotherapy and pharmacotherapy. *Mental Health Services Research*, 125–57.

Weisz, J., Sandler, I., Durlak, J. and Anton, B. (2005). Promoting and protecting youth mental health through evidence-based prevention and treatment. *American Psychologist*, **60**, 628–48.

Yates, P., Kramer, T. and Garralda, M. E. (2006). Use of a routine mental health measure in an adolescent secure unit. *British Journal of Psychiatry*, **188**, 583–4.

Young, A. S., Grusky, O., Jordan, D. and Belin, T. R. (2000). Routine outcome monitoring in a public mental health system: the impact of patients who leave care. *Psychiatric Services*, **51**, 85–91.

12

Outcome measurement in adult mental health services

Tom Trauer

Of the three age groups considered in this book, it is in the adult area that the greatest amount of material and literature lies. Several of the other chapters in this book present detailed descriptions of outcome measurement (OM) systems in other countries, special settings and particular groups of consumers. Therefore in this chapter we shall not attempt to cover everything that has been reported on OM with adults world-wide. Rather, we shall outline routine outcome measurement (ROM) in adult clinical services in Australia.

History

The chapter by Jane Pirkis and Tom Callaly (Chapter 2) in this book has described the history and policy background to ROM in Australia. It had been anticipated that ROM would be introduced gradually, and a number of preparatory activities were undertaken prior to full national implementation across all age groups. In order to keep the process manageable, these activities were limited to the adult area.

Following the policy decision to introduce ROM (Australian Health Ministers, 1992) a review of existing adult measures was commissioned. Following a review of over 100 measures, against the criteria of applicability, acceptability, practicality, reliability, validity and sensitivity to change, Andrews et al. (1994) recommended six as potentially suitable for ROM and worthy of further attention. These were the Health of the Nation Outcome Scales (HoNOS, Wing et al., 1998), the Life Skills Profile (LSP, Rosen et al., 1989); the Role Functioning Scale (RFS, Goodman et al., 1993), the Behaviour and Symptom Identification Scale (BASIS, Eisen et al., 1986), the Mental Health Inventory (MHI, Veit and Ware, 1983) and the Medical Outcomes Study – Short Form (SF-36, Ware et al., 1993). All of these measures were subsequently field-tested in Queensland by Stedman et al. (1997) and most were found to be suitable for routine use. Around the same time, significant experience was gained in the use of two of the 'short-listed' instruments (HoNOS and LSP) in a large national project funded to develop a casemix classification for mental health services (Buckingham et al., 1998).

Given the likelihood that the HoNOS would figure significantly in the future, a field trial of the instrument was conducted in Victoria in 1996 (Trauer et al., 1999b). Over 2000 adult consumers in five services were assessed once and about half were reassessed after a few months. Psychometric aspects were reported, as well as associations with demographic, diagnostic and service use variables.

Following a plan to introduce ROM into Australian mental health services in a staged fashion, the next step was a State-funded project to: produce an OM training package; deliver training in the full range of adult measures in four selected pilot agencies; develop proprietary software for the entry and reporting of OM data; develop a framework for the analysis and reporting of OMs; and conduct a consumer consultation project designed to identify consumer views regarding self-assessment and the process of outcome measurement. This

Outcome Measurement in Mental Health: Theory and Practice, ed. Tom Trauer. Published by Cambridge University Press.
© Cambridge University Press 2010.

resulted in a training manual (Eagar et al., 2000) and two training videos; experience with train-the-trainer and direct training in OM (Coombs et al., 2002, Trauer et al., 2002); specialized OM software for use at the local level (Callaly et al., 2000); a reporting framework that distinguished individual and aggregate-level reporting (Eagar et al., 2001); and a report detailing that consumers supported ROM as potentially contributing to the treatment they receive, that there is a wide range of content areas and life domains of importance to them, and that they are as concerned with the process by which they are involved in OM as by the selection and details of the instruments used (Graham et al., 2001). More detail of this work is presented in the chapter on skills and training by Tim Coombs and myself (Chapter 21).

The collection protocol

This preparatory work led the way to the specification of the implementation of ROM in public mental health services throughout the nation, and this commenced formally in 2003. Covering the three age groups of child and adolescent, adult, and older persons, the specification, known as the National Outcomes and Casemix Collection (NOCC, Commonwealth Department of Health and Ageing, 2002), set out the details of which patients should be rated, using which scales, at what time points, by whom, and covering what periods. For adults, the 'suite' of instruments to be used include the HoNOS, a short form of the LSP (Rosen et al., 2006), a consumer self-report measure (one of the BASIS, MHI, or the K10; Kessler et al., 2002), and the Focus of Care. Both the LSP-16 and the Focus of Care had been developed for the Australian mental health casemix project (Buckingham et al., 1998). The other data items in the collection serve primarily casemix purposes. With some exceptions for highly specialized services, the NOCC protocol for adults is as presented in Table 12.1.

As is explained in more detail in the chapter by Jane Pirkis and Tom Callaly (Chapter 2), the NOCC protocol is organized around the concept of the episode, and recognizes three service settings (inpatient, community residential and ambulatory) and three collection occasions (admission, review and discharge). 'Ambulatory' is roughly synonymous with 'Community', and 'Admission' and 'Discharge' correspond to 'Intake' and 'Closure' respectively. There are two kinds of reviews: standard reviews occur after 3 months of care in an episode, while ad hoc reviews may be conducted at the discretion of the clinician for any reason.

Table 12.1 shows that the HoNOS is required to be completed at all collection occasions in all settings. The period covered by the HoNOS is the previous 14 days. One exception is made to this: at discharge from acute inpatient settings the HoNOS ratings are based on the past 3 days

Table 12.1 National Outcome and Casemix Collection protocol for adults

Mental health service setting	Inpatient			Community residential			Ambulatory		
Collection occasion	A	R	D	A	R	D	A	R	D
HoNOS	•	•	•	•	•	•	•	•	•
LSP-16				•	•	•		•	•
Consumer self-report				•	•	•	•	•	•
Psychiatric diagnoses	•		•	•	•			•	•
Focus of care								•	•
Mental health legal status	•	•		•	•			•	•

A = admission; R = review; D = discharge.

(including the day of discharge). The LSP-16, whose period covered in the last 3 months, is not required in inpatient settings, where length of stay is usually very brief, nor at admission to ambulatory episodes, where it may be difficult to assess the consumer's functioning that far back.

The HoNOS and LSP-16 are completed by the clinician, but the consumer self-report is a self-assessment. The review of instruments in 1994 by Andrews et al. recommended several such instruments, and to these the K-10 (Kessler et al., 2002) was later added. States and Territories were given the option of which of the BASIS, MHI and K-10 they would use, and currently all three are in use in the different jurisdictions. While policy can make clinician-completed measures mandatory, a consumer self-assessment is necessarily voluntary. Clinician training aims to encourage them to invite consumers to complete a self-report at the points designated in the protocol, while recognizing that there will be situations where it will be inappropriate. Such situations include the consumer being too ill or having insufficient understanding or concentration, and the possibility that completing a measure might cause distress. Clinicians are expected to use their clinical judgement in this regard. There are some good practice principles for the offering of the self-report measure.

- Invite the consumer to self-rate their own health status and be genuinely interested in the responses that the consumer gives.
- Follow up the self-rating with an invitation to the consumer to discuss their answers, elaborate on how they feel, and discuss how it might impact on their individual treatment plan.
- Identify any discrepancies between consumer and clinician ratings and use this information to reassess perceptions.
- Share the knowledge gained from both single and multiple ratings with the consumer themselves and integrate the results into the individual treatment plan.

(Buckingham and Casey, 2000)

Subsequent activity

Since the implementation of ROM throughout public mental health services in Australia in 2003, assessments have been used at various levels for various purposes. Some of these, such as using ratings at the clinical level, are comparatively 'invisible' in the clinical literature, in the sense that services have incorporated ROM into their standard operating practices and culture. Admittedly, the penetration of ROM into service cultures has not been uniform across the country. In this section, we shall document some of the specific areas of work involving adult OMs that have been reported.

(a) Completion of the measures

For outcome measures to be 'routine' implies that they are applied at all, or at least most, of the specified occasions. The interests of the individual consumer are not promoted when the measures that could inform his/her treatment and management are absent, and aggregated uses of measures are impaired when they are completed in only a patchy fashion. Averages based on incomplete data may lack credibility on account of biases, i.e. important differences between the outcomes of consumers from whom measures were obtained and those from whom they were not. Speer and Newman (1996) noted:

> There is now considerable evidence indicating that clients who provide follow-up data generally are more functional, are healthier, and have more resources than clients who either choose not to, or are unable to provide follow-up data. Clients who participate in follow-up are those who are generally most likely to benefit from psychosocial interventions. Conclusions based on cohorts with large attrition rates are likely to overestimate the positive effects of the interventions. We recommend aiming to obtain a 90% data completion rate; findings based on completion rates of less than 70% should be viewed with considerable caution. (p. 123)

In order to compute completion rates one needs to divide the numbers actually completed by the number that should have been completed. The former figure is easy to obtain, but the latter is more difficult, since it depends on an accurate count of the occasions when measures should have been completed, according to the prevailing protocol. A further complication is that completion rates for consumer self-report measures will depend on the measure being offered or presented by the clinicians, and then being accepted by the consumer, this acceptance always being necessarily voluntary.

Such evidence that exists suggests that completion rates can be extremely different between services, and often quite variable within services over time. Trauer (2004) compared completion rates at the introduction of ROM in four adult mental health services in Victoria, Australia. Rates varied between 0% and 80%, depending primarily on agency. One agency had recorded discharge assessments, but no admission assessments, possibly an artefact of their data entry system. Another agency began with high rates which dropped rapidly over the first 6 months, while another started slowly but escalated equally rapidly over the same period. The study was unable to determine the reasons for these large differences, but local knowledge suggested that senior and middle management support and the information technology systems were probably relevant.

The New Zealand mental health classification and outcomes study (CAOS) required clinicians to collect measures over a 6-month study period. Most (80% to 97%) episodes of care had a measure of some kind completed at some stage, but many fewer (53% to 61%) had matching assessments at the start and end of the episode (Trauer et al., 2004, p. 16), a necessity for using the measures to calculate change.

A survey of the use of the HoNOS in mental health trusts in the UK found that, despite it being part of a mental health minimum data set, the overall completion rate was only 9.5% (Office of Health Economics, 2008, p. 35). Consistent with other interpretations, the cause was thought to be antipathy to the instrument itself ('HoNOS has been recommended by the Department of Health, which apparently makes it an unpopular instrument with clinicians') and a strong preference among policy-makers and academics for self-rated measures over clinician measures such as HoNOS 'which are by definition based on a medical model of mental health problems'.

Similar conclusions were drawn from a joint consumer/clinician-led project (Black et al., 2009) conducted a few years later in one of the agencies studied earlier by Trauer (2004). It concluded that 'the major barrier to completion of the measures is not the consumers' willingness to engage, but the continued resistance of clinicians to embrace the measures in their clinical practice' (p. 98).

(b) Training

As with the other age groups, there has been activity to develop and extend training resources, and to explore issues around training. Much of this activity has been undertaken by the Training and Service Development section of the Australian Mental Health Outcomes and Classification Network (AMHOCN). While numerous and high-quality training resources have been developed in the past, there has been a recognition that new materials need to be produced in order to incorporate new developments and changes. Although questions have been raised about the need for formal training in the use of HoNOS (Rock and Preston, 2001), all staff who will use OMs are expected to receive training. Further details of training and other workforce development issues are to be found in the chapter by Tim Coombs and myself (Chapter 21) in this book.

(c) Length of stay in acute inpatient units

A number of studies have appeared in which the relationship between HoNOS scores and length of stay (LOS) in acute inpatient units has been examined. Boot et al. (1997) looked at LOS in a number of public and private psychiatric inpatient units across Australia. They noted the very different diagnostic mix seen in public and private settings, and found that, while there were comparable reductions in HoNOS scores between admission and discharge, LOS was longer in the private units. Shortly thereafter, Goldney et al. (1998) reported a study that encompassed six private psychiatric hospitals; they found a negligible relationship between HoNOS scores and LOS, although in a later study some of the same authors (Smith et al., 2002) found that consumers who were rated higher on HoNOS scale 2 (self-harming thoughts and behaviours) had a significantly shorter LOS than those who were rated lower. Trauer et al. (1999a) compared the finding from the Boot et al. and Goldney et al. studies with new HoNOS data collected in a public inpatient unit. Combining the results from the various sources, they concluded that public facilities tended to show greater improvement, owing to higher admission severities, and their lengths of stay tended to be shorter, thus rendering public facilities more 'efficient' in terms of reduction in HoNOS score per hospital day. They also found that scores on HoNOS scale 2 (self-harm) were significantly higher in the public facilities. They proposed that since self-harm is a criterion for involuntary admission, and since private hospitals in Australia do not take involuntary admissions, these differences might account for the apparent difference in 'efficiency'. This was followed by a study by Hugo (2000), who examined the change in HoNOS scores between admission and discharge in relation to symptom severity, admission medico-legal status (i.e. whether involuntary or not) and LOS. He found that involuntary hospitalization was associated with higher admission severities and longer LOS, which led him to conclude that factors unrelated to admission legal status affect differences in efficiency ratings found between public and private acute psychiatric inpatient facilities. A later study (Trauer, 2008) showed that higher scores at admission on the HoNOS Hallucinations/delusions item were associated with longer lengths of stay, while higher scores on the Deliberate self-harm and Depressed mood items were associated with shorter lengths of stay. It was speculated that a reason for the absence of a relationship between HoNOS total score and LOS was that item associations with longer and shorter LOS were cancelling out.

(d) Demonstration of service effectiveness

Related to studies of length of stay are those that seek to use routinely collected measures to evaluate the overall effectiveness of mental health services. These approaches have relied on computing the differences in scores between collection occasions (see Table 12.1) and aggregating these (for more details see the chapter on assessing change (Chapter 20)). Most such reports deal with the difference between admission and discharge, partly because the data tend to be more complete at these points, and because changes between admission and discharge represent a natural interval for judging the effect of the intervening service delivery. In adult inpatient settings, several studies, in Australia (Trauer, T., Callaly, T. and Herrman, H.. 2005, Evaluation of adult mental health services using routine outcome measures; unpublished report) and around the world (McClelland et al., 2000, Trauer et al., 2006), have shown that on average HoNOS total scores decline by about half between admission and discharge. Burgess et al. (2006) analysed the nationally collected Australian HoNOS data and also found 50% admission–discharge reductions in inpatient settings, as well as somewhat lower reductions (30%) in community settings. These reductions, which represent effect sizes of 1.0 (large) and 0.5 (medium) respectively, led them to conclude that people in contact with public-sector mental health services generally do get better, and that the evidence is supportive of the quality and effectiveness of mental health services.

(e) Use of outcome measures in clinical team meetings

There have been a few reports showing how OMs can be used at the level of the adult clinical team. There are several potential benefits in this. First, the OM results can directly assist the team in its deliberations and decision-making and, second, expertise and skill in the use of the measures can be shared.

Slattery and Anstey (2008) described a unit that had established a system of collecting and discussing consumers' HoNOS scores during their multi-disciplinary ward rounds. This activity helped the team to formulate effective management plans and contributed to decisions regarding a consumer's readiness for discharge. They found that visual projection of the information enabled the most up-to-date data to be accessed, improved efficiency and created an infrastructure supportive of the instrument's clinical use.

Trauer et al. (2009) reported on a project in which OM experts and trainers attended the team meetings of four adult community teams fortnightly over about 3 months. During these meetings, the visitors contributed to the team discussion of OMs during routine clinical reviews, using local and national outcome measurement data and tools, and their own expertise. Attitudes of clinicians toward ROM in general and the specific instruments were assessed at the beginning and end of the period, and again after about 5 months. On average, team members felt that OMs were more useful and easier to use between the beginning and end of these attendances, and most of these improvements were maintained at follow-up. Team members appeared to appreciate the assistance provided to them, and felt more confident in using the OM information. A positive attitude in the most senior clinician in the meeting, plus the availability of data projection technology, assisted the process. Contrasting with the fairly unstructured approach adopted by Trauer et al. (2009), Stewart (2008) outlined a five-stage process whereby HoNOS results can be considered systematically in a team meeting.

A section in Chapter 18 (Outcome measurement – applications and utility) of this book describes how levels and thresholds of scores on the HoNOS and LSP-16 have been developed to assist clinical teams to make decisions about reducing levels of contact, discharge and transfer.

(f) Outcome measurement and the recovery model

Lakeman (2004), critiquing an exposition of OM in adult services by Coombs and Meehan (2003), asserted that ROM had 'only a limited capacity to capture the richness of people's recovery journeys or provide information that can usefully inform care', is seriously flawed in its failure to capture the subtlety of individual differences, and may 'dumb down' clinical research. To the extent that it does not attempt to capture concepts such as coping, hope, social connectedness, self-efficacy, empowerment or self-esteem, it neglects, and may be antithetical to, the true meaning and spirit of recovery. Coombs and Meehan (2005) responded by pointing out that the consumer self-rating measure, which is a mandatory measure so long as the consumer can complete it, affords the kind of participation that the recovery perspective requires. Browne (2006), commenting on the above interchange, concurred with Lakeman, and expressed doubts whether outcome measures assess the kinds of things that are of importance to consumers in the 'new culture' of recovery. In a similar vein, Happell felt that ROM fails to involve the consumer in the design of instruments, fails to reflect those aspects of treatment consumers consider to affect their recovery (2008b) and that the government-endorsed systems of ROM 'are little more than tokenistic' (2008a, p. 120).

Whether any form of ROM is compatible with a recovery paradigm is both a philosophical and an empirical question. In this regard it is interesting to note that an early version of an Australian measure of stage of recovery was found to correlate significantly with the HoNOS and the K-10, both standard OM instruments in the Australian context (Andresen et al., 2006).

(g) Relationships between instruments

As explained earlier, OM was conceived as being based on a set of measures, no single measure being deemed sufficient to capture the range of important aspects of outcome. For adult services the main instruments were the HoNOS, aimed at assessing overall illness severity, the LSP-16, to assess disability and functional impairment, and a self-rating instrument, to ensure that the consumer's perspective was included. It is apparent from the collection protocol (see Table 12.1) that there are many situations where several instruments are meant to be collected at the same time, and this affords the opportunity to examine their inter-relationships. One fairly consistent finding has been that scores on instruments completed by the provider tend to be quite strongly correlated, while the correlation between those instruments and that completed by the consumer is much lower. For example, Stedman et al. (1997), Trauer (2004, Analysis of outcome measurement data from the four Victorian 'Round One' agencies; unpublished report) and Trauer et al. (2004) all found correlations between 0.65 and 0.69 between HoNOS and LSP-16, but the first two of these studies found correlations between 0.13 and 0.36 between these two instruments and the BASIS, a consumer self-report measure. A further demonstration of the low correspondence between provider and consumer perceptions came from a study by Trauer and Callaly (2002) that compared provider ratings on the HoNOS with consumer self-ratings on its parallel form (HoNOS-SR, College Research Unit, 1996). Consumer ratings were significantly higher (worse) than case manager ratings on four of the 12 HoNOS scales, and significantly lower on one. Overall, agreement levels were slight to moderate, but particularly low for depressed mood. Despite these differences, case managers tended to overestimate the actual degree of similarity between their own ratings and those of their clients. In a similar study Stewart (2009) compared ratings by clinicians, consumers and their significant others (family/friends) on specially adapted versions of the instrument. Contrary to Trauer and Callaly, he found generally satisfactory levels of agreement between all three parties. The findings have generally been interpreted as signifying that the different stakeholders' perspectives are typically quite dissimilar, and represent differing information sources. The implications are that they both need to be collected, and that it is unsafe to infer one from the other.

Some have studied the relationship between HoNOS, the most widely used instrument in clinical services, and the Camberwell Assessment of Need (CAN, Phelan et al., 1995), which is most widely used in non-government organizations (NGOs; see the chapter by Glen Tobias (Chapter 16)). Consistent with the conclusions of the previous paragraph, Issakidis and Teesson (1999) found that consumers' rating of need on the CAN and clinicians' rating on the HoNOS were only moderately correlated ($r = 0.35$), while Gallagher and Teesson (2000), using the HoNOS and the staff version of the CAN, found that consumers receiving assertive case management were rated as having higher levels of disability and need than patients receiving standard case management, and concluded that both instruments were promising contenders for routine use. These results are compatible with two studies from the Institute of Psychiatry in London. Slade et al. (1999) found that HoNOS was good for tracking changes in social functioning over time, but the Camberwell Assessment of Need Short Appraisal Schedule (CANSAS) was more suitable for treatment planning, and Salvi et al. (2005) concluded that 'When a detailed characterisation of clinical and social needs of the patient and outcomes is required, HoNOS and CANSAS should be used' (p. 151).

References

Andresen, R., Caputi, P. and Oades, L. (2006). Stages of recovery instrument: development of a measure of recovery from serious mental illness. *Australian and New Zealand Journal of Psychiatry*, **40**, 972–80.

Andrews, G., Peters, L. and Teesson, M. (1994). *The Measurement of Consumer Outcome in Mental Health: A Report to the National Mental Health Information Strategy Committee*. Sydney: Clinical Research Unit for Anxiety Disorders.

Australian Health Ministers (1992). *National Mental Health Policy*. Canberra: Australian Government Publishing Service.

Black, J., Lewis, T., McIntosh, P., et al. (2009). It's not that bad: the views of consumers and carers about routine outcome measurement in mental health. *Australian Health Review*, **33**, 93–9.

Boot, B., Hall, W. and Andrews, G. (1997). Disability, outcome and casemix in acute psychiatric inpatient units. *British Journal of Psychiatry*, **171**, 242–6.

Browne, G. (2006). Outcome measures: do they fit with a recovery model? *International Journal of Mental Health Nursing*, **15**, 153–4.

Buckingham, B. and Casey, D. (2000). *Australian plans and progress in implementing routine outcome measures in mental health*. Mental Health Research & Development Strategy: Outcomes Conference. Wellington, New Zealand.

Buckingham, W., Burgess, P., Solomon, S., Pirkis, J. and Eagar, K. (1998). *Developing a Casemix Classification for Mental Health Services*. Canberra: Department of Health and Ageing.

Burgess, P., Pirkis, J. and Coombs, T. (2006). Do adults in contact with Australia's public sector mental health services get better? *Australia and New Zealand Health Policy*, **3**, 9.

Callaly, T., Trauer, T. and Hantz, P. (2000). *HBL: HoNOS, BASIS-32 and LSP16* [computer software]. Geelong: Barwon Health.

College Research Unit (1996). *HoNOS: Health of the Nation Outcome Scales: Report on Research and Development July 1993-December 1995*. London: Department of Health.

Commonwealth Department of Health and Ageing (2002). *National Outcomes and Casemix Collection: Technical specification of State and Territory reporting requirements for the outcomes and casemix components of 'Agreed Data' under National Mental Health Information Development Funding Agreements*. Canberra.

Coombs, T. and Meehan, T. (2003). Mental health outcomes in Australia: issues for mental health nurses. *International Journal of Mental Health Nursing*, **12**, 163–4.

Coombs, T. and Meehan, T. (2005). Standardized routine outcome measurement: response to Lakeman. *International Journal of Mental Health Nursing*, **14**, 215–17.

Coombs, T., Trauer, T. and Eagar, K. (2002). Training in mental health outcome measurement: evaluation of the Victorian experience. *Australian Health Review*, **25**, 74–82.

Eagar, K., Buckingham, B., Coombs, T., et al. (2000). *Outcome Measurement in Adult Area Mental Health Services: Implementation Resource Manual*. Melbourne, Victoria: Department of Human Services Victoria.

Eagar, K., Buckingham, B., Coombs, T., et al. (2001). *Victorian Mental Health Outcomes Measurement Strategy Framework For Agency-Level Standard Reports*. Wollongong.

Eisen, S. V., Grob, M. C. and Klein, A. A. (1986). BASIS: The development of a self-report measure for psychiatric inpatient evaluation. *Psychiatric Hospital*, **17**, 165–71.

Gallagher, J. and Teesson, M. (2000). Measuring disability, need and outcome in Australian community mental health services. *Australian and New Zealand Journal of Psychiatry*, **34**, 850–5.

Goldney, R. D., Fisher, L. J. and Walmsley, S. H. (1998). The Health of the Nation Outcome Scales in psychiatric hospitalisation: a multicentre study examining outcome and prediction of length of stay. *Australian and New Zealand Journal of Psychiatry*, **32**, 199–205.

Goodman, S. H., Sewell, D. R., Cooley, E. L. and Leavitt, N. (1993). Assessing levels of adaptive functioning: the Role Functioning Scale. *Community Mental Health Journal*, **29**, 119–31.

Graham, C., Coombs, T., Buckingham, W., et al. (2001). *Consumer Perspectives of Future Directions for Outcome Self-Assessment*. Report of the Consumer Consultation Project, Wollongong.

Happell, B. (2008a). Determining the effectiveness of mental health services from a consumer perspective: Part 1: enhancing recovery. *International Journal of Mental Health Nursing*, **17**, 116–22.

Happell, B. (2008b). Determining the effectiveness of mental health services from a consumer perspective: Part 2: barriers to recovery and principles for evaluation. *International Journal of Mental Health Nursing*, **17**, 123–30.

Hugo, M. (2000). Comparative efficiency ratings between public and private acute inpatient facilities. *Australian and New Zealand Journal of Psychiatry*, **34**, 651–7.

Issakidis, C. and Teesson, M. (1999). Measurement of need for care: a trial of the Camberwell Assessment of Need and the Health of the National Outcome Scales. *Australian and New Zealand Journal of Psychiatry*, **33**, 754–9.

Kessler, R. C., Andrews, G., Colpe, L. J., et al. (2002). Short screening scales to monitor population prevalences and trends in nonspecific psychological distress. *Psychological Medicine*, **32**, 959–76.

Lakeman, R. (2004). Standardized routine outcome measurement: pot holes in the road to recovery. *International Journal of Mental Health Nursing*, **13**, 210–15.

McClelland, R., Trimble, P., Fox, M. L., Stevenson, M. R. and Bell, B. (2000). Validation of an outcome scale for use in adult psychiatric practice. *Quality in Health Care*, **9**, 98–105.

Office of Health Economics (2008). *NHS Outcomes, Performance and Productivity*.

Phelan, M., Slade, M., Thornicroft, G., et al. (1995). The Camberwell Assessment of Need: the validity and reliability of an instrument to assess the needs of people with severe mental illness. *British Journal of Psychiatry*, **167**, 589–95.

Rock, D. and Preston, N. (2001). HoNOS: is there any point in training clinicians? *Journal of Psychiatric and Mental Health Nursing*, **8**, 405–9.

Rosen, A., Hadzi-Pavlovic, D. and Parker, G. (1989). The Life Skills Profile: a measure assessing function and disability in schizophrenia. *Schizophrenia Bulletin*, **15**, 325–37.

Rosen, A., Hadzi-Pavlovic, D., Parker, G. and Trauer, T. (2006). *The Life Skills Profile: Background, Items and Scoring for the LSP–39, LSP–20 and the LSP–16*, Sydney, available at: http://www.blackdoginstitute.org.au/docs/LifeSkillsProfile.pdf.

Salvi, G., Leese, M. and Slade, M. (2005). Routine use of mental health outcome assessments: choosing the measure. *British Journal of Psychiatry*, **186**, 146–52.

Slade, M., Beck, A., Bindman, J., Thornicroft, G. and Wright, S. (1999). Routine clinical outcome measures for patients with severe mental illness: CANSAS and HoNOS. *British Journal of Psychiatry*, **174**, 404–8.

Slattery, T. and Anstey, S. (2008). Clinical utility of HoNOS in an inpatient setting. *Australian and New Zealand Journal of Psychiatry*, **42**, A6.

Smith, D., Fisher, L. and Goldney, R. (2002). Do suicidal ideation and behaviour influence duration of psychiatric hospitalization? *International Journal of Mental Health Nursing*, **11**, 220–4.

Speer, D. C. and Newman, F. L. (1996). Mental health services outcome evaluation. *Clinical Psychology: Science and Practice*, **3**, 105–29.

Stedman, T., Yellowlees, P., Mellsop, G., Clarke, R. and Drake, S. (1997). *Measuring Consumer Outcomes in Mental Health*. Canberra: Department of Health and Aged Care.

Stewart, M. (2008). Making the HoNOS(CA) clinically useful: a strategy for making HonOS, HoNOSCA, and HoNOS65+ useful to the clinical team. *Australian and New Zealand Journal of Psychiatry*, **42**, A5.

Stewart, M. (2009). Service user and significant other versions of the Health of the Nation Outcome Scales. *Australasian Psychiatry*, **17**, 156–63.

Trauer, T. (2008). Are HoNOS scores related to length of stay in acute inpatient units? *Australian and New Zealand Journal of Psychiatry*, **42**, A10.

Trauer, T. and Callaly, T. (2002). Concordance between mentally ill clients and their case managers using the Health of the Nation Outcome Scales (HoNOS). *Australasian Psychiatry*, **10**, 24–8.

Trauer, T., Callaly, T. and Hantz, P. (1999a). The measurement of improvement during hospitalisation for acute psychiatric illness. *Australian and New Zealand Journal of Psychiatry*, **33**, 379–84.

Trauer, T., Callaly, T., Hantz, P., et al. (1999b). Health of the Nation Outcome Scales (HoNOS): results of the Victorian field trial. *British Journal of Psychiatry*, **174**, 380–8.

Trauer, T., Coombs, T. and Eagar, K. (2002). Training in routine mental health outcome assessment: the Victorian experience. *Australian Health Review*, **25**, 122–8.

Trauer, T., Eagar, K., Gaines, P. and Bower, A. (2004). *New Zealand Mental Health Consumers and their Outcomes*. Auckland: Health Research Council of New Zealand.

Trauer, T., Eagar, K. and Mellsop, G. (2006). Ethnicity, deprivation and mental health outcomes. *Australian Health Review*, **30**, 310–21.

Trauer, T., Pedwell, G. and Gill, L. (2009). The effect of guidance in the use of routine outcome measures in clinical meetings. *Australian Health Review*, **33**, 144–51.

Veit, C. T. and Ware, J. E. (1983). The structure of psychological distress and well-being in general populations. *Journal of Consulting and Clinical Psychology*, **51**, 730–42.

Ware, J., Snow, K. K., Kosinski, M. and Gandek, B. (1993). *SF-36 Health Survey: Manual and Interpretation Guide*. Boston, MA: New England Medical Center, The Health Institute.

Wing, J. K., Beevor, A. S., Curtis, R. H., et al. (1998). Health of the Nation Outcome Scales (HoNOS). Research and development. *British Journal of Psychiatry*, **172**, 11–18.

13 Outcome measurement in older persons

Rod McKay and Regina McDonald

Introduction

For health and community service providers, caring for older people with mental health disorders can be both challenging and rewarding. Older people have a diverse array of life experiences contributing to their individuality. The older person with a mental health problem commonly has social, medical or functional problems associated with ageing and life events. Consequently, optimal management of their mental health issues requires a coordinated approach from different professional service providers, with different intervention foci and different ways of measuring 'outcomes'. In this situation there are also different ways of conceptualizing what constitutes an older person, and what a mental health disorder is. The answers to these questions may have a significant impact upon how an individual with a 'mental health' problem can access help, what outcomes are sought and how they are measured. This chapter will attempt to look at the challenges this brings to outcome measurement in older persons with mental health disorders, and some of the ways these challenges have been addressed.

Is outcome measurement different in older people?

Outcomes may be measured for a number of reasons. The importance of issues that make outcome measurement different in older people may vary across these reasons. Attribution of change for the older person with a mental health problem is often complicated by multiple concurrent interventions addressing issues such as living conditions, availability of family and social networks, physical functioning and comorbid physical illness.

Treatment programmes in mental health should aim to achieve a positive outcome for the older person. There should ideally be an improvement in some physical conditions but specifically improvements in mental health problems and general functioning (Glendinning et al., 2006) related to activities of daily living and the capacity to relate to others more effectively. This will potentially result in an improvement in the health and well-being and quality of life for the older person. However, the goal may be to maximize remaining skills and reduce disability (Kennedy, 2000). How does one distinguish whether no measurable change is evidence of an effective preventative strategy or of an ineffective attempt to improve a condition? It is suggested that the presence of such complex factors results in a lack of confidence by service providers that measurement within mental health services for older people will demonstrate an impact (Macdonald, 2005).

Interpretation or introduction of outcome measurement in older people requires consideration of what outcomes are important, how frequently they are measured and what associated data must be collected to interpret them. Key associated data required to interpret outcome measure results will be similar to those required for other populations. However, the relative importance of items is likely to be different in older people. For instance, it may

Outcome Measurement in Mental Health: Theory and Practice, ed. Tom Trauer. Published by Cambridge University Press.
© Cambridge University Press 2010.

be more desirable to collect detailed information about residential type, cognitive status and behavioural and social interventions. If outcome measures are intended to guide funding decisions, different factors may be important, such as physical functional needs or access to relevant aged care services.

A particular challenge for service providers of mental health care for older people is that consumers are likely to be in contact with multiple service providers. Ideally, outcomes in mental health are measured in a manner that is:

- the same as the methods used by other service providers (Macdonald, 2002) and
- similar enough to the outcomes measured by service providers in key comparison populations.

In establishing a system to measure the outcomes of older consumers in mental health care, compromise will be required. But by working systematically through the issues below it is possible to establish a system that can meet a significant proportion of the desirable attributes of outcome measurement, and improve the utilization of existing measurement systems.

Issues include:

(1) the characteristics of the population whose outcomes are to be measured;
(2) the outcome domains that are most important to measure from the perspective of mental health services, funders, consumers and carers;
(3) other key service providers to this population, and how they measure 'outcomes';
(4) other populations it is desirable to be able to compare aspects of outcomes with; and
(5) how, and why, consumer and carer input will occur.

Population being measured

Internationally, there is significant variability in the structure of mental health services for older people. Thus, services planning to measure the outcomes of 'mental health' care for 'older people' may be serving quite different populations. In particular these may vary in terms of:

- what is considered a mental health disorder, with the greatest variability regarding the inclusion of consumers with dementia, and
- whether 'older' is considered in a chronological or functional sense. The meaning of old age differs in terms of functionality, employment and political and economic situations within different cultures (World Health Organization, no date).

Within this chapter the population of 'older persons in mental health care' is considered to be divisible into three, overlapping, groups:

(1) those who are 65 years or older with a primary non-dementia-related mental illness,
(2) those mostly 65 years or older with a primary dementia-related illness, and
(3) those 65 years and older with mental illness of earlier onset complicated by significant functional impairment related to ageing.

It is proposed that the optimal measurement and interpretation of outcomes may vary between these groups.

What is the evidence base?

Published literature on routine outcome measurement for older people is not as extensive as for other age groups. Differing approaches to outcome measurement are likely to benefit from using different tools, or using tools in different ways. It has been stated (Wiger and Solberg,

2001) that there is 'individualized outcome assessment', which relates to the measuring of progress against agreed criteria in a consumer's care plan, and 'normative outcome assessment', which compares the progress of an individual consumer relative to a larger population using pre-existing instruments with known normative data. Individualized outcome measurement may, but does not always, involve the use of specific measures. We review some of the available instruments in a later section. Individualized and normative approaches have been brought together to some degree with a clinometric (de Vet et al., 2003) methodology using Goal Attainment Scaling (Rockwood et al., 2003). Goal Attainment Scaling measures achievement of individualized goals of consumers in a standardized manner that allows comparison of results between different populations. In a frail elderly population, the rating of outcomes using Goal Attainment Scaling was found to be more responsive to clinical change than alternative psychometric measures.

The HoNOS instruments are reported (Pirkis et al., 2005) to 'have adequate or good validity, reliability, sensitivity to change and feasibility/utility'. These authors concluded, 'that collectively, the HoNOS family of measures can assess outcomes for different groups on a range of mental health-related constructs, . . . and can be regarded as appropriate for routinely monitoring consumer outcomes, with the view to improving treatment quality and effectiveness'. The HoNOS does not unfortunately assess spiritual elements. Spirituality is important to many mental health patients (Epstein and Olsen, 2001), particularly older people, and people of certain cultural and ethnic backgrounds.

The HoNOS has been found to predict 12-month outcomes in the elderly mentally ill (Ashaye et al., 1999), and be useful for comparing populations of older consumers with those with learning difficulties to inform service planning (Ashaye et al., 1997); but was also found to benefit from adaptation for older people (Turner, 2004).

The HoNOS65+ was developed specifically for older people and, like the other HoNOS scales, measures behaviour, impairment, symptomatology and social functioning in the older person. However, it was amended to include specific aspects of older persons' mental health such as 'the phenomenology of depression, delusions occurring in the presence of dementia, incontinence and agitation/restlessness' and is able to differentiate between those suffering from organic and functional illnesses (Burns et al., 1999). All items of the HoNOS65+ have been found to be equally important in making an overall judgement of clinical severity (Burgess et al., 2009). The HoNOS65+ has been found (Cheung and Strachan, 2007) to demonstrate consumer change in an acute psychogeriatric inpatient unit and the HoNOS65+ was regarded as meeting the criteria for a clinical outcome measure for community mental health services for older people in a study examining its acceptability to clinicians, validity, reliability and sensitivity to change (Spear et al., 2002). However, it was found to be of limited utility in a memory clinic service (Cheung and Williams, 2009).

It has been proposed that effective implementation of routine outcome measurement also requires development of a minimum dataset, intervention codes and appropriate information technology support (Macdonald, 2002). Macdonald also describes methods of analysis of HoNOS65+ data from such collections, provides illustrative findings and discusses the positive impact of the process of analysis and feedback.

Whilst often used in a normative manner, adaptation of the use of the HoNOS65+ for individualized outcome assessment has been described (McKay and McDonald, 2008) through identifying the 'key item' for each consumer. This is the individual HoNOS65+ item that best relates to the clinical issue that will be the main clinical focus for change during an episode of care. These authors also described the process of service review that was necessary to make routine outcome measurement meaningful within clinical care.

The Camberwell Assessment of Need for the Elderly (CANE, Reynolds et al., 2000) is a 24-item (plus two carer need items) scale designed to provide consumer, staff and carer views of the needs of older people with mental health disorders, and the degree to which they are met. The CANE has been used to assess the effectiveness of interventions for residents with dementia in residential aged care facilities (Orrell et al., 2007) and psychiatric day hospital care for older people (Ashaye et al., 2003). It has also highlighted the difference in perceptions by consumers, staff and carers regarding needs, and the importance of gaining these different perceptions (Hancock et al., 2003).

Potential outcome domains

There have been many different schema defining outcome domains relevant to mental health and aspects of aged care (World Health Organization, 2001) but unfortunately no schema specifically for older consumers of mental health services. A review of adult mental health schema (Slade, 2002b) concluded that most domains fitted into the categories of well-being, cognition/emotion, behaviour, physical health, interpersonal, society and services. Although using different terms, similar domains have been proposed for consumers with dementia (Sansoni et al., 2007), as well as 'stage of illness', 'health-related quality of life', function and 'patient and carer satisfaction'.

As older people are often seen across a variety of aged care and mental health service settings there can be a lack of conformity in what outcome domains are expected to be collected and therefore what assessment instruments would be required. As for younger adults, outcomes for older adults 'should be considered multidimensionally by measuring multiple outcome domains' (Slade, 2002a). What must be decided is which domains are most important to focus upon for a specific consumer population and how this is feasible given available resources and relevant systems of key partners. Consideration must be given to consumer and carer views of what functional domains are important to focus upon and what changes are significant, both in general, and for individual consumers (Hancock et al., 2003). An example of different goals for older people in a domain is within social functioning: return to work is a common goal in younger adults, but restoration of 'roles' and re-engagement with family and social networks may be more relevant for many older people.

Key associated service providers

Where multiple service providers are involved there are significant issues that need consideration and negotiation regarding what measures are to be used, who will collect them and which services will be responsible for collating them. There are also likely to be differences in what information is collected routinely about patients, and the rules defining this collection. These must be understood to allow appropriate use of outcome measures.

Key service providers, other than mental health services specializing in services for older persons, include public and private mental health service providers, medical aged care services, general practice, emergency departments, residential aged care providers and providers of community services to older people.

Key comparison populations

A further issue requiring consideration is what other population groups older people with mental health problems should be compared with. Key associated service providers will each serve overlapping, but differing, populations. It may be more important to compare outcomes with some of these than others. For instance, if an older persons' mental health service focuses upon people with non-dementia-related illness, a key group to compare outcomes with may be younger people with mental illness,. There would be limited purpose in comparing outcomes with older people with dementia in aged care services. However, if a service sees people with dementia-related illnesses, or focuses on older people with significant functional impairment related to ageing, the importance of particular comparison groups will change.

How, and why, consumer and carer input will occur

Patient-rated outcomes have become increasingly important in the evaluation of treatments and interventions in mental health care (Hanson et al., 2007) and service delivery. These have particular challenges for older people. Some older consumers, such as those with moderate to severe dementia, will have a limited capacity to complete self-rated instruments (Sansoni et al., 2007). Whilst some instruments used in general populations may be suitable for older people, this will not be the case for all instruments in all settings (Hill et al., 1996). There is also significant debate about the greatest priority for carer measures. Potentially, carer measures may be used to assess and monitor carer burden (or stress), carer satisfaction or aspects of the consumer by the carer acting as a proxy for a consumer who cannot complete a self-report measure (Sansoni et al., 2007).

What tools are available?

It is recommended that someone embarking upon outcome measurement with older people with mental health disorders first familiarize themselves with assessment instruments routinely collected in relevant local services and consider their suitability for the needs of the potential consumer population. If these do not at first appear suitable for the intended local uses, consideration can be given to adapting methods used elsewhere, using measures already used in relevant populations internationally, or consulting the numerous reviews of assessment instruments suitable for clinical practice within aged care (Sansoni et al., 2007), aged care psychiatry (Burns et al., 2002, Moriarty, 2002, Reilly et al., 2004) and mental health services in general (Slade, 2002b). However, it must be noted that not all assessment instruments are suitable for routine outcome measurement (Slade, 2002b). Instruments for outcome measurement of specific domains that may be particularly suited for older consumers of mental health services have also been reviewed (Perlis et al., 2002).

Additional factors for consideration are:

- potential assessors' competence, and need for training,
- the time required to complete the measures if accurate outcomes are to be achieved, and
- the potential influences of particular aspects of the likely consumer population upon the use or validity of instruments, e.g. cognitive status, educational background, language and cultural or indigenous status. This may be particularly relevant to consumer- and carer-rated measures (Sansoni et al., 2007).

Selected clinician-rated scales nominated for use in older persons' mental health care in Australia are the Health of the Nation Outcome Scales for Elderly People (HoNOS65+, Burns et al., 1999), the Resource Utilization Groups Activities of Daily Living subscale (RUG-ADL, Fries et al., 1994), the Life Skills Profile (LSP, Parker et al., 1991) for community care and a consumer-rated scale, either the Kessler 10 (K10, Kessler et al., 2002) or the Behaviour and Symptom Identification Scale (BASIS-32, Eisen et al., 2000) or the Mental Health Inventory

(MHI, Veit and Ware, 1983). The most widely used of these measures is the HoNOS65+ as it can be used to gather information about key areas of mental health and social functioning (Meadows and Fossey, 2007).

However, as well as assessment instruments other resources that may be worthwhile considering to improve the utilization of measures are:

- information resources regarding outcome assessment for professionals, consumers and carers (Australian Mental Health Outcomes and Classification Network (AMHOCN), 2009, Ohio Department of Mental Health, 2009, Royal College of Psychiatrists, 2009)
- publicly available outcome measure reference data and protocols describing how and when to collect outcome measures in large-scale systems (Australian Mental Health Outcomes and Classification Network (AMHOCN), 2009, Ohio Department of Mental Health, 2009)
- texts with specific discussion of outcome measurement in older people (Macdonald, 2002, Perlis et al., 2002)
- potential intervention codes that allow standard recording of relevant actions by health care providers and minimum data sets that provide appropriate contextual information (Macdonald, 2002).

Attitudes to outcome measurement

There is limited literature that describes the attitude to outcome measurement of older consumers, their carers or service providers. However, it has been suggested (Glendinning et al., 2006) that the outcomes most desired by older adults were related to change, maintenance or prevention and the process of receiving service. In small studies quite varied views have been expressed about staff attitudes to the HoNOS65+ (Spear et al., 2002, Cheung and Williams, 2009). Significant variation exists between services, with leadership and clinical application of measures probably key variables. It is also worth noting the importance of systemic service factors in the use of assessment instruments in old-age psychiatry services (Reilly et al., 2004).

Using outcome measures to improve practice

Outcome measures may be used at a number of levels to improve practice. These may include:

- direct care with the consumer and their family
- communication between professionals involved in care
- assisting improvements in practice within clinical teams
- benchmarking between clinical units, in service management, and
- policy-making, research or funding.

In considering how outcome measures may improve practice, a feature that is not always explicitly stated, but usually present, is a clear focus upon what aspects of practice are intended to be improved. To improve outcomes, outcome measures need to be linked to practice, and interpreted in conjunction with other information. Once these linkages are established, the question of 'how outcome measures can improve practice' is, in some ways, self-limiting in that it can be interpreted as suggesting that outcome measurement may only be relevant to specific aspects of mental health care, rather than to all practice. It may be more productive to ask: 'What aspect of practice requires assessment or improvement; and how can outcome measures assist this?'

To improve practice using outcome measures it is necessary to cope with the complexity of data that is produced through their routine administration. It may be worth considering how methods explored to use complex data from quality-of-life instruments in other settings (Guyatt et al., 2002) may be applied to data in mental health services for older people. Systems issues that facilitate successful clinical utilization of outcome measurement in relevant services have been described (Macdonald, 2002, McKay and McDonald, 2008).

Within benchmarking activities between mental health services for older people in Australia, outcome measures have been used in a number of ways. Analysis of HoNOS65+ items, either as mean scores or as percentage 'significant' (scoring 2 or more), has been used, together with other data such as diagnosis, to understand variation in severity and outcome in clinical populations served. Analysis of changes from admission to discharge in individual items has also been used to generate discussions regarding discharge thresholds and decisions, which aspects of consumers needs are most responsive to interventions, what aspects of consumers are vulnerable to deterioration, and differences between services in each of these issues. Unfortunately, to date there has not been any evaluation of the impact of such techniques.

Other uses of outcome measures have included:

- Utilizing the HoNOS65+ to improve workload distribution within a community older persons mental health team. This involved setting a threshold HoNOS65+ score at which the consumer would have a second outcome assessment by another clinician, then increased allocation of clinician hours if the rating was confirmed.
- Modelling the potential effects of introducing a new service component by using estimates of expected HoNOS65+ profiles at admission and discharge from different service components to model patient flow.
- Analysis of HoNOS65+ data in conjunction with demographic data to improve service understanding of consumers with markedly prolonged duration of inpatient admission.
- Utilizing repeated consumer self-report measures (e.g. Kessler 10) to monitor progress in depressed consumers, and to discuss this with them.

Methods of providing accessible statistics on collated outcome measures of older mental health consumers within large service systems can be found in both the USA (Ohio Department of Mental Health, 2009) and Australia (Australian Mental Health Outcomes and Classification Network (AMHOCN), 2009).

Challenges in implementing outcome measurement with older people

There are specific challenges in implementing and utilizing outcome measurement in older people, the foremost of these being the difficulties with incorporating consumer and carer viewpoints. Additionally the interface issues described earlier require significant negotiation, and compromise, to establish a meaningful system for consumers who will often be users of multiple services. This may sometimes mean using instruments that are not specifically designed for use in older people, and so require careful interpretation. Interpretation can be limited by the restricted research and development focus upon mental health services for older people. Gaining sufficient resources and research focus for these needs is likely to be an ongoing challenge.

However, many challenges are similar to those in other populations. These include all the issues associated with any significant systems change, and in particular gaining an awareness that systems and practice must be adapted or sometimes changed significantly to make most use of outcome measurement. Weaknesses in activities such as the systematic collection of (any) data, monitoring of different aspects of a consumer's progress, care planning and systematic reflection upon practice and its outcomes are highlighted in implementing outcome measurement. Clinicians also require support to identify what adaptation of their practice may be desirable to both include the routine measurement of outcomes and improve their practice. Access to robust information systems, and to well-constructed, real-time reports from such systems is highly desirable. Such reports are likely to require ongoing evolution and to include 'core' reports useful in most settings, together with ones adapted to local needs or the needs of particular populations (such as older consumers). Importantly, if local leaders can be engaged and supported, and realistic timeframes adopted, these obstacles can be overcome.

Advice for those considering measuring outcomes in older people

A decision to commence outcome measurements, or change practice to utilize them, can be made at different levels of systems providing mental health care to older consumers, from a national policy level to a group of individual mental health clinicians seeing individual consumers. The factors that need to be considered and managed at different levels will vary in detail and execution, but be similar in concept.

Factors likely to aid success include to:

(1) have a clearly defined primary purpose for using outcome measures, supported by clinicians, senior management and/or policy makers;

(2) not assume systems, or outcome measures, used in non-elderly mental health consumers, or aged consumers without mental health disorders, will behave in the same manner for older mental health consumers; they may be useable, but their properties in the relevant population need to be understood;

(3) expect non-compliance and resistance, including exploiting differences between service systems; be clear about how this will be managed;

(4) expect full implementation to take a significant time; as this is often underestimated, plan how to use incomplete data in a meaningful way to keep stakeholders engaged, and measures collected;

(5) focus all key decisions, system design and communication to interested parties upon the primary purposes for introducing outcome measures; even whilst seeking to develop a flexible system with multiple potential uses;

(6) make a realistic appraisal of available, or potential, resources and design a system that is feasible within these resources; if resources are limited, either identify resources that can be diverted towards outcome measurement (e.g. by ceasing other data collection or identified activities), introduce a simplified system, or defer introduction until resources are available;

(7) avoid establishing 'outcome measures' as a separate (clinical or managerial) workflow or information system, but rather either incorporate them into existing systems or use the introduction of outcome measures to redesign existing systems; initiatives that link outcome data with demographic and clinical data in information systems are likely to improve utilization;

(8) ensure adequate staff training, focused upon how to use outcome measures to meet their primary purpose;

(9) support staff who are responsible for leading, managing or supervising other staff to be able to extract information formats that meet their needs;

(10) support clinical champions or staff expected to manage the introduction of outcome measures to find at least one 'partner'; this both assists maintaining momentum and maintaining morale through the stresses of change management;

(11) finally, but not least importantly, ensure that system design, planning and implementation includes consumers and carers; if outcome measurements are meaningful to consumers and carers they will expect clinicians and managers to use them.

The future

Areas where mental health services appear to have particular challenges, but also particular opportunities to improve consumer outcomes, are in developing decision-support systems such as those used in other populations (Lambert et al., 2005, McKay et al., 2008) and developing more effective systems to capture, analyse and utilize input from consumers and carers. The integration of such input with clinicians' assessments, supported by systems that encourage evidence-based practice, would appear to have significant potential. The challenges of capturing appropriately interventions for consumers with multiple care providers must also be overcome.

The ageing of populations in developed countries is a major challenge to their healthcare systems, and there is significant focus in most such countries on how this challenge can be met. This is associated with an increasing demand that health services demonstrate their effectiveness in order to justify their funding. Although the demand to demonstrate effectiveness has been felt by mental health services, there appears to have been less focus within such services on the impact of an ageing population. However, services providing mental healthcare for older people must expect that the demand to demonstrate effectiveness, and efficiency, will increase. With research currently being undertaken investigating a range of issues related to mental illness in older people, future treatment options will develop. This will lead to a demand for new treatment options and better outcomes, from an elderly cohort with different characteristics from those previously and currently receiving mental health and aged care services (Ames and Richie, 2007).

Outcome measurement has significant potential to assist in managing these demands. More importantly, it has significant potential to improve consumer outcomes; but a potential that requires research, skilful management and clinical innovation.

References

Ames, S. and Richie, R. (2007). Psychiatric disorders affecting the elderly in Australia. In G. Meadows, B. Singh and M. Grigg, eds., *Mental Health in Australia. Collaborative Community Practice.* Melbourne: Oxford University Press.

Ashaye, O., Mathew, G. and Dhadphale, M. (1997). A comparison of older longstay psychiatric and learning disability inpatients using the Health of the Nation Outcome Scales. *International Journal of Geriatric Psychiatry*, **12**, 548–52.

Ashaye, K., Seneviratna, K., Shergill, S. and Orrell, M. (1999). Do the Health of the Nation Outcome Scales predict outcome in the elderly mentally ill? A 1-year follow-up study. *Journal of Mental Health*, **8**, 615–20.

Ashaye, O. A., Livingston, G. and Orrell, M. W. (2003). Does standardized needs assessment improve the outcome of psychiatric day hospital care for older people? A randomized controlled trial. *Aging & Mental Health*, **7**, 195–9.

Australian Mental Health Outcomes and Classification Network (AMHOCN) (2009). National Outcomes and Casemix Collection, retrieved 21 May 2009 from www.mhnocc.org.

Burgess, P., Trauer, T., Coombs, T., McKay, R. and Pirkis, J. (2009). What does 'clinical significance' mean in the context of the Health of the Nation Outcome Scales? *Australasian Psychiatry*, **17**, 141–8.

Burns, A., Beevor, A., Lelliott, P., et al. (1999). Health of the Nation Outcome Scales for Elderly People (HoNOS 65+). *British Journal of Psychiatry*, **174**, 424–7.

Burns, A., Lawlor, B. and Craig, S. (2002). Rating scales in old age psychiatry. *British Journal of Psychiatry*, **180**, 161–7.

Cheung, G. and Strachan, J. (2007). Routine 'Health of the Nation Outcome Scales for elderly people' (HoNOS65+) collection in an acute psychogeriatric inpatient unit in New Zealand. *New Zealand Medical Journal*, **120**, U2660.

Cheung, G. and Williams, G. (2009). Clinical utility of Health of the Nations Outcome Scales for older persons in a memory clinic. *Australasian Psychiatry*, **17**, 149–55.

de Vet, H. C. W., Terwee, C. B. and Bouter, L. M. (2003). Current challenges in clinometrics. *Journal of Clinical Epidemiology*, **56**, 1137–41.

Eisen, S. V., Dickey, B. and Sederer, L. I. (2000). A self-report symptom and problem rating scale to increase inpatients' involvement in treatment. *Psychiatric Services*, **51**, 349–53.

Epstein, M. and Olsen, A. (2001). Mental illness: responses from the community. In G. Meadows and B. Singh, eds., *Mental Health in Australia*. Melbourne: Oxford University Press.

Fries, B. E., Schneider, D. P., Foley, W. J., et al. (1994). Refining a casemix measure for nursing homes. Resource Utilisation Groups (RUG-III). *Medical Care*, **32**, 668–85.

Glendinning, C., Clarke, S., Hare, P., et al. (2006). *Outcomes-focused services for older people*. London: Social Care Institute for Excellence.

Guyatt, G. H., Osoba, D., Wu, A. W., Wyrwich, K. W., Norman, G. R. and the Clinical Significance Consensus Meeting Group (2002). Methods to explain the clinical significance of health status measures. *Mayo Clinic Proceedings*, **77**, 371–83.

Hancock, G., Reynold, T., Woods, B., Thornicroft, G. and Orrell, M. (2003). The needs of older people with mental health problems according to the user, the carer, and the staff. *International Journal of Geriatric Psychiatry*, **18**, 803–11.

Hanson, L., Bjorkman, Y. and Priebe, S. (2007). Are important patient-rated outcomes in community mental health care explained by only one factor? *Acta Psychiatrica Scandinavica*, **116**, 113–18.

Hill, S., Harries, U. and Popay, J. (1996). Is the short form 36 (SF-36) suitable for routine health outcomes assessment in health care for older people? Evidence from preliminary work in community based health services in England. *Journal of Epidemiology and Community Health*, **50**, 94–8.

Kennedy, G. (2000). *Geriatric Mental Health Care: A Treatment Guide for Health Professionals*. New York: Guildford Press.

Kessler, R. C., Andrews, G., Colpe, L. J., et al. (2002). Short screening scales to monitor population prevalences and trends in non-specific psychological distress. *Psychological Medicine*, **32**, 959–76.

Lambert, M. J., Harmon, C., Slade, K., Whipple, J. L. and Hawkins, E. J. (2005). Providing feedback to psychotherapists on their patients' progress: clinical results and practice suggestions. *Journal of Clinical Psychology*, **61**, 165–74.

Macdonald, A. J. D. (2002). The usefulness of aggregate routine clinical outcomes data: the example of HoNOS65+. *Journal of Mental Health*, **11**, 645–56.

Macdonald, A. (2005). Evaluation of service delivery. In B. Draper, P. Melding and H. Brodaty, eds., *Psychogeriatric Service Delivery: An International Perspective.* Oxford: Oxford University Press.

McKay, R. and McDonald, R. (2008). Expensive detour or a way forward? The experience of routine outcome measurement in an aged care psychiatry service. *Australasian Psychiatry*, **16**, 428–32.

McKay, R., Coombs, T., Burgess, P., et al. (2008). *Development of Clinical Prompts to Enhance Decision Support Tools Related to the National Outcomes and Casemix Collection (Version 1.0).* Brisbane/Sydney/ Melbourne: Department of Health and Ageing.

Meadows, G. and Fossey, E. (2007). A structured assessment instrument as a guide to essential skills: The HoNOS. In G. Meadows, B. Singh and M. Grigg, eds., *Mental Health in Australia. Collaborative Community Practice.* Melbourne: Oxford University Press.

Moriarty, J. (2002). *Assessing the mental health needs of older people: Systematic Review on the Use of Standardised Measures to Improve Assessment Practice.* Kings College London.

Ohio Department of Mental Health (2009). Consumer Outcomes, retrieved 23 April 2009 from www.mh.state.oh.us/what-we-do/protect-and-monitor/consumer-outcomes/index.shtml.

Orrell, M., Hancock, G., Hoe, J., et al. (2007). A cluster randomised controlled trial to reduce the unmet needs of people with dementia living in residential care. *International Journal of Geriatric Psychiatry*, **22**, 1127–34.

Parker, G., Rosen, A., Emdur, N. and Hadzi-Pavlov, D. (1991). The Life Skills Profile: psychometric properties of a measure assessing function and disability in schizophrenia. *Acta Psychiatrica Scandinavica*, **83**, 145–52.

Perlis, R., Davidoff, D., Falf, W., et al. (2002). Outcome measurement in geriatric psychiatry. In W. IsHak, T. Burt and L. Sederer, eds., *Outcome Measurement in*

Psychiatry: A Critical Review. Washington DC: American Psychiatric Publishing.

Pirkis, J. E., Burgess, P. M., Kirk, P. K., et al. (2005). A review of the psychometric properties of the Health of the Nation Outcome Scales (HoNOS) family of measures. *Health and Quality of Life Outcomes*, **3**, 76.

Reilly, S. D., Challis, D., Burns, A. and Hughes, J. (2004). The use of assessment scales in old age psychiatry services in England and Northern Ireland. *Aging & Mental Health*, **8**, 249–55.

Reynolds, T., Thornicroft, G., Abas, M., et al. (2000). Camberwell Assessment of Need for the Elderly (CANE); development, validity, and reliability. *British Journal of Psychiatry*, **176**, 444–52.

Rockwood, K., Howlett, S., Stadnyk, K., et al. (2003). Responsiveness of goal attainment scaling in a randomized controlled trial of comprehensive geriatric assessment. *Journal of Clinical Epidemiology*, **56**, 736–43.

Royal College of Psychiatrists (2009). Health of the Nation Outcome Scales, retrieved 23rd April 2009 from www.rcpsych.ac.uk/crtu/healthofthenation.aspx.

Sansoni, E., Senior, K., Kenny, P. and Low, L. (2007). *Final Report: Dementia Outcomes Measurement Suite Project: Centre for Health Service Development.* University of Wollongong.

Slade, M. (2002a). Routine outcome assessment in mental health services. *Psychological Medicine*, **32**, 1339–43.

Slade, M. (2002b). What outcomes to measure in routine mental health services, and how to assess them: a systematic review. *Australian and New Zealand Journal of Psychiatry*, **36**, 743–53.

Spear, J., Chawla, S., O'Reilly, M. and Rock, D. (2002). Does the HoNOS65+ meet the criteria for a clinical outcome indicator for mental health services for older people? *International Journal of Geriatric Psychiatry*, **17**, 226–30.

Turner, S. (2004). Are the Health of the Nation Outcome Scales (HoNOS) useful for measuring outcomes in older people's mental health services? *Aging & Mental Health*, **8**, 387–96.

Veit, C. T. and Ware, J. E. (1983). The structure of psychological distress and well-being in general populations. *Journal of Consulting and Clinical Psychology*, **51**, 730–42.

Wiger, D. and Solberg, K. (2001). *Tracking Mental Health Outcomes: A Therapist's Guide to Measuring Client Progress, Analyzing Data, and Improving Your Practice*. New York: Wiley.

World Health Organization (2001). *The World Health Organisation Report 2001. Mental Health: New Understanding*. New Hope, Switzerland: World Health Organization.

World Health Organization (no date). Definition of an older or elderly person, retrieved 10 February 2009 from www.who.int/healthinfo/survey/ageingdefi nolder/en/index.html.

14

Outcome measurement with indigenous consumers

Tricia Nagel and Tom Trauer

Introduction

The need to monitor outcomes is nowhere more pressing than in those areas where systems appear to be least effective. For Indigenous[1] peoples of Australia there has been delayed recognition of the dire mental health consequences of many aspects of colonization and development (Human Rights and Equal Opportunity Commission, 1997, Calma, 2007). High suicide rates and community concern have begun to attract national attention and intervention after decades of procrastination (Zubrick et al., 1995, Australian Bureau of Statistics, 2005, Brown and Brown, 2007). 'While some have argued that it is necessary to develop Indigenous-specific tools to assess status and outcomes with sufficient validity, others recognize the potential loss to Indigenous consumers if they are not included in the national datasets. However, comparability in the use of mainstream measures with Indigenous consumers is highly under-researched' (Haswell-Elkins et al., 2007).

The lack of research and development can be attributed to complexity as well as to political will. In terms of complexity, many of the challenges are similar to those of the non-Indigenous setting. There is tension in outcome measurement (OM) between the needs and perspectives of the different stakeholders who collect and use this information. The multi-dimensional framework for health performance indicators in Australia recognizes the need to measure outcomes at population and service level as well as at the level of the individual consumer. Nevertheless individual consumer outcome measures are collected for diverse purposes (Durie and Kingi, 1997, NMHWG Information Strategy Committee Performance Indicators Drafting Group, 2005). Three main uses of consumer outcomes data are: macro-level service planning, service provider treatment planning, and client- and carer-level feedback about individual status and progress and burden of care.

There is immediate disparity in the nature of the information needed. Good treatment planning revolves as much around the residual strengths within a person and the supports in their environment as around their deficits. Issues of individual family support and social inclusion will be paramount as clinician and client and family work together to promote good outcomes. On the other hand service planners will be interested in the deficits in functioning which point to general service needs, and will seek to categorize and diagnose in order to compare those outcomes with other populations and other settings.

The cross-cultural setting of Indigenous clients brings greater complexity to the process of OM. Social disadvantage which is beyond the scope of the service to change will nevertheless complicate presentations and progress (Vos et al., 2004). Cultural diversity, which may or may not be recognized, will impact upon access, engagement, communication and treatment

---

[1] For the purpose of this paper 'Indigenous' refers to Australia's Aboriginal and Torres Strait Islander peoples and acknowledges their rich diversity of culture.

Outcome Measurement in Mental Health: Theory and Practice, ed. Tom Trauer. Published by Cambridge University Press.
© Cambridge University Press 2010.

effectiveness (Eley et al., 2006, Paradies, 2006). Literacy, language and worldview differences will influence the Indigenous person's experience of treatment pathways (Cass et al., 2002, Nagel et al., 2009). Similar issues arise in the assessment of ethnic and cultural groups generally (Bhui, 2001). These differences will have direct impact on the way in which treatment is experienced and the outcomes that result.

One pivotal difference in the Indigenous setting is that of the 'whole of life' worldview. Indigenous perspectives draw much stronger connections between 'mental health' and 'physical', 'spiritual' and 'family' ways of being (Durie and Kingi, 1997, National Aboriginal and Torres Strait Islander Health Council, 2003). Indigenous peoples have argued that culture is not simply one aspect on a continuum of how they might rate their progress, it is central (Smylie et al., 2006).

In addition, Indigenous peoples in Australia have diverse cultures and languages, rendered more so in response to dominant society influences, political interventions and generational change (Eades, 2005). Despite multiple national and local frameworks and recommendations, best practice in terms of access, assessment and OM is far from routine in Australia, and the evidence base for what constitutes best practice remains weak (Social Health Reference Group, 2004).

> Indigenous health-care performance measurement systems in Canada, Australia, and New Zealand are underdeveloped locally and hence deficient in their support of local service development. Rather, they are essentially government-driven systems that are intended to assess progress towards state-defined objectives for Indigenous health. Additionally, Indigenous concepts of health are marginalised at all levels of health care measurement. (Smylie et al., 2006)

Maori and Australian Indigenous peoples face similar challenges and have sought similar solutions in OM. They have sought to develop holistic cultural frameworks that guide adaptation of existing tools or development of new tools and that celebrate cultural difference and cultural identity (Smylie et al., 2006). This chapter will explore issues, challenges and solutions to OM in Indigenous peoples, primarily of Australia.

Approaches to outcome measurement with indigenous peoples

The development and use of tools that will yield valid results with cultural and ethnic subpopulations recognizes the need for internationally standardized and reliable measures which can describe and compare patients, services, costs and outcomes across language and cultural boundaries (Bhui et al., 2003). While recognizing that a single measure cannot address all of the desirable properties, this challenge has been approached in several different ways.

One approach has been to simply use or adapt existing tools. Adaptations have included language changes to improve readability and relevance, and changes to the process of assessment to include other Indigenous informants. This approach has been applied to mental health outcome measures (Trauer et al., 2004), substance misuse screening tools (Schlesinger et al., 2007) and depression measures (Esler et al., 2007, Lee et al., 2008).

A second approach is to develop new measures within the particular cultural paradigm, which incorporate cultural values and measure outcome according to cultural criteria. Examples of this approach are seen in the development of the Maori outcome measure (Kingi and

Durie, 1997) and, in the Australian Indigenous context, development of a screening tool for youth at risk (Westerman, 2000) and a child well-being tool (Harrison, 2008).

A third approach has been to take a number of existing tools and items and gather them into one broad module of 'well-being' that may be used in social or population surveys. An example of this approach is the social and emotional well-being module of the national Indigenous health survey. This approach takes into account 'deficits' in functioning and also gathers information about strengths, cultural identity and social context, as well as making language changes to improve readability, and process changes to include Indigenous interviewers.

An example of each of these approaches is described in detail below.

Use of existing outcome measures

The rationale for the use of mainstream assessment measures with Indigenous consumers is that they allow comparison across services and cultures. Generic tools will simplify needs for service provider training and information system requirements, and will facilitate the development of the culture and processes related to performance indicators so that benchmarking becomes the norm (NMHWG Information Strategy Committee Performance Indicators Drafting Group, 2005). It can be argued that only by comparing 'like with like' can the relative disadvantage of cultural and ethnic minority consumers be identified and quantified.

A project whose broad aim was to investigate the feasibility of using mainstream outcome assessment tools, the HoNOS (Wing et al., 1998) and LSP (Rosen et al., 1989, Buckingham et al., 1998), with adult Indigenous consumers in North Queensland was initiated in 2003 (Mental Health Branch, 2009, Outcome measurement in adult indigenous mental health consumers; Brisbane: Queensland Health, unpublished report). In particular, the project explored whether the instructions for use of these standard measures needed to be adjusted for use with Indigenous consumers. Two hundred and seventy-one Indigenous consumers were assessed a total of 496 times. Despite the advice to providers to include additional informants, over half of assessments involved neither a family member nor a local health practitioner. Scores on HoNOS and LSP assessments in the community were consistently higher the more additional informants were involved, probably because clinicians could better appreciate the severity and extent of consumers' problems. The HoNOS and LSP appeared to perform well from a technical point of view, and cultural informants were positively disposed toward their use. Comparison with national, predominantly non-Indigenous, HoNOS data revealed comparable mean ratings on Behavioural items, lower ratings on Impairment and Depressive items, and higher ratings on the 'environmental' items of Accommodation and Occupation.

Four principles guiding the use of outcome measures with Indigenous consumers were developed. In abbreviated form, Principle 1 recommended the use of additional informants, Principle 2 advised that ratings should objectively reflect underlying disadvantage, Principle 3 advised that ratings should reflect behaviours that are not sanctioned or accepted within the local culture, and Principle 4 warned against rating phenomena that were socially and culturally accepted.

Another study that used mainstream OMs with Indigenous consumers was the New Zealand Classification and Outcomes Study (CAOS, Gaines et al., 2003), whose main objectives were to develop the first version of a national casemix classification for specialist mental health services and to trial the introduction of OM into routine clinical practice. Over a 6-month study period, child and adolescent and adult consumers in eight of the country's 21 District Health Boards were assessed on a variety of standard outcome measures (see New Zealand chapter (Chapter 3) by Graham Mellsop and Mark Smith for more details).

In comparing the scores of the Indigenous and non-Indigenous consumers, there were three broad findings (Trauer et al., 2004, 2006). First, there were large differences on the routine measures between the three ethnicity groupings, with Maori and Pacific Island consumers being rated as having greater severity overall than the All Other group, and significantly different on several HoNOS items. Second, changes in scores between start and end of episodes of care tended to be quite similar across the three groups once starting scores were taken into account – that is, they were quite similar in percentage terms. Third, ethnicity differences did not appear to be a simple function of social deprivation, since they were present, but to different degrees, across the different levels of deprivation.

The Queensland and New Zealand studies were able to show consistent differences between their respective Indigenous consumers and corresponding non-Indigenous consumers through the use of mainstream instruments. In both cases the severity and disability levels of the Indigenous consumers were worse than their non-Indigenous counterparts.

Development of culturally valid measures

The rationale for the development of culture-specific instruments lies in the need to recognize the often very large gulf between Indigenous and non-Indigenous concepts of health. There is a danger, or fear, that by using measures based on alien concepts of health, the assessment process will lack credibility and face validity with those being assessed.

There have been few attempts in Australia to develop culturally specific tools for mental health OM or to translate standard tools for use in Indigenous settings. Nevertheless there is recognition of the impact of differing social and cultural schemas on psychiatric diagnosis and assessment (Sheldon, 2001). This has led to calls for culturally appropriate engagement of Indigenous people (Westerman, 2004, Nagel and Thompson, 2007), for cultural competence within mental health services (Australian Indigenous Doctors Association, 2004, Social Health Reference Group, 2004), and to warnings about the risks to individuals when practitioners are unaware of their cultural frameworks and the assumptions they bring to their role (Hunter, 2002, Kirmayer et al., 2003, Kowanko et al., 2004, Paradies, 2006).

Westerman (2004) proposed that culturally appropriate engagement would acknowledge cultural disparity, gender differences and communication style differences and would involve effective use of cultural consultants. The cultural consultant, an Aboriginal person nominated by the client and validated by the community, is essential to culturally safe engagement (Vicary and Westerman, 2004, Westerman, 2004). The call for culturally competent services recommends tailoring delivery of services to meet patients' social, cultural and linguistic needs to increase access to quality care for all patient populations. These recommendations are supported by increasing evidence that failure to acknowledge cultural difference is linked not only with limited access to services and limited effectiveness of services which are received, but also with poorer outcomes as a specific result of this failing (Kirmayer et al., 2003, Kowanko et al., 2004).

The 'Hua Oranga' Maori outcome measure is an example of the development of a new cultural measure. The aim of the 'Hua Oranga' initiative was to develop a Maori mental health outcomes measure, a consumer-focused tool appropriate for routine use in clinical and other care situations. The research was undertaken on the premise that any measure of effectiveness is dependent on the validity of the tools used and their capacity to accurately consider Maori perspectives of outcome and Maori approaches to treatment and care (Durie and Kingi, 1997, Kingi and Durie, 1997). The measure was developed through application of an existing model of Maori concepts of health and wellness, 'Te Whare Tapa Wha', comprising four dimensions:

spiritual, mental, physical and family. Three outcome perspectives – client, family member and clinician – are collected and combined. The development and testing work has involved the identification of key individuals who commented on the measure and framework, resulting in certain modifications and enhancements, and selection of a diverse range of test sites, reflecting urban, rural and residential mix, as well as a wide range of clinical settings and varying degrees of acculturation and de-culturation. This tool allows consideration of Maori perspectives in terms of outcome and approaches to treatment and care and provides an important model for combining cultural values and OM. At the time of writing, there have been no published results of the use of this instrument in the field.

One down-side to the development of any new instrument is that it is time-intensive, particularly in cross-cultural settings (De Vellis, 1991). Key steps in scale development such as engagement of experts to determine the item set, pilot testing and careful evaluation will founder if common ground cannot be found. The scale developers need to integrate the heterogeneity of Indigenous cultures and languages and manage the need to consult broadly with Indigenous communities to ensure representative views have been sought.

Thus translation of established tools becomes an attractive option. Tool translation, however, is also time-consuming, requiring (a) a proper translation process, (b) cross-cultural verification and adaptation and (c) verifying the psychometric properties of the instrument in the target language (Knudsen et al., 2000). Again the complexity of multiple languages and heterogeneity of Indigenous cultures challenges this activity.

Perhaps the most demanding element of either tool development or translation is to overcome the stigma which research and related activities has engendered within the Indigenous community. Researchers have often failed to engage with the Indigenous community, have enhanced their own careers rather than Indigenous research capacity, have taken and revealed sensitive information, have used insensitive methodologies, and have failed to feed findings back in ways that are accessible to the Indigenous peoples from whom the information was gathered (The Aboriginal and Torres Strait Islander Research Agenda Working Group (RAWG) of the NHMRC, 2002, Schnarch, 2004). In addition, the often resource-poor settings of Indigenous health demand brevity, practicality and high face validity (Bailey et al., 2002).

The development of culture-specific measures is typically restricted to self-report instruments, since providers, who are more frequently non-Indigenous, cannot be expected to validly assess their Indigenous consumers according to Indigenous health concepts.

Indigenous-specific surveys of health and well-being

An example of the third approach, that of developing a well-being module, is seen in the approach taken in the development of the National Aboriginal and Torres Strait Islander Health Survey (NATSIHS). Three organizations have worked collaboratively since 2003 to develop accurate measures of social and emotional well-being among Indigenous Australians from a community perspective: the Australian Institute of Health and Welfare (AIHW), the National Aboriginal Community Controlled Health Organization (NACCHO) and the Australian Bureau of Statistics (ABS).

The design of the programme involved expert consultation to determine a draft tool, pilot testing of that tool and modification, and implementation of the module in the 2004–05 NATSIHS in which 5,757 adults were surveyed. The interim module has eight domains: psychological distress, impact of psychological distress, positive well-being, anger, life stressors, racial discrimination, cultural identification and removal from natural family. The choice of these domains reflects the need for a multi-dimensional approach to mental health. The items were chosen from pre-existing measures such as the K-5, a modified version of the Kessler Psychological Distress Scale-10 (K-10, Kessler et al., 2000) with addition of specific questions (Australian Institute of Health and Welfare, 2009, NSW Health Department, no date).

The analysis of the module involved an internal and external validation process comparing the results from the domains in the module with each other, and with other relevant variables in the survey (such as chronic disease) and comparing results with other data sets such as hospitalization rates. For example, Indigenous Australians were hospitalized for mental health problems at 1.8-times the rate of non-Indigenous Australians and the rate of mental health service contacts for Indigenous Australians was double that of non-Indigenous Australians. These findings are consistent with findings from the NATSIHS, which showed that Indigenous adults were twice as likely as non-Indigenous adults to report high or very high levels of psychological distress (Australian Institute of Health and Welfare, 2009).

Issues in the assessment of outcome in Indigenous consumers

We have described three different approaches to the assessment of mental health status at the personal or societal level. While they are quite different in their philosophical underpinnings, and in their practical applications, there are certain themes that pervade all three to different degrees. These are the need (a) to engage with family members, (b) to acknowledge social and cultural context and (c) to ensure culturally appropriate communication and feedback. We now examine each of these in turn.

Engagement of family members

For Indigenous people health is interpreted in terms of relationship through spiritual connections to the land and ancestors, and relationships within the community such as those with the elders (McLennan and Khavarpour, 2004). The need to understand relationship has been emphasized in many landmark reports and frameworks (Swan and Raphael, 1995, Social Health Reference Group, 2004). One strategy for greater understanding is engagement with the family of mental health clients. This was explicitly acknowledged in the first of the 'good practice' principles arising from the Queensland study (Mental Health Branch (2009)) described earlier.

Acknowledgement of social and cultural context

Not only family relationships, but the broader societal context, are important in understanding Indigenous health. The explanation and understanding of the frequently worse health status revealed by OM needs to acknowledge the potential origin of problems in terms of the impact of colonization: trauma, loss and grief, separation of families and children, taking away of land, loss of culture and identity, and the impact of social inequity, stigma and racism (Swan and Raphael, 1995). Others have emphasized that maintenance of wellness, not solely management of illness, should be the goal:

> I have observed that mental health services separate mental health from health and they have compartmentalised it into another body. It is this model that does not work for Aboriginal people. We do not need to be fragmented or torn apart any further. Mental health services for Indigenous people need to reflect our world view and vision of how we see things at the moment … (Garvey, 2008)

This focus on wellness is echoed in calls for tools which strengthen cultural identity and celebrate cultural difference, adopt a holistic framework and incorporate social, spiritual and cultural perspectives (Murray et al., 2002, Kirmayer et al., 2003, Ypinazar et al., 2007), and acknowledges the importance of spirituality and traditional rituals in helping Indigenous healing and well-being (McLennan and Khavarpour, 2004).

Indigenous peoples of Canada, First Nations, Metis and Inuit, face similar challenges to those of the Indigenous Australian population (Young, 2003). Poor health outcomes are complicated by limited cross-cultural understanding within the health system, and limited access to services (Smye et al., 2001).

In common with Australian Indigenous people there are varied acculturation histories and health beliefs of First Nations and other Aboriginal people across Canada. Despite this heterogeneity many hold to the view that health refers to a person's whole being, including physical, mental, emotional and especially spiritual being (Smye et al., 2001).

The difference of world view is further complicated by practical differences of communication. Language, literacy and response to direct questions differ in Indigenous people and vary in context around Australia. In terms of direct questions they may be experienced as intrusive, they may lead to long delays in response which are culturally appropriate yet misinterpreted, and they may result in affirmative responses which are 'polite' rather than accurate (Eades, 2005).

Many of these differences can be overcome if the workforce is culturally competent and trained and supported to deliver cross-cultural assessment and treatment. Development of the workforce is thus another challenge to culturally valid OM. Apart from training of non-Indigenous service providers (Johnstone and Read, 2000) one of the obvious strategies for promotion of cultural competence is that of development of the Indigenous workforce. As yet in Australia the Indigenous mental health workforce is outnumbered and overwhelmed by dominant values and the monoculture of dominant health frameworks (Royal Australian and New Zealand College of Psychiatrists, 2003, Brideson, 2004, Robinson and Harris, 2005).

Culturally appropriate communication and feedback

Another challenge for service delivery and OM for Indigenous people is the need to communicate and feed back those outcomes in ways that are understood by the individuals concerned, and their community. The meaning of OM for delivery of service is of most import to the population whose outcomes they represent. Until the 'outcomes literacy' and shared understandings of Indigenous practitioners and clients is enhanced the important principle of ethical research of feedback of research findings cannot be met (The Aboriginal and Torres Strait Islander Research Agenda Working Group (RAWG) of the NHMRC, 2002).

These same issues have been of concern in other countries. The development of the 'OCAP' principles (Ownership, Control, Access and Possession) in Canada, for example, represents a strategy adopted by First Nations organizations to bring self-determination to research. 'It is a political response to tenacious colonial approaches to research and information management' (Schnarch, 2004). The principles arose from a long list of grievances including that 'Research results are not returned to the community or they are returned in a form or language that is inaccessible'. (Schnarch, 2004).

Conclusions

In conclusion, there are a number of challenges to ensuring valid and culturally sensitive assessment and outcome measurement for Indigenous people in Australia, and there is much work yet to be done.

Specific solutions involve promotion and expansion of the Indigenous mental health workforce, development of cultural competence within services and careful adaptation of measures or development of new tools. Culture-specific measures will take differences of world view into account, including attention to strengths as well as deficits, while generic measures, some of which have some regard to strengths as well, will enable a standardized assessment of severity, which will facilitate comparison with the mainstream. This comparison can identify the 'health gap', and lead to focused action to reduce it.

References

Australian Bureau of Statistics (2005). *The Health and Welfare of Australia's Aboriginal and Torres Strait Islander Peoples*. Canberra.

Australian Indigenous Doctors Association (2004). An introduction to cultural competency, available at: www.racp.edu.au.

Australian Institute of Health and Welfare (2009). *Measuring the Social and Emotional Wellbeing of Aboriginal and Torres Strait Islander Peoples*. Canberra.

Bailey, R., Siciliano, F., Dane, G., et al. (2002). *Atlas of health related infrastructure in discrete indigenous communities*. Melbourne: Aboriginal and Torres Strait Islander Commission.

Bhui, K. (2001). Mental health needs assessment for ethnic and cultural minorities. In G. Thornicroft, ed., *Measuring Mental Health Needs*. London: Gaskell.

Bhui, K., Mohamud, S., Warfa, N., Craig, T. J. and Stansfeld, S. A. (2003). Cultural adaptation of mental health measures: improving the quality of clinical practice and research. *The British Journal of Psychiatry*, **183**, 184–6.

Brideson, T. (2004). Moving beyond a 'Seasonal Work Syndrome' in mental health: service responsibilities for Aboriginal and Torres Strait Islander populations. *Australian e-Journal for the Advancement of Mental Health*, **3**.

Brown, A. and Brown, N. (2007). The Northern Territory intervention: voices from the centre of the fringe. *MJA*, **187**, 621–3.

Buckingham, W., Burgess, P., Solomon, S., Pirkis, J. and Eagar, K. (1998). *Developing a Casemix Classification for Mental Health Services*. Canberra: Department of Health and Aging.

Calma, T. (2007). 40 years on: what does the 'Yes' vote mean for Indigenous Australians? available from: http://www.hreoc.gov.au/about/media/speeches/social_justice/2007/40_years_on20070822.html, retrieved October 2007.

Cass, A., Lowell, A., Christie, M., et al. (2002). Sharing the true stories: improving communication in indigenous health care. *eMJA*, **176**, 466–70.

De Vellis, R. (1991). *Scale Development: Theory and Applications*. Newbury Park: Sage.

Durie, M. and Kingi, T. K. (1997). *A Framework for Measuring Maori Mental Health Outcomes*. A report prepared for the Ministry of Health, Palmerston North.

Eades, D. (2005). *Aboriginal English*. Aboriginal Literacy Resource Kit, North Sydney, available at: http://www.une.edu.au/langnet/aboriginal.htm, retrieved May 2007.

Eley, D., Hunter, K., Young, L., et al. (2006). Tools and methodologies for investigating the mental health needs of Indigenous patients: it's about communication. *Australasian Psychiatry*, **14**, 33–7.

Esler, D., Johnston, F. and Thomas, D. (2007). The acceptability of a depression screening tool in an urban, Aboriginal community-controlled health service. *Australian and New Zealand Journal of Public Health*, **31**, 259–63.

Gaines, P., Bower, A., Buckingham, W., et al. (2003). *New Zealand Mental Health Classification and Outcomes Study: Final Report*. Auckland: Health Research Council of New Zealand.

Garvey, D. (2008). A review of the social and emotional wellbeing of Indigenous Australian peoples – considerations, challenges and opportunities, available at: http://www.healthinfonet.ecu.edu.au/sewb_review, retrieved April 2009.

Harrison, J. (2008). *Aboriginal children's wellbeing and the role of culture: Outcomes of an Australian research project into measurements and assessment tools for Aboriginal and Islander children.* Association of Childrens Welfare Agencies Conference, 18–20 August, Sydney.

Haswell-Elkins, M., Sebasio, T., Hunter, E. and Mar, M. (2007). Challenges of measuring the mental health of Indigenous Australians: honouring ethical expectations and driving greater accuracy. *Australasian Psychiatry*, 15, S29–S33.

Human Rights and Equal Opportunity Commission (1997). Bringing them Home. Report of the National Inquiry into the Separation of Aboriginal and Torres Strait Islander Children from Their Families, available at: http://www.austlii.edu.au/au/special/rsjproject/rsjlibrary/hreoc/stolen/prelim.html, retrieved October 2007.

Hunter, E. (2002). 'Best intentions' lives on: untoward health outcomes of some contemporary initiatives in Indigenous affairs. *Australian and New Zealand Journal of Psychiatry*, 36, 575–84.

Johnstone, K. and Read, J. (2000). Psychiatrists' recommendations for improving bicultural training and Maori mental health services: a New Zealand survey. *Australian and New Zealand Journal of Psychiatry*, 34, 135–45.

Kessler, R. C., Wittchen, H.-U., Abelson, J. and Zhao, S. (2000). Methodological issues in assessing psychiatry disorders with self-reports. In A. A. Stone, J. S. Turkkan, C. A. Bachrach et al., eds., *The Science of Self-Report: Implications for Research and Practice.* London: Lawrence Erlbaum.

Kingi, T. K. and Durie, M. (1997). *'Hua Oranga' A Maori Measure of Mental Health Outcome.* Palmerston North: Te Pūmanawa Hauora, School of Māori Studies, Massey University.

Kirmayer, L., Simpson, C. and Cargo, M. (2003). Healing traditions: culture, community and mental health promotion with Canadian Aboriginal peoples. *Australasian Psychiatry*, 11 Supplement, S15–S23.

Knudsen, H., Vasques-Barquero, J., Welcher, B., et al. (2000). Translation and cross-cultural adaptation of outcome measurements for schizophrenia. *The British Journal of Psychiatry*, 177, s8–s14.

Kowanko, I., de Crespigny, C., Murray, H., Groenkjaer, M. and Emden, C. (2004). Better medication management for Aboriginal people with mental health disorders: a survey of providers. *Australian Journal of Rural Health*, 12, 253–7.

Lee, K., Clough, A., Jaragba, M., Conigrave, K. and Patton, G. (2008). Heavy cannabis use and depressive symptoms in three Aboriginal communities in Arnhem Land, Northern Territory. *MJA*, 188, 605–8.

McLennan, V. and Khavarpour, F. (2004). Culturally appropriate health promotion: its meaning and application in Aboriginal communities. *Health Promotion Journal of Australia*, 15, 237–9.

Murray, R., Bell, K., Elston, J., et al. (2002). *Guidelines for development, implementation and evaluation of national public health strategies in relation to ATSI peoples.* Melbourne: National Public Health Partnership.

Nagel, T. and Thompson, C. (2007). AIMHI NT 'Mental Health Story Teller Mob': developing stories in mental health. *Australian e-Journal for the Advancement of Mental Health (AeJAMH)*, 6.

Nagel, T., Thompson, C., Robinson, G., Condon, J. and Trauer, T. (2009). 'Two-way' approaches to Indigenous mental health literacy. *Australian Journal of Primary Health*, 15, 50–5.

National Aboriginal and Torres Strait Islander Health Council (2003). *National strategic framework for Aboriginal and Torres Strait Islander health – framework for action by governments.* Canberra: Commonwealth of Australia.

NMHWG Information Strategy Committee Performance Indicators Drafting Group (2005). *Key Performance Indicators for Australian Public Mental Health Services.* ISC discussion paper No. 6, Canberra.

NSW Health Department (no date). Report on the 1997 and 1998 NSW Health Surveys, Sydney, available at: http://www.health.nsw.gov.au/publichealth/, retrieved April 2009.

Paradies, Y. (2006). A systematic review of empirical research on self-reported racism and health. *International Journal of Epidemiology*, **35**, 888–901.

Robinson, G. and Harris, A. (2005). *Aboriginal Mental Health Worker Program*. Final Evaluation Report. Darwin.

Rosen, A., Hadzi-Pavlovic, D. and Parker, G. (1989). The Life Skills Profile: a measure assessing function and disability in schizophrenia. *Schizophrenia Bulletin*, **15**, 325–37.

Royal Australian and New Zealand College of Psychiatrists (2003). Position Statement No. 50, Aboriginal and Torres Strait Islander Mental Health Workers. *Aboriginal and Islander Health Worker Journal*, **27**.

Schlesinger, C., Ober, C., McCarthy, M., Watson, J. and Seinen, A. (2007). The development and validation of the Indigenous Risk Impact screen (IRIS): a 13 item screening instrument for alcohol and drug mental health risk. *Drug and Alcohol Review*, **26**, 109–17.

Schnarch, B. (2004). Ownership, Control, Access, and Possession (OCAP) or self-determination applied to research a critical analysis of contemporary First Nations research and some options for First Nations communities. *Journal of Aboriginal Health*, **1**, 80–95.

Sheldon, M. (2001). Psychiatric assessment in remote Aboriginal communities. *Australian & New Zealand Journal of Psychiatry*, **35**, 435–42.

Smye, V., Mussell, B. and Mussell, B. (2001). Aboriginal mental health:'what works best'. A discussion paper. British Columbia.

Smylie, J., Anderson, I., Ratima, M., Crengle, S. and Anderson, M. (2006). Indigenous health performance measurement systems in Canada, Australia, and New Zealand. *The Lancet*, **367**, 2029.

Social Health Reference Group (2004). *Social Health Reference Group for National Aboriginal and Torres Strait Islander Health Council and National Mental Health Working Group: A national strategic framework for Aboriginal and Torres Strait Islander People's mental health and social and emotional well being 2004–2009*. Canberra.

Swan, P. and Raphael, B. (1995). *Report on Indigenous and Torres Strait Islander Mental Health: 'Ways Forward', Part I & Part II*. Canberra.

The Aboriginal and Torres Strait Islander Research Agenda Working Group (RAWG) of the NHMRC (2002). *The NHMRC Road Map: A Strategic Framework for Improving Aboriginal and Torres Strait Islander Health Through Research*. Canberra.

Trauer, T., Eagar, K., Gaines, P. and Bower, A. (2004). *New Zealand Mental Health Consumers and their Outcomes*. Auckland: Health Research Council of New Zealand.

Trauer, T., Eagar, K. and Mellsop, G. (2006). Ethnicity, deprivation and mental health outcomes. *Australian Health Review*, **30**, 310–21.

Vicary, D. and Westerman, T. (2004). 'That's just the way he is': some implications of Aboriginal mental health beliefs. *Australian e-Journal for the Advancement of Mental Health (AeJAMH)*, **3**, 1–10.

Vos, T., Haby, M. M., Barendregt, J. J., et al. (2004). The burden of major depression avoidable by longer-term treatment strategies. *Archives of General Psychiatry*, **61**, 1097–103.

Westerman, T. (2000). *Psychological assessment and working with suicide and depression in Aboriginal people: Participant workbook*. Indigenous Psychological Services.

Westerman, T. (2004). Engagement of Indigenous clients in mental health services: What role do cultural differences play? *Australian e-Journal for the Advancement of Mental Health*, **3**.

Wing, J. K., Beevor, A. S., Curtis, R. H., et al. (1998). Health of the Nation Outcome Scales (HoNOS). Research and Development. *British Journal of Psychiatry*, **172**, 11–18.

Young, T. K. (2003). Review of research on aboriginal populations in Canada:

relevance to their health needs. *BMJ*, **327**, 419–22.

Ypinazar, V., Margolis, S., Haswell-Elkins, M. and Tsey, K. (2007). Indigenous Australians' understandings regarding mental health and disorders. *Australian*

and New Zealand Journal of Psychiatry, **41**, 467–78.

Zubrick, S. R., Silburn, S. R., Garton, A., et al. (1995). *Western Australian Child Health Survey: Developing Health and Well-being in the Nineties*. Perth.

Routine measurement of outcomes by Australian private hospital-based psychiatric services

Allen Morris-Yates and Andrew C. Page

Introduction

Routine outcome measurement has been widely embraced by Australian private hospitals with psychiatric beds. Generally, treatment providers welcomed the prospect of measurement as it provided an opportunity to demonstrate what they believe are efficient and effective services, and to identify best practice to facilitate benchmarking and thereby improve services. The present chapter will outline the context and history of routine outcome measurement in the Australian private mental health sector and describe some of the initiatives.

The context

In Australia, mental health services are delivered by a mix of public and private service agencies and providers. In collaboration with a Federal Government, State and Territory Governments manage specialized public mental health services. Private-sector mental health services include the range of mental health services provided by psychiatrists in private practice, and inpatient and day-only services provided by private hospitals, for which private health insurers and other agencies, such as the Australian Government Department of Veterans' Affairs, pay benefits. In 2008 Australia had 27 stand-alone private psychiatric hospitals and 22 psychiatric units located within private general hospitals. Together these hospitals had approximately 1,700 designated psychiatric beds. Private-sector services also include those provided in general hospital settings and by general practitioners, clinical psychologists, mental health nurses and other allied health professionals.

Private psychiatric hospitals provide services predominantly within the overnight inpatient setting. Table 15.1 provides statistics regarding overnight inpatient care provided in private hospitals, public acute hospitals and public psychiatric hospitals (Australian Institute of Health and Welfare, 2008). A comparison of patients admitted to private hospital-based psychiatric services with those admitted to public-sector psychiatric units or hospitals clearly indicates that different groups of people receive care in each sector. Unlike some other areas in Australian health care, the private psychiatric hospital sector provides care to a group of patients who are mostly not being cared for in public psychiatric units.

For the remainder of this chapter we will use the term 'Hospitals' to refer to private hospitals with psychiatric beds and the term 'Payers' to refer to Health Insurers, the Australian Government Department of Veterans' Affairs, State and Territory Workcover Authorities and other agencies that pay benefits in respect of the psychiatric care provided by Hospitals.

The development of a National Model

The Strategic Planning Group for Private Psychiatric Services (SPGPPS) was formed in 1996 under the auspices of the Australian Medical Association (AMA) to address issues such as funding, classification, quality of care and outcome measurement as they affected the private sector. The group comprised representatives of the AMA, the Royal Australian and New Zealand College of Psychiatrists, the Australian Health Insurance Association, the Australian Private Hospitals Association, the National Community Advisory Group on Mental Health and the Australian Government Department of Health and Family Services.

In its early discussions the SPGPPS came to the view that there should be a long-term commitment to the use of outcomes data within the private sector. Accordingly, in 1998 the SPGPPS initiated a project to develop a national model for the collection and analysis of data which could better inform all stakeholders about the quality and effectiveness of care provided in Hospitals. Development of the model involved two parallel strands. At the technical level, a practical and affordable model for an information infrastructure needed development and documentation. A second and parallel process of thorough consultation with and education of key stakeholders was needed. Significant resources were devoted to consultation, both to ensure that those groups were informed and committed, and to obtain their input into the technical development.

Table 15.1 Comparison of public and private psychiatric hospitals casemix during the most recent period for which published data is available (July 2005 to June 2006).

		Private hospitals	Public acute hospitals	Public psychiatric hospitals
Number of overnight separations		31,363	117,948	11,948
Sex	Male	36.1%	51.5%	60.8%
	Female	63.9%	48.5%	39.2%
Age	0–14 years	0.9%	2.6%	1.6%
	15–24 years	10.6%	16.0%	15.2%
	25–44 years	33.6%	44.7%	54.7%
	45–64 years	36.5%	21.9%	20.4%
	65 and older	18.5%	14.9%	8.1%
Principal diagnoses (ICD-10-AM)				
Schizophrenia, schizoaffective and delusional disorders (F20–F29)		8.1%	25.7%	40.4%
Major depression, bipolar disorder and other mood disorders (F30–F39)		47.3%	24.1%	20.9%
Neurotic, stress-related and somatoform disorders (F40–F48)		16.9%	15.2%	12.5%
Mental and behavioural disorders due to psychoactive substance use (F10–F19)		17.2%	19.7%	16.5%
Disorders of adult personality and behaviour (F60–F69)		2.1%	4.1%	4.8%
Organic, including symptomatic, mental disorders (F00–F09)		4.8%	7.1%	2.7%
Other mental and behavioural disorders (F50–F59, F70–F99)		3.7%	4.1%	2.2%
Involuntary legal status		0.8%	24.7%	62.0%

With hindsight it is clear that full and open consultation with stakeholders was critical to the success of the project. First, it would have been foolhardy to attempt to develop and implement a data collection and analysis system without taking account of existing practices and current developments. Second, the collection and analysis of detailed data on services and outcomes raised (and continues to raise) many issues for all stakeholders (Shahian et al., 2001, Hermann et al., 2007, Liptzin, 2009). These included:

- Who would have access to the data collected?
- How would the data be collated?
- What case classification and risk adjustment, if any, would be employed?
- Who would have access to the resulting statistical information?
- How would those results be presented?

In some instances, those concerns could be addressed by identifying current best practice. In other cases, the concerns related to procedural issues that had not yet been fully defined. Both kinds of issues needed to be aired, their implications and possible responses worked through, and each group given the opportunity to understand and appreciate the concerns of others. Indeed, given the potential for abuse of the data collected, any approach which did not clearly address consumers', service providers' (both psychiatrists and Hospitals) and Payers' genuine concerns regarding data collection and use would not have been accepted. The technical development process was informed by a strategy whose objective was to identify and fully document comprehensive answers to the following questions.

- What are the key stakeholders' information needs (what questions) and what concerns do they have regarding the use of information?
- What data must be collected in order to address those questions?
- What protocols should guide the ascertainment and collection of that data?
- Once collected, how can the data be transformed into useful, accessible information?
- Having acquired the information requested, how can we ensure that it is used effectively and appropriately?

In 2000 the final report on the National Model was published (Morris-Yates and The Strategic Planning Group for Private Psychiatric Services Data Collection and Analysis Working Group, 2000). It included agreed guidelines and recommendations regarding the data to be collected, the protocol for the collection of data, the submission and central management of the data collected, the analysis of data and dissemination of information, and access to data and information at all stages in its processing and dissemination. These are summarized below.

The data to be collected

Data needed to be collected for two main purposes: (a) to describe and explain the reasons for the utilization of services during the episode of care, and (b) to enable evaluation of the outcomes of the episode of care.

(a) The minimum data set

Since 1995 all private hospitals in Australia are required to regularly submit to their Payers an agreed patient episode-level data set under what is known as the Hospitals Casemix Protocol

(HCP).[1] The data items constituting the HCP data set address issues of needs for care, service utilization and costs.

Given that the HCP data set was designed to address the first of the purposes identified above, it was agreed that the Minimum Data Set be limited to the existing HCP Data Set. Whilst the HCP data did not meet all requirements, its use had and continues to have many practical advantages. First, Hospitals' and Payers' existing data collection and submission processes could be used. Second, because the HCP data are strongly tied to the payment models employed by Payers and are used by many of them to monitor Hospitals' performance, the data set is generally reliable and complete.

At present, the HCP data set consists of unit records defined at the level of an episode of admitted patient care. For overnight inpatient care this means that there is generally one record for the whole episode. For care provided within the ambulatory care service setting the HCP records each same-day admission as a discrete record. This means that detailed information is captured about each occasion of service.

(b) Selection of measures of clinical status to enable evaluation of the outcomes of care

In selecting the measures to be collected the different needs of clinicians, Hospitals and Payers had to be considered and balanced. Hospitals and Payers need to know how the care provided affects the whole person – does it improve health and well-being? They require indicators that are related to generic concepts of functioning and well-being, rather than diagnosis- or treatment-specific concepts. In addition, managers need a very succinct statement of consumer outcome. Complex multi-dimensional data are difficult for them to interpret so ideal indicators of health outcome for both Hospitals and Payers:

- have few dimensions
- are widely applicable and widely used by all sections of the industry so that benchmark data from diverse sources are available and well understood, and
- are simple to collect and brief, minimizing burden on clinicians and Hospitals.

Clinicians need more detailed information than either Hospital managers or Payers. They need disease and treatment-specific information on changes in both symptoms and disability, so the generic measures most suitable for Payers are less likely to be suitable for clinical needs. It was concluded that the standardized measures selected for routine collection by all Hospitals should:

- not be diagnosis- or treatment-specific
- measure both distress and disability
- be very brief
- be easily administered
- be widely used with readily available, detailed benchmark data, and
- be either very low in cost or free.

The intention was that the chosen measures could be included within the clinical assessment process and any questionnaire battery a clinician may wish to use, without undue

---

[1] Further information regarding the HCP can be found on the Australian Government Department of Health and Ageing website at http://www.health.gov.au/internet/main/publishing.nsf/Content/health-casemix-data-collections-about-HCP (last accessed 3 June 2009).

impact. After reviewing the available options, it was agreed that Hospitals should collect two measures of patients' clinical status, the HoNOS and MHQ-14, at key points in the clinical path – at admission and discharge from episodes of care, and where episodes are of extended duration, at review every 91 days. The two measures and the specific reasons for their selection are outlined below.

(c) HoNOS – the clinician's perspective

The Health of the Nation Outcome Scales (HoNOS) is a clinician-rated measure developed by the Royal College of Psychiatrists (Wing et al., 1998). Its 12 scales provide a comprehensive, yet brief, summary of the clinician's assessment of the patient's clinical status over the preceding period (2 weeks at admission, 3 days at discharge). Ratings on each scale may range from 0 to 4 indicating the severity of problems during the period. Each scale is supported by a detailed glossary (Wing et al., 1999). Scales 1 to 10 address behavioural and symptomatic problems together with associated problems with relationships and activities of daily living; scales 11 and 12 are about the patient's domestic and occupational environment, particularly the extent to which it may help or hinder their recovery.

The selection of the HoNOS was based on four considerations. First, of the measures initially recommended by the Australian Government (Andrews et al., 1994), the HoNOS was the most comprehensive in its coverage and included ratings of problems relevant in both inpatient and ambulatory care settings. Second, the HoNOS was designed as a measure of health outcome for use by mental health service providers, and was brief, comprehensive and clinically relevant. Although it is clearly difficult to combine all these attributes in a single 12-item measure, the HoNOS, to a greater extent than any other available instrument, met those requirements. Third, at the time the National Model was under development the Australian Federal Government began directing funding towards encouraging the implementation of the HoNOS as a routine measure in public mental health services (Goldney et al., 1998). Collection of the same measure in the private sector would have many clear benefits. Fourth, also at that time, there existed a very substantial base of HoNOS data collected in Australia in both private and public-sector mental health services (Boot et al., 1997). With the implementation of HoNOS as the standard clinician-completed rating scale in both public mental health services and private hospital-based psychiatric services, that database has rapidly increased (Buckingham et al., 1998), facilitating benchmarking (Page et al., 2001) and other applied research in even the smallest of Hospitals.

(d) MHQ-14 – the patient's perspective

The identification of an appropriate self-report measure that met the requirements identified above was a significantly more difficult task. After reviewing many instruments against the stated criteria, it was concluded that the subset of 14 items that addressed symptoms of fatigue, anxiety and depression and the impact of those symptoms on social and role functioning from the Medical Outcomes Study questionnaire (SF-36, Ware and Sherbourne, 1992) used in the Rand Health Insurance Experiment (Manning et al., 1987) best met the requirements for a routinely collected self-report measure (Ware et al., 1998).

The measure, identified for convenience under the National Model as the Mental Health Questionnaire – 14-item version (MHQ–14), has a number of advantages (Newnham et al., 2007). First, it is very brief and easily administered and so will not impose an excessive burden on clinicians or Hospitals, or interfere with their existing data-collection regimens. Second, it enables the derivation of several important indicators of disability and distress related to mental disorders or problems and is easily interpreted by all stakeholders. Third, since the 14 items also constitute the mental health component of the SF-36, the most widely used patient-completed outcome measure in the general health sector, comparison data were readily available. In particular, the SF-36 had been used by the Australian Bureau of Statistics in the National Health Survey, thus providing Hospitals and Payers with general population-based norms (Australian Bureau of Statistics, 1995).

The submission and management of the data collected

Hospitals and Payers agreed that maximum benefit from the proposed collection would only be obtained if the data collected by participating Hospitals could be aggregated, and then analysed and reported to both Hospitals and Payers in accordance with agreed protocols. Hospitals agreed to submit the required data to a Centralized Data Management Service (CDMS) in a form that enabled linkage of records for the purposes of statistical analysis but which would not enable the personal identification of individual patients or their treating psychiatrists.

(a) The analysis of data and dissemination of information

The National Model specifies how key summary indicators and other derived data elements are calculated. A number of derived data elements, such as length of stay, were already defined in the Australian Institute of Health and Welfare's National Health Data Dictionary (Australian Institute of Health and Welfare, 1998). Many other important derived data elements, such as the summary scores derived from the clinical measures and the method for calculating a standardized measure of change, were specified within the National Model. Formally specified reports are limited to a basic set of analyses of:

- demographic and clinical profiles of those in care
- utilization and cost of services
- outcomes of care
- data quality.

As much of the benefit gained through access to this information would be lost if that access was not timely, it was agreed that Standard Reports should be prepared and distributed on a quarterly basis.

(b) Access to information

By the early 1990s, Australian protocols and standards governing access to personally identified information regarding patients were relatively well-developed. The Australian Government's Information Privacy Principles had provided a sound foundation for the development of the Australian Standard *AS4400 Personal Privacy Protection in Healthcare Information Systems* (Standards Australia, 1995). The major issues that had to be addressed in the development of the National Model related to access to aggregate statistical information regarding identified service providers (psychiatrists or Hospitals) and identified Payers. It was agreed that identified information regarding individual service providers or Payers must not be made generally available without the identified individual entity's explicit permission. Thus, the principles underlying *AS4400* were applied to all identified data, regardless of whether the subject of the record was an individual person or a business entity.

The analysis and reporting framework subsequently employed by the CDMS is based on a straightforward interpretation of those principles to ensure that the privacy and confidentiality of participating Hospitals and Payers are protected. For example, each Hospital's report is individualized so that they can identify themselves, but are unable to identify any other Hospital. Similarly, Payers receive aggregate statistics regarding their members' care at each participating Hospital, but cannot be provided with statistics regarding any identified Hospital's overall performance.

(c) The Private Mental Health Alliance's Centralized Data Management Service (CDMS)

After lengthy negotiations, in 2001 a Centralized Data Management Service was established under the auspices of the AMA on behalf of the primary financial stakeholders – the Australian Government Department of Health and Ageing, the Australian Private Hospitals Association and the Australian Health Insurance Association. As of July 2009, all private hospitals with psychiatric beds collect data in accordance with the National Model and subscribe to the services provided by the CDMS. For the 2009–2010 financial year the total cost of the CDMS was approximately \$270,000. For Hospitals, this means that the services cost them a little under \$100 per bed per annum.

The Private Mental Health Alliance (PMHA), the successor to the SPGPPS, is responsible for oversight of the operation of the CDMS. This arrangement enables clinicians, private health insurers, private hospitals, consumers and carers and the Australian Government to be actively engaged in its management. It ensures that problems or issues that may arise are dealt with openly and transparently.

The CDMS has three primary roles:

- support Hospitals' efforts to monitor, evaluate and improve the quality and effectiveness of the care they provide
- support Payers efforts to understand the quality, effectiveness and efficiency of the private Hospital-based psychiatric services that they fund, and
- support the Private Mental Health Alliance's members and their representatives' efforts to understand and make known the work of private-sector mental health services.

To fulfil those roles the CDMS provides the following materials and services:

- maintains and continuously improves the National Model for the collection and analysis of a minimum data set with outcome measures for private, hospital-based, psychiatric services (National Model)
- guides and references manuals for Hospital staff
- training resources
- Hospitals Standardised Measures database application (HSMdb, described below)
- standard quarterly reports to Hospitals and Payers as specified under the National Model, and
- provides the PMHA with an annual statistical report.

(d) Hospitals Standardized Measures database application (HSMdb)

The Hospital's Standardized Measures database (HSMdb) enables participating Hospitals to collect, submit and utilize data collected in accordance with the requirements of the National

Model. It was initially developed to help Hospitals avoid complex and costly changes that would be needed if they were to use their patient administration systems (PAS) to record the standardized measures. Since its initial development, the software has been substantially revised and expanded, with updates provided at least annually.

The routine data-entry functions in HSMdb are designed around the data-collection protocol and the basic standard data-collection formats defined by the National Model. This helps ensure that the data collected by Hospitals is recorded in a manner that is consistent with the National Model's requirements. HSMdb also enables Hospitals to import HCP data, which includes detailed coded information regarding service utilization, diagnoses and procedures, from their patient administration systems (PAS), and to link them with the standardized measures (HoNOS and MHQ-14) data recorded in HSMdb. This substantially reduces double entry of data. Hospitals then use HSMdb to create a compressed and encrypted data extract file that can be submitted quarterly to the CDMS via email. HSMdb also includes clinical review functions. These enable several different tasks to be completed, including:

- Quality improvement. For example, the clinical review function may be used to identify patients with specified characteristic patterns of service utilization or clinical profiles so that the details of their care may be more closely examined.
- Contractual reporting requirements. By selecting the appropriate administrative criteria (reference period and responsible payer) and then selecting the required aggregate statistical analyses, much of the information needed for a standard report that might be requested by a Payer can be obtained.
- Evaluation of new or existing clinical programmes. During data entry, one or more local data item fields may be used to identify episodes of care that involved patients' participation in a specific clinical programme. It is then possible to obtain aggregate statistics regarding that clinical programme.
- Provision of aggregate statistical information to treating psychiatrists. Patients' treating psychiatrists may be identified within HSMdb at each admission. Based on that, listings and aggregate statistics for each treating psychiatrist's patients can be obtained for any specified reference period.

An example of the primary format for the presentation of statistical information from the aggregate statistical report, created using the HSMdb software's Clinical Review functions, is shown in Figure 15.1.

(e) Provision of Standard Quarterly Reports

Under the National Model participating Hospitals submit their data to the CDMS quarterly, with submissions being due no later than 10 weeks following the end of the quarter. The CDMS aims to provide Hospitals with their Standard Quarterly Reports (SQR) within 13 weeks of the end of the quarter. Generally, it achieves that objective. Each Hospital's SQR provides information for the identified hospital in the current quarter and the current 12 months and also provides information regarding all hospitals for the current 12 months. The aggregate statistics contained in the report are partitioned by service setting (overnight inpatient care and ambulatory care) and stratified by a simple grouping based on principal diagnosis (Buckingham et al., 1998, Morris-Yates and The Strategic Planning Group for Private Psychiatric Services Data Collection and Analysis Working Group, 2000). The information is presented in a format similar to that shown in Figure 15.1. Similar SQRs are provided to each

Demographic Profile

Age Group:			0–14 yrs		15–24 yrs		25–44 yrs		45–65 yrs		65+ yrs	
Sex:	N	%	N	%	N	%	N	%	N	%	N	%
Male	193	26%	0	0%	27	4%	71	10%	73	10%	22	3%
Female	544	74%	0	0%	31	4%	243	33%	215	29%	55	7%
Total	737		0	0%	58	8%	314	43%	288	39%	77	10%

HoNOS (Clinician rating) Summary Scores

	N of available observations	Behavioural problems		Impairment		Symptomatic problems		Social problems		Total Score	
		mean / 95% c.i.	s.d.	mean / 95% c.i.	s.d.	mean / 95% c.i.	s.d.	mean / 95% c.i.	s.d.	mean / 95% c.i.	s.d.
Admission	737	2.8 / 2.6 2.9	2.1	1.7 / 1.6 1.8	1.6	5.2 / 5.1 5.3	1.4	1.8 / 1.7 1.9	1.4	11.6 / 11.4 11.9	3.5
Discharge	710	0.6 / 0.5 0.7	1.1	0.9 / 0.8 1.0	1.3	1.9 / 1.7 2.0	1.8	1.1 / 0.9 1.2	1.7	4.1 / 3.8 4.4	4.1
Change (E.S.)	710	0.93 / 0.86 1.00	0.93	0.48 / 0.42 0.55	0.88	1.54 / 1.47 1.61	1.01	0.51 / 0.46 0.57	0.78	1.45 / 1.38 1.51	0.91

MHQ-14 (Patient self-report) Summary Scores

	N of available observations	Vitality		Social Functioning		Role Functioning - Emotional		Mental Health	
		mean / 95% c.i.	s.d.	mean / 95% c.i.	s.d.	mean / 95% c.i.	s.d.	mean / 95% c.i.	s.d.
Admission	709	23 / 21 24	20	23 / 22 25	22	13 / 11 15	27	30 / 28 31	21
Discharge	654	49 / 47 50	25	57 / 54 59	29	54 / 51 58	44	57 / 55 59	24
Change (E.S.)	637	1.21 / 1.12 1.31	1.26	1.40 / 1.30 1.50	1.34	1.47 / 1.34 1.60	1.67	1.31 / 1.21 1.41	1.27

Service Utilisation

Number of Separations	737

Length of Stay	mean / 95% c.i.	s.d.	c.v.	Frequency distribution				
Days (minus Leave days and Days spent at home)				1–2	3–7	8–21	22–35	35+
	20 / 19 21	16	0.82	7%	16%	45%	19%	13%

Re-Admissions	28 days	91 days (3 months)	273 days (9 months)
% of episodes preceded by another within the specified interval (brief episodes excluded)	12%	32%	47%

Figure 15.1 An example of the primary table from the aggregate statistical report created using the HSMdb software's Clinical Review Functions.

participating Payer. The reports contain aggregate statistics regarding only their members' admissions to each participating Hospital, their members' admissions to all hospitals, and all patients' admissions to all hospitals. The SQRs for both Hospitals and Payers include detailed explanations of the statistics contained within the report's tables and figures but, as a matter of policy, do not contain any interpretation of specific similarities or differences between the report subject and any comparison groups. The CDMS provides clear advice on how similarities and differences may be interpreted and what contextual information may need to be taken into account in that interpretation, but does not offer opinions on specific matters. This reflects the very clearly defined role of the CDMS and allows it to retain a neutral, supportive stance towards both Hospitals and Payers.

Hospitals' progress with the implementation of routine outcomes measurement

Participating hospitals have made good progress implementing the National Model's data-collection requirements. The key indices used by the CDMS to monitor that progress are the pair-wise (i.e. at both admission and discharge) completion rates for the HoNOS and MHQ-14.

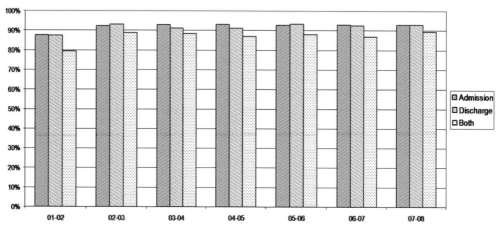

Figure 15.2 Median completion rates for the clinician-rated measure (HoNOS) at admission, discharge and both admission and discharge together (the pair-wise rate) obtained by participating Hospitals in each financial year since the initiation of the collection.

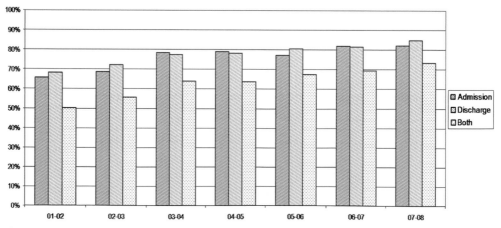

Figure 15.3 Median completion rates for the MHQ-14 at admission, discharge and both admission and discharge together (the pair-wise rate) obtained by participating Hospitals in each financial year since the initiation of the collection in 2001.

Due to the fact that participating Hospitals also provide the CDMS with accurate service utilization data, the CDMS is able to definitively ascertain each Hospital's completion rates. Figures 15.2 and 15.3 show the median completion rates for participating Hospitals in each financial year from the initiation of the collection in 2001.

After reviewing the performance of the best Hospitals and discussing the issues that might affect Hospitals' capacity to attain rates consistent with theirs, the CDMS indicated that the expected pair-wise completion rate would be 70%. The CDMS also set a benchmark, recommending Hospitals aim for a pair-wise completion rate of 90% for the HoNOS and 80% for the MHQ-14. In 2008, 15% of participating Hospitals did not meet the expected completion rate for the HoNOS and 49% attained the benchmark rate of 90%. For the MHQ-14, 40% did not meet the expected completion rate whilst 33% attained the benchmark of 80%. Although these high completion rates were not achieved overnight, they do demonstrate that through a process of stakeholder involvement, feedback, rebuke and encouragement, high completion rates are achievable.

Use of outcome measures data by Hospitals

The national data collection now implemented by Australian private hospitals with psychiatric beds has both extended their pre-existing outcome measurement programmes and fostered new initiatives. Before implementation of the National Model, information on outcomes, whilst collected by many Hospitals, was based on a range of different measures and was ascertained without reference to external mechanisms for ensuring consistency of ratings. Consequently it was hard to interpret. Some of the initiatives in the sector will now be described.

(a) Comparing outcomes across Hospitals

One early example was work by Boot and colleagues (Boot et al., 1997). They compared HoNOS admission ratings of patients in Australian private and public psychiatric hospitals to each other and to general public hospitals. Perhaps not surprisingly, patients in both public and private psychiatric hospitals exhibited higher scores than those in general hospitals, reflecting the presence of more psychopathology and associated disability. In addition, patients in private psychiatric hospitals were rated as having less severe scores than those in public psychiatric facilities. Again this is not a surprising result given that, as indicated in Table 15.1, the casemix is quite different across public and private facilities, with the former dealing with greater numbers of patients with chronic psychotic disorders, and private facilities with proportionally more patients with mood disorders. However, comparisons across published studies are difficult. Page and colleagues (Page et al., 2001) compared the results from another Australian private psychiatric hospital with the data from Boot et al. on the HoNOS and noted some differences; namely, the effect size per 10-day length of hospital stay was much larger than in the other hospitals. However, it was not clear whether the contrast arose because the hospital management was better, the hospital systems (e.g. bed numbers, models of care) varied, the patients were different (casemix) or the data-collection processes (e.g. scoring, inclusion and exclusion criteria, time of ratings) were dissimilar.

Soon after these data were collected, the majority of Hospitals began implementation of the National Model with the support of the CDMS, making it possible to address the above-mentioned issues. A national training programme addressed scoring issues; agreed protocols for data collection ensured consistency of measurement. Consistency of measurement has been particularly important in facilitating benchmarking between Hospitals.

For example, it is now possible for every participating hospital to compare its outcomes with the mean of all other hospitals across a range of common assessment measures, obtained under similar conditions, and coded and analysed in a comparable manner. Furthermore, hospitals can and do voluntarily 'benchmark' among themselves by combining their data to make detailed comparisons across facilities. In so doing, hospitals can increase the value (and the potential benefits to patients) they derive from the measurement of outcomes.

However, one limitation of regular reporting of outcomes has come to light, namely that for most Hospitals the outcomes in the present reporting period most often look very much like the outcomes in the preceding periods. Consequently, after the initial enthusiasm experienced by Hospitals that accompanied the demonstration that, on average, their patients are improving, there has been a sense of 'so now what?' Several avenues of investigation have been pursued now that outcomes measurement has become de rigueur. These include: investigations of the measures used, examination of longitudinal trends in outcomes, the use of outcomes data to inform clinical practice, and extension of the methods of measurement to improve outcomes.

(b) Illustrative investigations of the measures used

One instrument receiving substantial attention in Australia has been the HoNOS. The instrument has a scoring system in which the individual items are summed (to generate a total severity index) or four subscales are generated by summing the items relevant to behavioural problems, difficulties in basic functioning, distressing mental health symptoms and problems in social and environmental functioning. Within the public sectors of Australia and New Zealand, Trauer (1999) demonstrated the utility of the original scoring system for use in the Antipodes; however, he and his colleagues also validated an alternative five-factor scoring. Yet it was not clear the extent to which either of these scoring systems would generalize to the private psychiatric sector, where the majority of patients suffer from depressive disorders. To this end, data from a private hospital were examined and neither the original scoring method nor the revised five-factor model provided the best description of the observed data. Rather, a revised four-factor model generated the best fit, which corresponded to socio-economic factors, emotional symptoms, impairment associated with cognitive and physical problems, and anti-social or behavioural problems, and was able to provide the best description of the data in a private psychiatric sample (Newnham et al., 2009). Thus, the private sector in Australia has been active in examining the psychometric properties of the instruments being used (see also Page et al., 2007).

(c) Examination of longitudinal trends in outcomes

In addition to an examination of the measures, hospitals have begun to examine longitudinal trends in their data. Since the data are stored centrally, it has been possible for individual hospitals not only to examine trends in their data, but to compare those against the average of all Australian private psychiatric hospitals. This has proved a rich data source for comparisons, since quite powerful data analytic strategies, such as control charts (Carey, 2003), can be used to identify unexpected changes. For example, if a particular Hospital was to observe that its length of stay had changed in one direction over the past few reporting periods it might be tempted to make hospital-level attributions (e.g. the referral base has changed). However, if the trend was also observed across all Hospitals, then it would suggest that the reason might lie at another level (e.g. a shift in government policy). Such investigations have been useful in using data to alert Hospitals to important trends.

(d)   Use of outcomes data to inform clinical practice

One example of using data to inform practice has been the way that Hospitals have also been using the data to inform clinical decision-making, such as decisions about discharge from hospital. Clearly, this decision is best made by the health practitioner managing the hospitalization because, while a 'long' admission may be undesirable from the perspective of a hospital manager or insurer, from a clinical perspective a lengthy admission may be justifiable and good practice. However, Page and colleagues (2005) examined the degree to which clinical decision-making could be informed by information on the probability of discharge. They found that the probability of imminent discharge from hospital was not linear. That is, for the first couple of weeks the probability of an imminent discharge rose with each day in hospital, but then started to decline, rising again and falling around the 1-month period. On the basis of these data, it was decided to consider a hospital policy to review patients at the points when the probability of imminent discharge was declining. Reviewing a patient's admission at the point when the probability of a discharge was lower ensured that decisions were being taken at times when previously a discharge might not have been considered. The data showed that while overall patient outcomes were maintained, the length of stay reduced once the review process was instituted, showing that treatment could be delivered more efficiently without compromising patient care. However, it is one thing to use data to improve hospital procedures; it is another to use the data to enhance outcomes.

(e)   Use of outcomes data to improve practice

Australian private psychiatric hospitals are also using data to inform and improve clinical practice. For example, Newnham et al. (2010) evaluated the use of an existing instrument as a monitoring tool suitable for use in acute psychiatric service settings. The World Health Organization's Well-being Index (WHO-5, Bech et al., 1996) is a five-item self-report measure of positive well-being that has performed reliably and sensitively in psychiatric samples (Newnham et al., in press). Following the pioneering work of Lambert and colleagues (Lambert et al., 2005) a monitoring programme was developed that involved the regular administration of the WHO-5 to generate a measure of patient progress. Consistent with Lambert's original findings, patients who were 'not on track' were more likely to avoid a negative outcome when both staff and patient had access to the information about progress. In fact, the rate of negative outcomes, albeit low to begin with, was nearly halved by the inclusion of monitoring feedback.

Conclusions

The initiatives in particular hospitals in the Australian private sector have dove-tailed with the developments that have occurred nationally. The foundation provided by a national data-collection exercise provides a strong basis upon which individual hospitals can compare outcomes and evaluate quality improvement initiatives. Arguably the relative harmony within the private sector has arisen because of the care assigned to the processes involved in the establishment and maintenance of the data collection and dissemination. This is not to say that the process has been smooth, but that consultation and collaboration has facilitated incorporation of routine outcome measurement into private psychiatric care as service providers strive to provide excellence in mental health care.

References

Andrews, G., Peters, L. and Teesson, M. (1994). *The Measurement of Consumer Outcome in Mental Health: a Report to the National Mental Health Information Strategy Committee*. Sydney: Clinical Research Unit for Anxiety Disorders.

Australian Bureau of Statistics (1995). *National Health Survey: SF-36 Population Norms, Australia (ABS Catalogue No. 4399.0)*. Canberra: Australian Bureau of Statistics.

Australian Institute of Health and Welfare (1998). *National Health Data Dictionary Version 7.0*. Canberra: Australian Institute of Health and Welfare.

Australian Institute of Health and Welfare (2008). *Mental Health Services in Australia 2005–06*. Canberra: Australian Institute of Health and Welfare.

Bech, P., Gudex, C. and Johansen, K. S. (1996). The WHO (Ten) Well-being Index: validation in diabetes. *Psychotherapy and Psychosomatics*, **65**, 183–90.

Boot, B., Hall, W. and Andrews, G. (1997). Disability, outcome and casemix in acute psychiatric inpatient units. *British Journal of Psychiatry*, **171**, 242–6.

Buckingham, W., Burgess, P., Solomon, S., Pirkis, J. and Eagar, K. (1998). *Developing a Casemix Classification for Mental Health Services*. Canberra: Department of Health and Aging.

Carey, R. G. (2003). *Improving Healthcare with Control Charts*. Milwaukee, WI: ASQ Quality Press.

Goldney, R. D., Fisher, L. J. and Walmsley, S. H. (1998). The Health of the Nation Outcome Scales in psychiatric hospitalisation: a multicentre study examining outcome and prediction of length of stay. *Australian and New Zealand Journal of Psychiatry*, **32**, 199–205.

Hermann, R. C., Rollins, A., Caitlin K. and Chan, J. A. (2007). Risk-adjusting outcomes of mental health and substance-related care: a review of the literature. *Harvard Review of Psychiatry*, **15**, 52–69.

Lambert, M. J., Harmon, C., Slade, K., Whipple, J. L. and Hawkins, E. J. (2005). Providing feedback to psychotherapists on their patients' progress: clinical results and practice suggestions. *Journal of Clinical Psychology*, **61**, 165–74.

Liptzin, B. (2009). Quality improvement, pay for performance, and 'outcomes measurement': what makes sense? *Psychiatric Services*, **60**, 108–11.

Manning, W. G., Newhouse, J. P., Duan, N., et al. (1987). Health insurance and the demand for medical care: evidence from a randomized experiment. *American Economic Review*, **77**, 251–77.

Morris-Yates, A. and The Strategic Planning Group for Private Psychiatric Services Data Collection and Analysis Working Group(2000). *A National Model for the Collection and Analysis of a Minimum Data Set with Outcome Measurement for Private, Hospital-based, Psychiatric Services*. Canberra: Commonwealth of Australia.

Newnham, E. A., Harwood, K. E. and Page, A. C. (2007). Evaluating the clinical significance of responses by psychiatric inpatients to the mental health subscales of the SF-36. *Journal of Affective Disorders*, **98**, 91–7.

Newnham, E. A., Harwood, K. E. and Page, A. C. (2009). The subscale structure and clinical utility of the Health of the Nation Outcome Scale. *Journal of Mental Health*, **18**, 326–34.

Newnham, E. A., Hooke, G. R. and Page, A. C. (2010). Monitoring treatment response and outcomes using the World Health Organization's Wellbeing Index in psychiatric care. *Journal of Affective Disorders*, **122**, 133–8.

Page, A. C., Hooke, G. R. and Rutherford, E. M. (2001). Measuring mental health outcomes in a private psychiatric clinic: Health of the Nation Outcome Scales and Medical Outcomes Short Form SF-36. *Australian and New Zealand Journal of Psychiatry*, **35**, 377–81.

Page, A. C., Hooke, G. R. and Rampono, J. (2005). A methodology for timing reviews of inpatient hospital stay. *Australian and New Zealand Journal of Psychiatry*, **39**, 198–201.

Page, A. C., Hooke, G. R. and Morrison, D. L. (2007). Psychometric properties of the

Depression Anxiety Stress Scales (DASS) in depressed clinical samples. *British Journal of Clinical Psychology*, **46**, 283–97.

Shahian, D. M., Normand, S. L., Torchiana, D. F., et al. (2001). Cardiac surgery report cards: comprehensive review and statistical critique. *Annals of Thoracic Surgery*, **72**, 2155–68.

Standards Australia (1995). *AS 4400:1995, Personal Privacy Protection in Healthcare Information Systems, Homebush*. New South Wales: Standards Australia.

Trauer, T. (1999). The subscale structure of the Health of the Nation Outcome Scales (HoNOS). *Journal of Mental Health*, **8**, 499–509.

Ware, J. E. and Sherbourne, C. D. (1992). The MOS 36-item Short Form Health Status Survey (SF-36): I. Conceptual framework and item selection. *Medical Care*, **30**, 473–83.

Ware, J. E., Kosinski, M., Gandek, B., et al. (1998). The factor structure of the SF-36 Health Survey in 10 countries: results from the IQOLA Project. International Quality of Life Assessment. *Journal of Clinical Epidemiology*, **51**, 1159–65.

Wing, J., Curtis, R. H. and Beevor, A. (1999). Health of the Nation Outcome Scales (HoNOS): glossary for HoNOS score sheet. *British Journal of Psychiatry*, **174**, 432–4.

Wing, J. K., Beevor, A. S., Curtis, R. H., et al. (1998). Health of the Nation Outcome Scales (HoNOS). Research and development. *British Journal of Psychiatry*, **172**, 11–18.

16

Mental health outcome measurement in non-government organizations (NGOs)

Glen Tobias

Introduction

The scope of this chapter is confined to non-government organizations (NGOs) in Australia and New Zealand because of space limitations. There are considerable differences in how NGOs operate across the world and I will leave it to others to describe how they operate within the mental health service systems in their respective countries.

In the Australasian context, NGOs are a core component of specialist mental health services and complement clinical mental health services. While NGOs' roles and functions may vary slightly, they focus on addressing the impact of mental illness on a person's daily life and the social disadvantage resulting from illness. They work within a recovery and empowerment model to maximize people's opportunities to live successfully in the community (Mental Health and Drugs Division, 2009).

The Mental Health NGO sector is diverse, with services being provided by a variety of:

- stand-alone, mental-health-specific organizations
- organizations that provide a range of welfare and disability services
- organizations that provide a range of health and medical services
- peer support organizations, and
- church-affiliated organizations.

The general lack of documentation of a service delivery framework has resulted in further diversity in NGOs' approach and practices, and enormous inconsistencies both within and across states and countries.

In part this has been the result of governments prioritizing their attention on clinical mental health services, with NGOs being seen as a lower priority. While clinical services have been mandated by government to conduct and report routine outcome measurement (ROM), NGOs have largely been ignored. Where NGOs have been required to conduct ROM, it has not been required to be done with much rigour. For example, in Victoria, Australia, NGOs have been required by government to engage in ROM (Victorian Department of Human Services, 2004) but have been given a choice of three quite different outcome measures to use; the Behavior and Symptom Identification Scale (BASIS-32, Eisen et al., 1999), the Camberwell Assessment of Need Short Appraisal Schedule (CANSAS, Phelan et al., 1995) or the World Health Organization Quality of Life assessment (WHOQOL, The WHOQOL Group, 1995), and are not required to report the data they collect. In the absence of any accountability, some NGOs have simply ignored the directive.

How outcome measurement is practised in NGOs

As NGOs have generally not yet been required to conduct ROM by their government funding bodies, the motivation for NGOs to undertake ROM has been quite different compared to clinical services. While many have done nothing in relation to outcome measurement (OM) and are waiting until they are required to, some NGOs have decided to take the initiative and begin OM with the intention of being in a position to influence the process rather than just waiting for it to happen or be imposed. Organizations that fall into this latter group have also been motivated by a variety of other factors that have informed their approach to OM.

In a competitive funding environment some NGOs have focused on using OM to demonstrate their effectiveness and have chosen tools and processes that they hope will provide feedback on the service itself. This service evaluation approach often includes measures of consumer/carer satisfaction with service, measures of the 'recovery orientation' of the service and feedback on the service's outputs and processes.

The most common motivation, however, is dictated by what NGOs appear to have most in common: that is, a recovery-oriented, consumer-focused approach. This has resulted in NGOs looking to OM tools that:

- are self-assessed by consumers
- are holistic, covering a broad range of life issues, not just mental health
- assess a consumer's well-being or progress towards recovery
- can be used to engage consumers in a dialogue with their worker, and
- can be used in the goal setting and individual service planning process.

Additionally, a number of NGOs are planning more comprehensive, integrated systems that take a multi-faceted approach to OM, collecting a combination of subjective and objective evidence. This can include a consumer self-assessment of change, a methodology that records whether identified goals are being met and a system for collecting evidence of recovery through more objective indicators such as social connectedness. This includes collecting information from a variety of informants.

While the comprehensiveness of this holistic approach is commendable, it remains to be seen whether it is feasible or will provide the quantum of additional information to justify the resources invested in the system. As with any complex OM system, sustainability over time is certain to be a critical factor.

Outcome measurement tools and systems in use

When considering tools, many NGOs have begun with investigating the range of well-known, validated tools used in the clinical sector. This has resulted in the adoption by NGOs of some of the range of OM tools that are also used routinely by clinical mental health services. These include measures of illness and symptoms and measures of functioning and disability including the Health of the Nation Outcome Scales (HoNOS, Wing et al., 1998), the Life Skills Profile (LSP, Rosen et al., 1989), the BASIS-32 and the K10 (Kessler et al., 2002). The rationale for adopting tools from this range has been the ability to 'talk the same language' with clinical services, thus raising the profile of the NGOs and providing the opportunity to compare and contrast their work.

Another tool that is sometimes used in clinical settings and in routine use by NGOs is the Camberwell Assessment of Need (CAN, Phelan et al., 1995). The most commonly used version of the CAN is the Short Appraisal Schedule, CANSAS (Andresen et al., 2000, Trauer et al., 2008). Of all the outcome measures, CANSAS has had the strongest uptake by NGOs partly because as a needs assessment it can be used in a very practical way to assist in goal setting and also because it can be rated by a range of informants; consumer, key worker, clinician, carer/family member. It is also the tool most commonly mandated to be used in NGO settings.

A recent NGO study (Helyer et al., 2008) reporting the capacity of CANSAS to measure change in consumers' needs over time supports other studies (Wennström et al., 2008, Wiersma et al., 2009) that have noted its ability to function as an outcome measure. Unmet needs assessed by CANSAS have been found to be associated with quality of life (QoL) and reduction in unmet needs leads to improvements in QoL (Slade et al., 2004, Wiersma, 2006).

The CANSAS is also used as a needs assessment and precursor to goal setting by a growing number of Australian NGOs (Crowe et al., 2007) that are adopting the Collaborative Recovery Model (CRM, Oades et al., 2005) as their model of service delivery. CRM is also being implemented by a clinical mental health service in Ontario, Canada (Oades et al., 2009).

Beyond this range of tools are numerous other measures that are being used to a lesser or greater extent by NGOs. These are tools and methodologies that have been chosen by some NGOs precisely because they are regarded by those NGOs as being more holistic and/ or recovery-focused and not contaminated by a clinical paradigm. They range from well-known, validated tools to novel, locally developed instruments and evaluation methodologies. Some of the more commonly used tools in routine use by NGOs are the World Health Organization Quality of Life assessment (WHOQOL), the Recovery-Enhancing Environment scale (Ridgway and Press, 2004), Growing Well (St Luke's Anglicare Mental Health Services, 2007), the Recovery Assessment Scale (Giffort et al., 1995), the Role Functioning Scale (Goodman et al., 1993), the Psychosocial Rehabilitation Outcomes Toolkit (Arns et al., 2001), the Global Assessment of Functioning, (Jones et al., 1995) and the Avon Mental Health Measure (Markovitz, 1996).

How outcome measurement is viewed

Very little investigation has been done by NGOs into how ROM is viewed by those directly involved in it. Anecdotal evidence from a variety of NGOs suggests that managers and direct care staff are indeed keen to be able to track a consumer's changes over time. They are particularly interested in measuring a consumer's recovery path and want to know that they are making a difference. To achieve this they are more interested in the consumer's perspective and many are interested in measuring such things as relationships or a consumer's connections in the community. A recent NGO survey of 164 consumers and 57 staff found that both consumers and staff had overall positive attitudes towards ROM (Helyer et al., 2008).

Conflicting with these positive views towards ROM is the concern that the sector is becoming more bureaucratic and that OM adds to the administrative burden on staff, distracting them from the 'real work' of providing practical interventions that assist consumers in their recovery. While providers want tools that are comprehensive and meaningful, they necessarily have to balance this with instruments that are simple, brief and easy to use.

Many staff also dislike tools that focus on illness or deficits and believe that they do not have a place in a recovery, empowerment and strengths-based approach. In this respect there is often a strong focus on the actual tools rather than the processes that the tools should support. Within the sector a lot of energy is spent on searching for or wanting to develop a better tool, sometimes to the exclusion of the importance of OM processes – consumer engagement, discussion of perspectives, goal setting and tracking change.

In NGOs where staff have actively engaged in ROM and it has become part of the working culture, the focus is on consumer engagement and collaborative goal setting with less focus on the actual tools, which are viewed as a means to an end rather than being important in themselves.

Practice examples

The NGO sector does not have strong historical links with academic or research institutions and consequently the many examples of good practice remain, on the whole, unevaluated and unpublished. This, combined with the diversity of the sector, has resulted in a dearth of easily accessible information on practice across the sector. It must also be noted that ROM is relatively new to the NGO sector; only a small minority of organizations have more than 3 years of experience in ROM (Penrose-Wall, 2006, Te Pou, 2006).

The most significant effect of the implementation of ROM by NGOs has been that it has revolutionized how direct care staff frame their practice. NGOs have come from a position of being the 'non' sector and historically described themselves in terms of what they were not: non-government, non-profit, non-clinical and non-professional (Ronnau et al., 2008). OM has required staff in NGOs to think more critically about their role and function and NGOs are now more likely to describe themselves in terms of what they do rather than what they don't do.

Where staff working for NGOs may previously have felt unskilled and under-valued within the mental health system, ROM has brought more rigour to their work and provided a structure that has motivated and assisted the professional development of less skilful staff.

OM has also had a positive effect on the relationships between NGOs and clinical services. By clarifying their work and their role, NGO staff have been able to develop more empowered relationships with clinical staff based on improved understanding and mutual respect (Cornish et al., 2005).

An outstanding example of this is where a clinical service and an NGO have developed a database that allows a shared record for consumers that they both work with. NGO staff use the same OM tools as clinical staff and the results are entered into the database (Guthrie et al., 2008). This has resulted in a greater understanding of each other's work and a respect for and valuing of the differences. With the ability to analyse the data on the shared database these services also have the opportunity to plan and coordinate regional service provision more effectively.

Another example is where an NGO and a clinical service collaborated to use the same needs assessment tool in order to achieve a similar result. In this study, the CANSAS was rated by consumers, clinical and NGO staff. The three parties then met to discuss the similarities and differences and used this process to develop a joint individual service plan with the consumer (Cornish et al., 2005).

A further example of cooperation between NGOs and clinical services is where both services use the same consumer self-rated tool but, rather than both services offering the assessment to consumers multiple times a year, they take it in turns and share the data. In this and the preceding two examples, issues of confidentiality and privacy needed to be resolved and consumer consent obtained in order to allow the services to share data.

Most examples of good practice in the NGO sector arise where management has fully committed to leading the organizational change required to embed OM in the culture of the organization. Beyond the initial implementation, this has required an ongoing commitment to staff training and the development of IT systems to enable feedback of results to staff and consumers. Where outcome data have been entered into client databases, services have been able to extract population and outcomes data for use in service planning (Trauer and Tobias, 2004).

While there are only relatively few NGOs that have achieved this level of ROM, those that have report much higher OM completion rates compared with clinical services. It must be noted that consumers use NGO services entirely voluntarily so the quality of the relationship with consumers can be very different to what clinical services are able to achieve. NGOs also have much lower case loads than most clinical services, which increases their ability to engage with consumers and their capacity to undertake ROM.

Other factors that NGOs claim have contributed to high OM completion rates are that the practical relevance of ROM is reinforced when it is used in the goal-setting process with consumers and where the same tool is rated by consumers and staff in order to increase dialogue. One NGO study reports that more than 88% of consumers found that engaging in OM had improved communication with their key worker (Helyer et al., 2008).

A number of NGOs have plans to implement comprehensive OM systems that they have designed to collect both subjective and objective data from a range of sources. These typically include a consumer self-assessment of recovery or function, an assessment of goal achievement and an assessment of community participation or social connections. The more ambitious of these plans seek family/carer input and some intend to employ consumers to administer tools or collect information from service users.

While some of these systems have been trialled, to date none has been fully implemented.

Obstacles to outcome measurement

In considering the obstacles to OM that confront the NGO sector one must start with the diversity and lack of consistency that already exists. The one thing that would facilitate the implementation of a systematic approach to ROM by NGOs is leadership on the issue either from government funding departments or from the peak bodies of the sector. While currently we have a fertile ground for trialling OM, a point must come where the successes and failures of the various approaches are reviewed so that the sector as a whole can benefit. The current lack of research and reports could be overcome by leadership and consolidation within the sector.

Among the issues that need to be resolved is the lack of clarity about what exactly it is that we need to measure. Whose outcomes are they and who gets to define them? The debate on these fundamental issues has largely not occurred and it is probably naive to expect that these issues will be settled before further development of ROM by NGOs proceeds. However, this debate still needs to occur and it may be that the variety of practical OM experience in NGOs is able to enrich this debate.

Along with the lack of consistency in the NGO sector is the need for NGOs to integrate to a certain degree with clinical services in order that the two sectors function as a complementary system for consumers (Mental Health and Drugs Division, 2009). In considering implementation of ROM, NGOs should not fail to take into account what is currently occurring in the clinical sector. How an outcome measure in a clinical service would interface with an outcome measure in an NGO for a particular consumer is a question that remains unanswered (Te Pou, 2006). Choosing an OM tool that does not have a level of credibility or acceptance or is unfamiliar to the clinical sector may have ramifications for the NGO–clinical relationship.

The NGO sector is less well resourced than the clinical sector and lack of resources and funding is often cited as the inhibiting factor when it comes to being required to do different or additional work. This is even more acutely felt by small organizations that do not have the economies of scale of large NGOs or clinical services. NGOs generally do not have the level of IT infrastructure to support rapid and efficient input and output of outcomes data. In fact NGOs do not have access to a central database in the way that clinical services do and where they do have electronic client databases they are organization-specific and OM data from different NGOs cannot be compared.

Certainly, additional funding for staff training in order to develop OM skills and culture in the sector would provide an enormous impetus but it should also be acknowledged that requiring staff to undertake ROM can actually assist them to think more analytically about their role. Some organizations are concerned that their staff may not have the skills to rate OM tools and have cited this as a reason not to require staff ratings. This approach denies staff the opportunity to develop skills and expertise through practical experience of OM.

ROM does not currently hold a strong place in consumer culture and a challenge for NGOs is to maintain their established connection with consumers whilst being clear about the benefit of ROM for staff and consumers and ensuring it informs staff practice. This will require acknowledgement that OM is part of the *real work* with consumers, that OM in NGOs is about maintaining a focus on the social model of health rather than a medical model. It also requires a system to be put in place that ensures feedback is provided to staff and consumers and that the practice is kept fresh through training and supervision.

Simplistic thinking that OM *is* evaluation rather than incorporating OM into a broader evaluation system needs to be overcome, as does too much focus on the actual OM tools. When there is an over-emphasis on the tool rather than the process and practice that needs to be wrapped around it, workers can become distracted by constantly searching for a better tool.

The issues around attribution have remained problematic and unresolved. While ROM can contribute to the quality and rigour of their work, NGOs want to be able to use ROM to demonstrate their effectiveness. Many NGOs already collect a range of qualitative and quantitative information on service outputs and consumer outcomes; for example, Individual Service Plans, goal setting and attainment, case notes, attendance records, type of service use and hours of service provided. All of the above can contribute to a body of evidence of service effectiveness. ROM can form an important supplement to this evidence but given the complexity of the mental health system and of the needs of consumers, ROM should not be viewed as a 'quick fix' that enables a consumer outcome to be attributed to an NGO intervention.

Implementing outcome measurement in NGOs

NGOs that have implemented ROM have learned valuable lessons from the experience and many, given their time again, would do things differently. The following is a compilation of feedback and advice from NGOs who have been through the process of developing and implementing ROM in their services.

In contemplating the implementation of ROM, organizations should first assess and acknowledge what information they are already collecting that contributes to the overall picture and how this information can be used to track consumer outcomes, community outcomes, service outcomes and service outputs. Undertaking this process will require clarifying the aims of the service and deciding what effectiveness means in this context. This is a useful starting point for identifying what gaps exist and where ROM may best complement the current data set (Slade, 2002, Australian Institute for Primary Care, 2003).

Researching the literature and talking to other NGOs can assist in clarifying what tools are available and what it is that you want to measure. In contemplating designing and developing a new tool rather than using an existing one, NGOs should be aware of the enormous amount of time and resources required to achieve such an undertaking and ask themselves whether the additional expenditure is justified.

Many NGOs would recommend that consumers and staff are broadly consulted for any change process, including being involved in tool selection and the implementation process. Pragmatic decisions need to be made in selecting an appropriate tool and compromises need to be made between how comprehensive a tool is and choosing a tool that is concise and easy to use, is directly linked to the work and able to be integrated into everyday practice. It is also worth considering the acceptability and credibility of a tool for key partners and to the broader mental health sector.

Managers need to be prepared to drive the organizational change and to engage staff and consumers in the change process through the key messages that ROM is:

- about continuous quality improvement
- about evidence and credibility
- everyone's responsibility, and
- a core skill in contemporary mental health services.

The change needs to be supported by ongoing training, data collection and information systems (electronic databases) and mechanisms for the feedback of results to staff and consumers.

The future for outcome measurement in NGOs

Where it has actually been implemented, ROM in NGOs is mostly in its infancy. Very few NGOs have been conducting ROM for longer than 3 years. A survey of 232 New Zealand NGOs found that only 21 (9.1%) were using an OM tool (Te Pou, 2006) and in the state of New South Wales in Australia only 5% of NGOs are experienced in using validated outcome measures routinely (Penrose-Wall, 2006).

The NGO sector's lack of experience in and limited capacity to undertake research and lack of strong connections with research institutions severely reduce the likelihood that the diverse OM practices will be critically evaluated or the learning disseminated in a way that informs the sector. This in a sense simply mirrors the history of a sector that has felt undervalued, underfunded and overlooked in comparison to the clinical mental health sector.

While a general failure to mandate ROM in NGOs allows diversity and experimentation, it precludes the possibility of benchmarking and service system planning from data being collected. On the other hand there is a growing recognition by governments of the value and the capacity of the NGO sector and in many jurisdictions governments have a commitment to grow the sector. This must inevitably be accompanied by increased levels of accountability, including requirements to undertake and report on ROM.

While there is no reason to think that much will change in the immediate future, many NGOs hope for:

- more work and leadership to come from the sector on OM
- a holistic approach and greater sophistication in OM
- greater consistency in approach to OM
- OM to become accepted and embedded within the NGO culture
- agreed uniform tools to be mandated
- better integration of NGO OM with clinical OM, and
- resourcing from government for systems to enable reporting and analysis of OM data.

The Victorian Mental Health Reform Strategy requires the NGO sector to become more closely coordinated with clinical services, without losing its distinctive approach, and to become less fragmented and clearer about the scope of its activities (Mental Health and Drugs Division, 2009). While the literature suggests that mandating OM in mental health services does not necessarily achieve high levels of compliance (Trauer, 2004, Pirkis et al., 2005), a systematic approach to ROM across both the clinical and NGO sectors could assist the joint planning necessary to achieve the above agenda.

If government funding departments demand more from NGOs by mandating a uniform system for ROM, opportunities may be created to further develop and consolidate the NGO sector through the analysis and research that becomes possible with consolidated consumer outcome data.

References

Andresen, R., Caputi, P. and Oades, L. G. (2000). Interrater reliability of the Camberwell Assessment of Need Short Appraisal Schedule. *Australian and New Zealand Journal of Psychiatry*, **34**, 856–61.

Arns, P., Rogers, S., Cook, J., Mowbray, C. and Members of the IAPSRS Research Committee (2001). The IAPSRS Toolkit: Development, utility and relation to other performance measurement systems. *Psychiatric Rehabilitation Journal* **25**, 43–52.

Australian Institute for Primary Care (2003). *Improving Services through Consumer Population Outcome Measurement in PDRSS*. Melbourne: La Trobe University.

Cornish, D., Tobias, G., Farhall, J., Trauer, T. and Slade, M. (2005). Consumer/key worker/case manager/ perception of need – enhancing dialogue to improve outcomes. In K. Kellehear, M. Teesson, V. Miller et al., eds., *The Mental Health Services Conference, Gold Coast*. Sydney: TheMHS.

Crowe, T. P., Couley, A., Diaz, P. and Humphries, S. (2007). The adoption of recovery-based practice: the organisation's journey. *New Paradigm*, June, 51–7.

Eisen, S. V., Wilcox, M., Leff, H. S., Schaefer, E. and Culhane, M. A. (1999). Assessing behavioral health outcomes in outpatient programs: reliability and validity of the BASIS-32. *Journal of Behavioral Health Services & Research*, **26**, 5–17.

Giffort, D., Schmook, A., Woody, C., Vollendorf, C. and Gervain, M. (1995). *Construction of a scale to measure consumer recovery*, Springfield, IL: Illinois Office of Mental Health.

Goodman, S. H., Sewell, D. R., Cooley, E. L. and Leavitt, N. (1993). Assessing levels of adaptive functioning: the Role Functioning Scale. *Community Mental Health Journal*, **29**, 119–31.

Guthrie, D., McIntosh, M., Callaly, T., Trauer, T. and Coombs, T. (2008). Consumer attitudes towards the use of routine outcome measures in a public mental health service: a consumer-driven study. *International Journal of Mental Health Nursing*, **17**, 92–7.

Helyer, K., Tobias, G. and Trauer, T. (2008). Lessons learned from using routine outcome measurement in a psychiatric disability rehabilitation and support service. In K. Kellehear, V. Miller, L. Dunbar et al., eds., *The Mental Health Services Conference, Melbourne*. Sydney: TheMHS.

Jones, S. H., Thornicroft, G., Coffey, M. and Dunn, G. (1995). A brief mental health outcome scale: reliability and validity of the Global Assessment of Functioning (GAF). *British Journal of Psychiatry*, **166**, 654–9.

Kessler, R. C., Andrews, G., Colpe, L. J., et al. (2002). Short screening scales to monitor population prevalences and trends in nonspecific psychological distress. *Psychological Medicine*, **32**, 959–76.

Markovitz, P. (1996). *The Avon Mental Health Measure*. Bristol: Changing Minds.

Mental Health and Drugs Division (2009). *Because mental health matters: Victorian Mental Health Reform Strategy 2009-2019*. Melbourne: Department of Human Services.

Oades, L., Deane, F., Crowe, T., et al. (2005). Collaborative recovery: an integrative model for working with individuals who experience chronic and recurring mental illness. *Australasian Psychiatry*, **13**, 279–84.

Oades, L. G., Crowe, T. P. and Nguyen, M. (2009). Leadership coaching transforming mental health systems from the inside out.

International Coaching Psychology Review, **4**, 25–36.

Penrose-Wall, J. (2006). *Mapping the Difference We Make: Non-Government organisation use of routine consumer outcome evaluation in providing mental health care in NSW.* Sydney: Mental Health Coordinating Council of NSW.

Phelan, M., Slade, M., Thornicroft, G., et al. (1995). The Camberwell Assessment of Need: the validity and reliability of an instrument to assess the needs of people with severe mental illness. *British Journal of Psychiatry*, **167**, 589–95.

Pirkis, J., Burgess, P., Coombs, T., et al. (2005). Routine measurement of outcomes in Australia's public sector mental health services. *Australia and New Zealand Health Policy*, **2**, 8.

Ridgway, P. and Press, A. (2004). *Assessing the recovery-orientation of your mental health program: A user's guide for the Recovery-Enhancing Environment scale (REE). Version 1.* Lawrence, KS: University of Kansas, School of Social Welfare, Office of Mental Health Training and Research.

Ronnau, P., Papakotsias, A. and Tobias, G. (2008). 'Not for' sector in community mental health care defines itself and strives for quality. *Australian Journal of Primary Health*, **14**, 68–72.

Rosen, A., Hadzi-Pavlovic, D. and Parker, G. (1989). The Life Skills Profile: a measure assessing function and disability in schizophrenia. *Schizophrenia Bulletin*, **15**, 325–37.

Slade, M. (2002). What outcomes to measure in routine mental health services, and how to assess them: a systematic review. *Australian and New Zealand Journal of Psychiatry*, **36**, 743–53.

Slade, M., Gillard, M., Kuipers, E., Leese, M. and Thornicroft, G. (2004). The impact of mental health on the quality of life: are unmet needs the mediator? *Acta Psychiatrica Scandinavica*, **110** (S421), 57.

St Luke's Anglicare Mental Health Services (2007). *Growing Well Kit*, Bendigo, Victoria: La Trobe University Social Work & Innovative Resources.

Te Pou (2006). *NgOIT 2005 Landscape Survey.* Auckland: Te Pou o Te Whakaaro Nui, The National Centre of Mental Health Research and Workforce Development.

The WHOQOL Group (1995). The World Health Organization quality of life assessment (WHOQOL): position paper from the World Health Organization. *Social Science and Medicine*, **41**, 1403–9.

Trauer, T. (2004). Consumer and service determinants of completion of a consumer self-rating outcome measure. *Australasian Psychiatry*, **12**, 48–54.

Trauer, T. and Tobias, G. (2004). The Camberwell Assessment of Need and Behaviour and Symptom Identification Scale as routine outcome measures in a psychiatric disability rehabilitation and support service. *Community Mental Health Journal*, **40**, 211–21.

Trauer, T., Tobias, G. and Slade, M. (2008). Development and evaluation of a patient-rated version of the Camberwell Assessment of Need Short Appraisal Schedule (CANSAS-P). *Community Mental Health Journal*, **44**, 113–24.

Victorian Department of Human Services (2004). *Measuring Consumer Outcomes: Guidelines for PDRSS.* Melbourne: Mental Health and Drugs Division.

Wennström, E., Berglund, L., Lindbäck, J. and Wiesel, F. (2008). Deconstructing the 'black box' of the Camberwell assessment of need score in mental health services evaluation. *Social Psychiatry and Psychiatric Epidemiology*, **43**, 714–19.

Wiersma, D. (2006). Needs of people with severe mental illness. *Acta Psychiatrica Scandinavica Supplementum*, **113**, 115–19.

Wiersma, D., van den Brink, R., Wolters, K., et al. (2009). Individual unmet needs for care: are they sensitive as outcome criterion for the effectiveness of mental health services interventions? *Social Psychiatry and Psychiatric Epidemiology*, **44**, 317–24.

Wing, J. K., Beevor, A. S., Curtis, R. H., et al. (1998). Health of the Nation Outcome Scales (HoNOS). Research and development. *British Journal of Psychiatry*, **172**, 11–18.

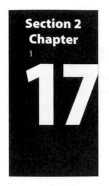

Outcome measurement in drug and alcohol services

Maree Teesson and Mark Deady

The primary aim of any health care service is to improve the health and functioning of the people it treats; it is no different in drug and alcohol services. Emphasis is increasingly being placed on the direct measurement of such health outcomes in drug and alcohol services across the world, using standard and agreed measures with proven reliability and validity. Indeed, the recent Institute of Medicine Committee on Quality of Health in America called for clinicians and organizations providing mental health and drug and alcohol services to increase their use of valid and reliable patient questionnaires or other patient-assessment instruments that are feasible for routine use to assess the progress and outcomes of treatment systematically (Institute of Medicine Committee on Quality of Health in America, 2006, p. 179).

Although outcome measurement is not new, at present there are few agreed consumer outcome measures in place in most fields, including in alcohol and drug treatment services. This chapter outlines the principles and issues of outcome measurement in the drug and alcohol field and reviews some of the most commonly used measures.

Drug and alcohol use disorders

Drug and alcohol use disorders (which include abuse and dependence of alcohol or other drugs) typically involve impaired control over the use of alcohol or drugs. Obtaining, using and recovering from drugs consume a disproportionate amount of the user's time, and the user continues to drink alcohol or use drugs in the face of problems that they know to be caused by it. Alcohol and drug abusers typically become tolerant to the effects of alcohol or drugs, requiring larger doses to achieve the desired psychological effect, and abrupt cessation of use often produces a withdrawal syndrome (Teesson et al., 2000b). Many alcohol or drug abusers experience other psychological and physical health problems, and their alcohol or drug use often adversely affects the lives of their spouses, children and other family members, friends and workmates.

The current Diagnostic and Statistical Manual of the American Psychiatric Association (DSM-IV-TR, American Psychiatric Association, 2000) has defined classes of drugs that may be part of a drug and alcohol use disorder. These are, in alphabetical order: alcohol, caffeine, cannabis, hallucinogens, heroin and other opiates, inhalants, nicotine, sedatives and stimulants (cocaine and amphetamines).

Drug and alcohol use disorders, from a public health perspective, are a significant risk factor for road traffic accidents, lost productivity, violence and diseases such as cancer, liver cirrhosis, brain damage and heart disease (Edwards et al., 1994). In developed countries, it is the second highest cause of disability in men aged 15–44 (Murray and Lopez, 1997). There are effective treatments available which will impact on these health consequences. The challenge is to apply the effective treatments efficiently.

Outcome Measurement in Mental Health: Theory and Practice, ed. Tom Trauer. Published by Cambridge University Press.
© Cambridge University Press 2010.

Who are the consumers of drug and alcohol treatment services?

A consistent picture on prevalence has emerged from the large US national epidemiological studies (Kessler et al., 1994, 2005) and the more recent world mental health survey consortium (Compton et al., 2007, Kessler and Wang, 2008), a picture that is congruent with available Australian data (Slade et al., 2009). In broad terms, 1 in 10 people in developed countries will have a drug and alcohol use disorder. The more severely affected of these people are the people toward whom effective treatments and outcome measurement should be directed. It is important to remember that only a minority of persons with drug and alcohol use disorders (fewer than one in five) seek treatment (Hall and Teesson, 2000).

Treatment can work for drug and alcohol use disorders

Despite the low treatment rates for alcohol and drug use disorders there is consistent evidence that treatments work (Teesson et al., 2002). The four largest studies conducted in the alcohol and drug field are the Drug and Alcohol Treatment Outcome Study (DATOS, Flynn et al., 2003), the California Drug and Alcohol Treatment Assessment project (CALDATA, Gerstein et al., 1994) in the United States, the National Treatment Outcome Study (NTORS, Gossop et al., 1998, Gossop et al., 2002) in the United Kingdom and the Australian Treatment Outcome Study in Australia (Teesson et al., 2006, 2008). These studies, which report on the treatment outcome of over 4000 individuals over 3 years, provide important information on the effectiveness of treatment under routine clinical conditions. The results of each study provide convincing support for the overall clinical and cost effectiveness of treatment for alcohol and other drug problems. Each study used commonly available measures of outcome, demonstrating the utility of such measures. The measures are all reviewed later in this chapter.

Why use standardized measures of outcome?

Clinicians use their clinical impressions as the main tool to continuously monitor and evaluate the outcome of their treatment for each patient. Similarly, consumers are constantly aware of their well-being. This informal assessment of outcome should guide clinicians towards desirable treatments and away from ineffectual treatments. The argument is therefore not 'why measure outcome', for everyone does at some level, but 'why attempt to introduce standardized measures of outcome?' The problem is that while clinical judgements are important and necessary, they have repeatedly been shown to be unreliable (Meehl, 1954).

Global judgements are equally fallible, simply because they are dominated by the clinician's recent experience of patients who they wrongly believe to be representative of all patients (Cohen and Cohen, 1984). In reality, the patients who are seen most often are those who are slow to improve, whilst assessment of the entire patient group would generally reveal a much better outcome. Having accurate information about outcome is therefore important to good clinical care. Standardizing the content and scoring of outcome measures ensures their validity and comparability across services and settings. Obtaining standardized responses to standardized questions is an efficient way to measure health, in part because results from many different studies and locations can be collated when standardized measures are used. The repeated measurement of symptoms, disability and risk factors using standardized measures is likely to improve treatment as well as provide the information necessary for identifying the outcome of treatment.

Our own research shows support for outcome measurement in the drug and alcohol field. Teesson and colleagues (2000a) surveyed 58 government and non-government alcohol and other drug treatment services across Australia regarding outcome measurement and 42 surveys were received completed. The survey covered three main questions: the importance of measurement of different areas of drug and alcohol treatment outcome, importance of methods of assessment, and the uses of outcome measurement. Importance is rated on a five-point scale from '1' (not important) to '5' (extremely important). Five assessment formats were rated covering questionnaires completed by the consumer, clinician or family member, an interview with the consumer and a rating scale completed by the clinician. A range of 'uses of information obtained from outcome measurement' were also assessed and include: to inform the clinician about progress of the consumer, to inform the consumer about their own progress, to assess the efficacy of treatment services, to make funding decisions about services, and an 'other' option. It was found that the use of alcohol and other drugs (quantity/frequency) and functioning were considered to be the most important areas for outcome evaluation. 'Clinician-rated questionnaire' or 'interview with the client' were rated as the preferred methods and respondents stated that the collection of such data would improve the effectiveness of treatment. Overall, outcome measurement on average was viewed as somewhat to extremely important (Teesson et al., 2000a).

Outcome measures in drug and alcohol

We have previously reviewed the literature on outcome measures (Teesson et al., 2000a). In this chapter we have updated that review and have presented the details of the four most prominent measures for routine outcome measurement in drug and alcohol services. Our assessment of the measures used the following criteria for rating of outcome measures:

Applicable and acceptable: the measures were assessed as to whether they address useful dimensions which are important to outcome and the consumer (drug use, disability, consumer satisfaction) and useful for the clinician in clinical treatment.

Brief and practical: the measure should be brief, there should be minimal cost involved in its use, the scoring and the interpretation of the data should be simple, training in the use of the measure and the interpretation of the data should be minimal and instructions should be available.

Reliable: measures should have acceptable psychometric properties so that sensible conclusions can be drawn from the results of measures at the level of the individual consumer and at the level of aggregated data. Reliability, validity and sensitivity to change are properties required by all outcome measures; the acceptable levels of each of these depend on the purpose of the measurement.

One particular issue for the drug and alcohol field is the reliability of self-reports of drug and alcohol use in the context of the stigma and discrimination associated with such use. Largely, concern relates to the accuracy of self-report among illicit drug users since there is a legal constraint that may be thought to bias truthful responding. However, there is really no other satisfactory or feasible method to attain such information relating to criminal and risk-taking behaviours and drug use. Darke (2010) suggests that there are two main concerns which are the cause of this apprehension. First, there is an anecdotal belief that all drug users are inherently pathological liars. Second, the illegal and socially stigmatized nature of the activities and behaviours being investigated is likely to discourage accurate reporting. In light of these obvious concerns, extensive research has been conducted in this area and self-report has been consistently found to be both highly valid and reliable (Weatherby et al., 1994, Harrison and Hughes, 1997, Darke, 1998, Welp et al., 2003, Jackson et al., 2004).

Valid: four types of validity are relevant: face validity, content validity, criterion related validity and construct validity.

Sensitivity to change: the measure is sensitive to change if change on the measure also reflects change in some external criterion.

In summary, measures which are suitable for use in routine clinical practice are likely to be brief, low-cost, multidimensional measures which require minimal training in their administration, scoring and interpretation, but which are sufficiently reliable, valid and sensitive to change to indicate outcome of the therapeutic intervention. Details of the four measures identified in the literature as best meeting these requirements are listed below; all are available in the public domain.

Opiate Treatment Index (OTI)

The Opiate Treatment Index (OTI) (Darke et al., 1991) is a structured interview primarily developed to allow comparability between research findings. It is an appropriate measure across all drug classes, including alcohol (Darke et al., 1992). The OTI can be administered without any specific training and takes approximately 20–40 minutes to complete. The OTI measures six independent outcome domains: drug use, HIV risk-taking behaviour, social functioning, criminality, health status and psychological adjustment as measured by the GHQ-28.

The OTI was originally validated in an Australian opiate treatment setting in 1992 and demonstrated high levels of test–retest reliability and validity (Darke et al., 1992). The OTI has also been found to be sensitive to changes in drug and alcohol behaviour over time (Baker et al., 2001, 2002, Shearer et al., 2001, Padaiga et al., 2007, Verthein et al., 2008).

Although initially developed for opioid use (Darke et al., 1992) the OTI is effective when used across licit (including alcohol) and illicit drugs (Mattick and Hall, 1993, Barrowcliff et al., 1999). It has been translated into a range of languages (e.g. Ruz et al., 1998, Swift et al., 1999, Liu et al., 2000) and has been used effectively with people with serious mental illness and substance use problems in inner-city Sydney (Teesson and Gallagher, 1999) and more widely across Australia (Baker et al., 2002). The OTI has also been used in adolescent and young adult populations (Spooner et al., 2001, Mills et al., 2004).

The Maudsley Addiction Profile (MAP)

The Maudsley Addiction Profile (MAP) (Marsden et al., 1998) was developed in the UK as a brief, multi-dimensional instrument for assessing treatment outcome for people with drug and/or alcohol problems. It is easily administered at intake, during and after an index treatment episode. It covers four domains of substance use, health risk behaviour, physical and psychological health and personal social functioning. The MAP consists of 60 questions and preliminary studies found the interviewer version to take approximately 12–25 minutes to complete.

In the initial sample of 60 drug users and 80 alcohol users, reliability and concurrent validity assessments of the scales were found to be moderate to good. Recently, the Treatment Outcomes Profile (TOP) was developed as a brief alternative to the MAP and has only 20 items and four sections (offending, health and social functioning, substance use and health risk behaviour). The preliminary report on the TOP has found the measure to have good reliability and validity and to show adequate sensitivity to client change (Marsden et al., 2008).

The MAP has been translated and validated in a number of different European countries (Marsden et al., 2000b, Mandersen et al., 2001, Gerevich et al., 2004, Hernández and Gómez,

2004, Bacskai et al., 2005). In a sample of 124 subjects in Italy, Spain and Portugal, the internal and test–retest reliabilities of the MAP were satisfactory (Marsden et al., 2000b).

The tool has also been used successfully in psychiatric/comorbid populations (Marsden et al., 2000a, Miles et al., 2003). One study has used the MAP on a population of adolescents aged between 14 and 16 years (Best et al., 2006).

The Addiction Severity Index (ASI)

The Addiction Severity Index (ASI, McLellan et al., 1980, 1992) was developed in the USA and is one of the most commonly used standardized assessment (rather than screening) instruments in the field of substance use disorders. The ASI is a 155-item multidimensional structured interview for assessing alcohol and drug dependence. Administration of the interview form takes between 30 and 60 minutes. While the ASI has been used frequently in research, its length has been a barrier to routine implementation. The ASI consists of seven sub-scales assessing past 30 day and lifetime alcohol use, drug use, medical problems, psychiatric problems, family/social problems, employment and legal problems.

A modified short version the ASI has also been developed and has shown promising results (Cacciola et al., 2007). A recently developed self-administered pen and paper version was found to have good internal consistency for the alcohol, drug, psychiatric and medical problem scales (Rosen et al., 2000). A computer program has been developed to assist with administration and scoring (McLellan et al., 1992).

The ASI has been generally found to have good reliability and validity; however, a recent review of 37 studies indicated that the psychometric performance of the ASI may be problematic (Mäkelä 2004). The authors of the ASI have pointed out that the omission of a number of studies may have led to somewhat biased conclusions in this review (McLellan et al., 2004).

The ASI has been validated and is frequently used across a variety of substance-abusing populations, including psychiatric patients, homeless people, pregnant women and incarcerated prisoners, and has been used to assess treatment outcome across a range of substances, including opiates, cocaine and alcohol (McLellan et al., 1992, Joyner et al., 1996). In psychiatric populations the general conclusion drawn from most individual studies and research summaries is that many of the sub-scales perform poorly with people who have severe mental illness (Carey et al., 1997). The ASI has been translated into a range of languages and evaluated across a range of countries (Krenz et al., 2004, Gerevich et al., 2005, Schmidt et al., 2007). An adolescent version of the ASI (the Teen-ASI) is available and preliminary studies show it to be a promising measure of adolescent drug abuse (Kaminer et al., 1991, 1993, Kaminer, 2008).

Brief Treatment Outcome Measure (BTOM)

The Brief Treatment Outcome Measure (BTOM) (Lawrinson et al., 2003) is a tool developed specifically to routinely assess outcomes of treatment for clients receiving opioid maintenance pharmacotherapy (OMP) services and for use in treatment evaluation research. The BTOM takes 10–20 minutes to complete. Treatment outcome is measured by scales developed or adapted from other instruments across the domains of drug dependence (measured by SDS), blood-borne virus exposure risk, drug use, health, psychological functioning and social functioning (Lawrinson et al., 2003). It has been adopted for routine AOD treatment outcome monitoring in Australia.

The evaluation of the BTOM took place in 37 metropolitan, rural and prison OMP services in Australia, among 160 OMP clients. The reliability and concurrent validity of the BTOM was found to be satisfactory (Lawrinson et al., 2005, 2006). The BTOM is now implemented throughout New South Wales, Australia.

A shorter version of the BTOM, the Brief Treatment Outcome Measure – Concise (BTOM-C), is also available. The recently designed Australian Alcohol Treatment Outcome Measure (AATOM) was developed as an equivalent alcohol tool. Two versions of the AATOM exist, one intended for use amongst clinicians for the purpose of routine treatment outcome monitoring (AATOM-C) and one for use amongst researchers (AATOM-R). In the initial sample of clients from AOD treatment agencies, the reliability of the AATOM-C was good to excellent for most scales. The results of the study demonstrate that the AATOM-C is, overall, a valid and reliable instrument, taking on average 10–15 minutes to administer (Simpson et al., 2007). The instrument also demonstrated the ability to measure change in client functioning over time (Simpson et al., 2009).

Simpson and colleagues (2007) emphasize the importance of comprehensive and consistent training of those who are to administer the AATOM-C and this is a limitation for routine implementation of this measure.

Summary

The measurement of outcome in drug and alcohol services is gaining increasing attention. We have reviewed the most frequently used and best performing outcome measures in this field. To date, no agreed measures of outcome have been implemented. However, new and promising development work towards outcome measurement on a national level in the UK and Australia has begun.

References

American Psychiatric Association (2000). *Diagnostic and Statistical Manual of Mental Disorders, Fourth Edition, Text Revision*. Washington DC: American Psychiatric Association.

Bacskai, E., Rozsa, S. and Gerevich, J. (2005). Clinical experiences with the Maudsley Addiction Profile (MAP) among heroin addicts. *Orvosi Hetilap*, **146**, 1635–9.

Baker, A., Boggs, T. G. and Lewin, T. J. (2001). Randomized controlled trial of brief cognitive-behavioural interventions among regular users of amphetamine. *Addiction*, **96**, 1279–87.

Baker, A., Lewin, T., Reichler, H., et al. (2002). Evaluation of a motivational interview for substance use within psychiatric in-patient services. *Addiction*, **97**, 1329–37.

Barrowcliff, A., Champney-Smith, J. and McBride, A. J. (1999). Use of a modified version of the Opiate Treatment Index with amphetamine users: validation and pilot evaluation of a prescribing service. *Journal of Substance Abuse*, **4**, 98–103.

Best, D., Manning, V., Gossop, M., Gross, S. and Strang, J. (2006). Excessive drinking and other problem behaviours among 14–16 year old schoolchildren. *Addictive Behaviors*, **31**, 1424–35.

Cacciola, J. S., Alterman, A. I., McLellan, A. T., Lin, Y.-T. and Lynch, K. G. (2007). Initial evidence for the reliability and validity of a 'Lite' version of the Addiction Severity Index. *Drug and Alcohol Dependence*, **87**, 297–302.

Carey, K. B., Cocco, K. M. and Correia, C. J. (1997). Reliability and validity of the Addiction Severity Index among outpatients with severe mental illness. *Psychological Assessment*, **9**, 422–8.

Cohen, P. and Cohen, J. (1984). The clinician's illusion. *Archives of General Psychiatry*, **41**, 1178–82.

Compton, W. M., Thomas, Y. F., Stinson, F. S. and Grant, B. F. (2007). Prevalence, correlates, disability, and comorbidity of

DSM-IV drug abuse and dependence in the United States: results from the national epidemiologic survey on alcohol and related conditions. *Archives of General Psychiatry*, **64**, 566–76.

Darke, S. (1998). Self-report among injecting drug users. *Drug and Alcohol Dependence*, **51**, 253–63.

Darke, S. (2010). Scales for research in the addictions. In P. G. Miller, J. Strang and P. M. Miller, eds., *Addiction Research Methods*. London: Wiley-Blackwell.

Darke, S., Ward, J., Hall, W., Heather, N. and Wodak, A. (1991). *The Opiate Treatment Index (OTI) Manual*. Sydney: Australia.

Darke, S., Hall, W., Wodak, A., Heather, N. and Ward, J. (1992). Development and validation of a multi-dimensional instrument for assessing outcome of treatment among opiate users: the Opiate Treatment Index. *British Journal of Addiction*, **87**, 733–42.

Edwards, G., Anderson, P., Babor, T. F., et al. (1994). *Alcohol Policy and the Public Good*. Oxford: Oxford University Press.

Flynn, P. M., Joe, G. W., Broome, K. M., Simpson, D. D. and Brown, B. S. (2003). Recovery from opioid addiction in DATOS. *Journal of Substance Abuse Treatment*, **25**, 177–86.

Gerevich, J., Bácskai, E. and Rózsa, S. (2004). Hungarian validation of Maudsley Addiction Profile (MAP). *Psychiatria Hungarica*, **19**, 123–30.

Gerevich, J., Bácskai, E., Kó, J. and Rózsa, S. (2005). Reliability and validity of the Hungarian version of the European Addiction Severity Index. *Psychopathology*, **38**, 301–9.

Gerstein, D. R., Johnson, R. A., Harwood, H. J., et al. (1994). *Evaluation Recovery Services: The California Drug and Alcohol Treatment Assessment (CALDATA)*. Sacramento, CA.

Gossop, M., Marsden, J., Stewart, D., et al. (1998). Substance use, health and social problems of service users at 54 drug treatment agencies. Intake data from the National Treatment Outcome Research Study. *British Journal of Psychiatry*, **173**, 166–71.

Gossop, M., Marsden, J., Stewart, D. and Treacy, S. (2002). Change and stability of change after treatment of drug misuse: 2 year outcomes from the National Treatment Outcome Research Study (UK). *Addictive Behaviors*, **27**, 155–66.

Hall, W. and Teesson, M. (2000). Alcohol-use disorders: who should be treated and how? In G. Andrews and S. Henderson, eds., *Unmet Need in Psychiatry: Problems, Resources, Responses*. Cambridge: Cambridge University Press.

Harrison, L. and Hughes, A. (1997). *The Validity of Self-Reported Drug Use: Improving the Accuracy of Survey Estimates*. Rockville, MD: US Department of Health and Human Services: National Institutes of Health.

Hernández, M. Á. T. and Gómez, C. F. (2004). Spanish validation of the Maudsley Addiction Profile (MAP). *Adicciones*, **16**, 267–75.

Institute of Medicine Committee on Quality of Health in America (2006). *Improving the Quality of Health Care for Mental and Substance Use Conditions*. Washington DC: National Academies Press Report.

Jackson, C. T., Covell, N. H., Frisman, L. K. and Essock, S. M. (2004). Validity of self-reported drug use among people with co-occurring mental health and substance use disorders. *Journal of Dual Diagnosis*, **1**, 49–63.

Joyner, L. M., Wright, J. D. and Devine, J. A. (1996). Reliability and validity of the addiction severity index among homeless substance misusers. *Substance Use & Misuse*, **31**, 729–51.

Kaminer, Y. (2008). The Teen Addiction Severity Index around the globe: the Tower of Babel revisited. *Substance Abuse*, **29**, 89–94.

Kaminer, Y., Bukstein, O. and Tarter, R. E. (1991). The Teen-Addiction Severity Index: rationale and reliability. *International Journal on Addictions*, **26**, 219–26.

Kaminer, Y., Wagner, E., Plummer, B. and Seifer, R. (1993). Validation of the Teen Addiction Severity Index (T-ASI). Preliminary findings. *American Journal on Addictions*, **2**, 250–4.

Kessler, R. C. and Wang, P. S. (2008). The descriptive epidemiology of commonly occurring mental disorders in the United States. *Annual Review of Public Health*, **29**, 115–29.

Kessler, R. C., McGonagle, K. A., Zhao, S., et al. (1994). Lifetime and 12-month prevalence of DSM-III-R psychiatric disorders in the United States. Results from the National Comorbidity Survey. *Archives of General Psychiatry*, **51**, 8–19.

Kessler, R. C., Chiu, W. T., Demler, O. and Walters, E. E. (2005). Prevalence, severity, and comorbidity of 12-month DSM-IV disorders in the National Comorbidity Survey Replication. *Archives of General Psychiatry*, **62**, 617–27.

Krenz, S., Dieckmann, S., Favrat, B., et al. (2004). French version of the Addiction Severity Index (5th Edition): validity and reliability among Swiss opiate-dependent patients. *European Addiction Research*, **10**, 173–9.

Lawrinson, P., Copeland, J. and Indig, D. (2003). *The Brief Treatment Outcome Measure: Opioid Maintenance Pharmacotherapy (BTOM) Manual*. Sydney.

Lawrinson, P., Copeland, J. and Indig, D. (2005). Development and validation of a brief instrument for routine outcome monitoring in opioid maintenance pharmacotherapy services: the brief treatment outcome measure (BTOM). *Drug and Alcohol Dependence*, **80**, 125–33.

Lawrinson, P., Copeland, J. and Indig, D. (2006). Regional differences in injecting practices and other substance use-related behaviour among entrants into opioid maintenance pharmacotherapy treatment in New South Wales, Australia. *Drug and Alcohol Dependence*, **82**, S95–S102.

Liu, Z., Lian, Z., Zhou, W., et al. (2000). A preliminary study on the severity of drug addiction in drug abusers. *Chinese Mental Health Journal*, **14**, 231–4.

Mäkelä, K. (2004). Studies of the reliability and validity of the Addiction Severity Index. *Addiction*, **99**, 398–410.

Mandersen, J., Nizzoli, U., Corbelli, C., et al. (2001). Reliability of the Maudsley Addiction Profile ERIT Version (MAP) and the Treatment Perceptions Questionnaire (TPQ) in Italy, Spain and Portugal for the evaluation of treatments. *Adicciones*, **13**, 217–27.

Marsden, J., Gossop, M., Stewart, D., et al. (1998). The Maudsley Addiction Profile (MAP): a brief instrument for assessing treatment outcome. *Addiction*, **93**, 1857–68.

Marsden, J., Gossop, M., Stewart, D., Rolfe, A. and Farrell, M. (2000a). Psychiatric symptoms among clients seeking treatment for drug dependence. Intake data from the National Treatment Outcome Research Study. *British Journal of Psychiatry*, **176**, 285–9.

Marsden, J., Nizzoli, U., Corbelli, C., et al. (2000b). New European instruments for treatment outcome research: reliability of the Maudsley Addiction Profile and treatment perceptions questionnaire in Italy, Spain and Portugal. *European Addiction Research*, **6**, 115–22.

Marsden, J., Farrell, M., Bradbury, C., et al. (2008). Development of the treatment outcomes profile. *Addiction*, **103**, 1450–60.

Mattick, R. P. and Hall, W. (1993). *A Treatment Outline for Approaches to Opioid Dependence*. Canberra: AGPS.

McLellan, A., Luborsky, L., Woody, G. and O'Brien, C. (1980). An improved diagnostic evaluation instrument for substance abuse patients. The Addiction Severity Index. *Journal of Nervous and Mental Disease*, **168**, 26–33.

McLellan, A. T., Kushner, H., Metzger, D., et al. (1992). The fifth edition of the Addiction Severity Index. *Journal of Substance Abuse Treatment*, **9**, 199–213.

McLellan, A. T., Cacciola, J. S. and Alterman, A. I. (2004). Commentaries on Mäkelä: the ASI as a still developing instrument: response to Mäkelä. *Addiction*, **99**, 411–12.

Meehl, P. E. (1954). *Clinical versus Statistical Prediction: A Theoretical Analysis and a Review of the Evidence*. Minneapolis: University of Minnesota Press.

Miles, H., Johnson, S., Amponsah-Afuwape, S., et al. (2003). Characteristics of subgroups of individuals with psychotic illness and a comorbid substance use disorder. *Psychiatry Services*, **54**, 554–61.

Mills, K. L., Teesson, M., Darke, S., Ross, J. and Lynskey, M. (2004). Young people with heroin dependence: findings from the Australian Treatment Outcome Study (ATOS). *Journal of Substance Abuse Treatment*, **27**, 67–73.

Murray, C. J. L. and Lopez, A. D. (1997). Alternative projections of mortality and disability by cause 1990–2020: global burden of disease study. *Lancet*, **349**, 1498–504.

Padaiga, Z., Subata, E. and Vanagas, G. (2007). Outpatient methadone maintenance treatment program. Quality of life and health of opioid-dependent persons in Lithuania. *Medicina (Kaunas, Lithuania)*, **43**, 235–41.

Rosen, C. S., Henson, B. R., Finney, J. W. and Moos, R. H. (2000). Consistency of self-administered and interview-based Addiction Severity Index composite scores. *Addiction*, **95**, 419–25.

Ruz, F. I., Gonzalez, S. F. and Ruiz, A. F. (1998). Drug dependent patients in the methadone maintenance program: evaluation in primary care of psychosocial and organic severity. *Aten Primaria*, **21**, 384–8.

Schmidt, P., Küfner, H., Hasemann, S., et al. (2007). Ist der European Addiction Severity Index ein sinnvolles disgnoseinstrument bei alkhollabhängigkeit? [Is the European Addiction Severity Index a useful tool in the diagnostic routines of alcohol dependence?] *Fortschritte der Neurologie, Psychiatrie*, **75**, 541–8.

Shearer, J., Wodak, A., Mattick, R. P., et al. (2001). Pilot randomized controlled study of dexamphetamine substitution for amphetamine dependence. *Addiction*, **96**, 1289–96.

Simpson, M., Lawrinson, P., Copeland, J. and Gates, P. (2007). *The Australian Alcohol Treatment Outcome Measure (AATOM-C): Psychometric Properties*. Sydney: National Drug and Alcohol Research Centre.

Simpson, M., Lawrinson, P., Copeland, J. and Gates, P. (2009). The Alcohol Treatment

Outcome Measure (ATOM): a new clinical tool for standardising outcome measurement for alcohol treatment. *Addictive Behaviors*, **34**, 121–4.

Slade, T., Johnston, A., Oakley Browne M. A. , Andrews, G. and Whiteford, H. (2009). 2007 National Survey of Mental Health and Wellbeing: methods and key findings. *Australian and New Zealand Journal of Psychiatry*, **43**, 594–605.

Spooner, C., Mattick, R. P. and Noffs, W. (2001). Outcomes of a comprehensive treatment program for adolescents with a substance-use disorder. *Journal of Substance Abuse Treatment*, **20**, 205–13.

Swift, W., Maher, L. and Sunjic, S. (1999). Transitions between routes of heroin administration: a study of Caucasian and Indochinese heroin users in south-western Sydney, Australia. *Addiction*, **94**, 71–82.

Teesson, M. and Gallagher, J. (1999). Evaluation of a treatment programme for serious mental illness and substance use in an inner city area. *Journal of Mental Health*, **8**, 19–28.

Teesson, M., Clement, N., Copeland, J., Conroy, A. and Reid, A. (2000a). *The Measurement of Outcome in Alcohol and Other Drug Treatment: A Review of Available Instruments*. Sydney: National Drug and Alcohol Research Centre.

Teesson, M., Hall, W., Lynskey, M. and Degenhardt, L. (2000b). Alcohol- and drug-use disorders in Australia: implications of the National Survey of Mental Health and Wellbeing. *Australian and New Zealand Journal of Psychiatry*, **34**, 206–13.

Teesson, M., Degenhardt, L. and Hall, W. (2002). *Addiction: Clinical Psychology Module*. Taylor Routledge.

Teesson, M., Ross, J., Darke, S., et al. (2006). One year outcomes for heroin dependence: Findings from The Australian Treatment Outcome Study (ATOS). *Drug and Alcohol Dependence*, **83**, 174–80.

Teesson, M., Mills, K., Ross, J., et al. (2008). The impact of treatment on 3 year outcomes for heroin dependence: findings from the Australian Treatment Outcome Study (ATOS). *Addiction*, **103**, 80–8.

Verthein, U., Bonorden-Kleij, K., Degkwitz, P., et al. (2008). Long-term effects of heroin-assisted treatment in Germany. *Addiction*, **103**, 960–6; discussion 967–8.

Weatherby, N. L., Needle, R., Cesari, H., et al. (1994). Validity of self-reported drug use among injection drug users and crack cocaine users recruited through street outreach. *Evaluation and Program Planning*, **17**, 347–55.

Welp, E. A., Bosman, I., Langendam, M. W., et al. (2003). Amount of self-reported illicit drug use compared to quantitative hair test results in community-recruited young drug users in Amsterdam. *Addiction*, **98**, 987–94.

Section 3

Current Issues in Outcome Measurement

18 Outcome measurement – applications and utility

Tom Trauer

Outcome measures (OMs) are collected in order to be used and to be useful. This chapter will survey the main uses to which OMs can be or have been put. One way to think of the applications and utility of OMs is by identifying who stands to benefit from them. There is at least potential utility to individuals in the following four groups:

- consumers, and their carers
- direct care providers, including clinicians
- service team leaders and managers, and
- policy makers and funders.

Consumers and carers

The areas in which OMs can be of most use and relevance to consumers and carers are in promoting dialogue with service providers, tracking the consumer's progress, identifying hidden problems and needs, and in promoting self-efficacy, empowerment and recovery.

(a) Promoting dialogue

Several studies have shown that many consumers are positive about OMs insofar as they promote communication and thereby enhance the quality of their care. Stedman et al. conducted focus groups with consumers, who thought OM could improve communication between mental health professionals and consumers (1997, p. 54). Graham et al. (2001) also reported on a series of focus groups, primarily around the issue of consumer self-assessment. There was general support for routine outcome assessments, which were seen as having potential to contribute to the treatment they receive. Key issues included 'how the consumer is approached for information, how outcome measurement is used to strengthen therapeutic dialogue and the use of consumer ratings in treatment planning' (p. 1). More specific concerns included: how their self-ratings will improve the treatment they receive; whether they will have access to the clinician's ratings; whether anonymity and confidentiality can be guaranteed; and how the possible negative impact of completing an assessment of one's own health will be dealt with. Similar concerns were raised in focus groups conducted by Bickman et al. (1998, p. 62 ff) in relation to OM with children and adolescents.

In a study spanning six countries (Priebe et al., 2007), keyworkers asked their patients with severe mental illness to rate their satisfaction with quality of life and treatment at regular intervals. Responses were fed back immediately on screen displays, compared with previous ratings and discussed. Patients receiving this intervention had better subjective quality of life, fewer unmet needs and higher treatment satisfaction after 12 months than patients who were randomized not to receive it. The authors concluded that:

> Gathering outcome data from a procedure that is meaningful to patients and clinicians and beneficial for the individual patient is more likely to be successful than conventional methods of routine outcome measurement in which outcomes are rated by patients outside clinical consultations and the results later made available to clinicians … The latter approach makes it difficult to determine whether the process of outcomes management had an impact on what clinicians and patients did in clinical consultations. Incorporating the assessment and feedback of outcomes into routine clinical encounters makes it more likely to have a direct impact on what happens in practice when clinicians and patients interact. (p. 425)

Guthrie et al. (2008) interviewed 50 consumers about their experiences with OMs. One-third felt they had not played an active part in the process, and about half of those who completed a self-rating instrument reported that their case manager had not discussed their responses with them. Nevertheless, two-thirds to three-quarters of the consumers felt that completing a self-rating instrument helped their case manager to understand them better and led to them receiving better care. Even though the instrument used (the Behaviour and Symptom Identification Scale: BASIS, Eisen, 1996) contains several intrusive questions, most consumers denied feeling afraid to answer any questions. Most of the consumers were unaware that their case managers were completing separate measures on them, and of those who were aware, two-thirds said that those results had not been discussed with them. The majority of those with whom those separate, clinician-rated, measures had been discussed said that they had found it useful.

(b) Tracking progress

The serial and systematic assessment of mental health status involved in routine OM is ideally suited to the tracking of progress, and most consumers have a keen interest in this, as have their carers and service providers. However, the different parties to a consumer's treatment may have different concepts of what constitutes progress, and even when they agree on which problem areas or life domains should be considered, they may perceive different degrees of change in the consumer.

Numerous studies attest to the low correlation between consumers' and service providers' assessments of illness severity and personal functioning. In two studies comparing adult consumer self-rated measures and provider measures, the correlations between the provider measures were 0.65 and 0.69, while the correlations between the consumer and the provider measures were much lower, between 0.13 and 0.36 (Stedman et al., 1997, Trauer, 2004, Analysis of outcome measurement data from the four Victorian 'Round One' agencies; unpublished report). Tobias and Trauer (2008) found that consumers identified significantly fewer unmet needs than their case managers or key workers. Hansson et al. (2001) and Hansen et al. (2002) reported similar findings. Since agreement between consumers and clinicians on simultaneous assessments tends to be modest, the chances that they will agree on changes in assessments between time points are likely to be as modest, or worse. Perhaps for this reason, most of the uses of OMs to track progress have relied on consumer measures, or clinician measures, but rarely both.

The most comprehensive and sophisticated system using a consumer measure to track progress in treatment was developed by Michael Lambert (see Chapter 6 in this book). Over an extensive programme of clinical research he and his colleagues have demonstrated that when routine self-assessments by consumers are fed back to their treating clinicians with indications of whether the progress is 'on track' or 'not on track', failing or problematic treatment can be quickly identified, and remedied. A similar system was described by Miller et al. (2005). Implementations of OM systems where consumers receive directly structured reports of their progress, however, are uncommon.

(c) Identifying hidden problems and needs

The identification of hidden problems and needs can occur when two or more parties independently rate the same consumer on the same instrument, and discrepancies arise. Certain instruments, such as the Strengths and Difficulties Questionnaire (SDQ, Goodman, 2001) and the Camberwell Assessment of Need (CAN, Phelan et al., 1995) are available in versions suitable for completion by children/youths, parent and teachers (SDQ) and consumers and service providers (CAN). Some limited work has also been done comparing the regular, provider-completed Health of the Nation Outcome Scales (HoNOS, Wing et al., 1998) with consumer-completed versions of the same scales (Trauer and Callaly, 2002, Stewart, 2009). Whenever one person identifies a particular problem or need and another does not, the possibility exists that the area that is a concern to one is hidden or out of the awareness of the other. While OMs can reveal differences in perception or understanding between consumers themselves and others, they cannot determine whose perception or understanding is correct. Indeed, it is unhelpful to think that when parties disagree one (or maybe both) is mistaken. Quite separately from where any objective truth might lie, the unmasking of the discrepancy can contribute to a more realistic dialogue, and can make for more sensible and achievable targets in personal service plans.

Slade et al. (1999), comparing HoNOS and the short form of the CAN, found different levels of agreement in different domains of needs, while Issakidis and Teesson (1999), using the same pair of instruments, found generally weak levels of agreement. Trauer and Callaly (2002) also found weak levels of agreement between consumers and case managers, which were consistently overestimated by the case managers.

Specific instances of OMs shedding light on previously undetected problems are infrequently reported. Nevertheless, Trauer et al. (2009) reported a few instances of consumers rating themselves, on self-report measures, as having problems with alcohol or drugs, while their clinicians had not rated any problem on the corresponding scale of the HoNOS.

(d) Promoting self-efficacy, empowerment and recovery

The Ohio Mental Health Consumer Outcome System (for details see Chapter 5 by James Healy and Dee Roth) explicitly links OM to empowerment and recovery, thus: 'A consumer/ family member uses Outcomes information to empower him/herself in the Recovery process. He/she completes the appropriate Outcomes instrument and uses the results of this self-assessment to help develop his/her treatment plan' (The Ohio Department of Mental Health, 2008, p. 4-2). Whether, and to what extent, OMs actually promote higher-order aspirations of consumers is a debated point, on which there is comparatively little hard evidence at present. Some (Coombs and Meehan, 2003) contend that they do, while others (e.g. Lakeman, 2004) argue the opposite. Hasler et al. (2004) examined the outcome domains deemed important by patients following outpatient treatment for non-psychotic and non-substance-related conditions. While changes in mood states were judged to be particularly important, they found that areas such as personal growth, purpose in life and positive relations with others were relevant therapeutic achievements in certain patients, especially those with adjustment and personality disorders. Such current evidence as is available suggests that the consumer self-rated outcome is more likely to enhance self-efficacy, empowerment and recovery than the provider-completed measures.

Direct care providers, clinicians

Some uses of OMs for clinicians, such as tracking progress and identifying hidden problems, are essentially the same as for consumers, so the earlier discussion will not be repeated here. Furthermore, anything that benefits the consumer should, in principle at least, benefit the clinician as well. Other uses of OMs more specific to clinicians are providing a standardized method for monitoring changes over time, contributing to individual treatment plans and assisting with clinical decisions.

(a) Standardized method for monitoring changes over time

Gradual changes can be imperceptible. When dealing with long-standing conditions, clinicians can easily form the view that the consumer's status is essentially static, a situation that can easily lead to therapeutic pessimism. Also, standardized assessments are helpful when there is a change of clinicians involved with a consumer, because they have all used the same yardstick. In services that have been using OM for several years, the opportunity exists to view variations in health status over a protracted period. Of course, when this information can be shared with the consumer and carers, they can benefit as well.

Figure 18.1 shows OM assessments on a single consumer over a period of more than 4 years.

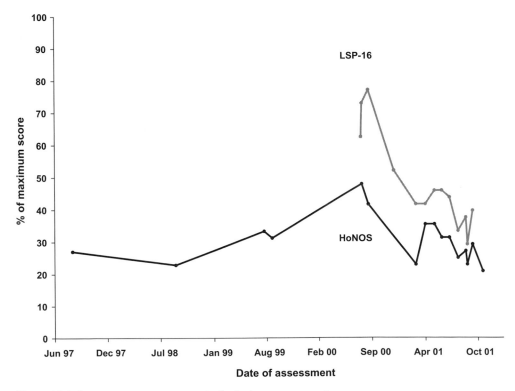

Figure 18.1 Outcome measure assessments of a single consumer over time.

The first HoNOS assessment was in 1997 and assessments with the Life Skills Profile (Rosen et al., 1989, 2006) only commenced in 2000. The multiple LSP assessments over about 1 year show a rapid improvement in personal functioning, alongside more limited changes in the more symptom-oriented HoNOS.

(b) Contributing to individual service plans

Many outpatient and community services will have, as part of their standard or recommended practice, individualized documents, variously known as Individual Service Plans (ISPs), Individual Treatment Plans, Care Plans, and the like. It has been proposed (Department of Human Services, 2003, Mellsop and Wilson, 2006) that OMs can contribute directly to the development of these plans. A survey of clinicians by Callaly et al. (2006, p. 167) found that 'The most commonly mentioned clinical value of outcome measures was their potential to show the broader picture of the client's progress over time. Possible uses included improving the dialogue between clinicians and consumers, helping to identify goals for service planning, using the total score as a general rule of thumb to gauge the severity of consumers' problems and giving feedback to the client which demonstrates progress'. The rationale of ISPs is that they are negotiated, with both parties contributing their view on what could and should be aimed for. The inclusion of OMs in the process of developing the ISP can ensure that (a) both voices are heard, (b) there is a relatively objective means of determining whether aspirations have been met and (c) important domains are covered.

(c) Informing clinical decision-making

There are several reports of clinicians within services using routinely collected OMs to help them make clinical decisions. Prowse and Hunter (2008) described how a service used the LSP to assist in the assignment of consumers to particular forms of treatment, while Slattery and Anstey (2008), working in the same service, showed how HoNOS scores assisted the multidisciplinary team to formulate effective management plans and aided in decisions regarding consumer's readiness for discharge. Prowse and Coombs (2009) described the development of thresholds of HoNOS total scores ('flags') to assist community mental health teams to make decisions regarding discharge or transfer. Keppich-Arnold (2005) similarly showed how lower scores on the older-person version of the HoNOS (HoNOS65+) were used as a guide to lower contact, with total scores of less than 4 raising the question of suitability for discharge.

The Decision Support Tool (DST) developed by the Australian Classification and Outcomes Network (AMHOCN) enables a clinician to compare a given consumer's score on an OM with the distribution of scores of similar consumers in the national database. In Figure 18.2 the clinician has entered a HoNOS score of 15 from a 27-year-old male consumer with a principal diagnosis of anxiety disorder; the assessment was made at a review in a community setting.

The output that accompanies the chart indicates that there are 544 HoNOS assessments matching this consumer's supplied details, and their median is 9.0. The chart shows the position of a score of 15, and accompanying text explains that his score is at the 85th percentile, i.e. 85% of assessments of similar consumers are 15 or lower. Feedback like this enables a clinician to evaluate and contextualize the score obtained from OMs.

Service team leaders and managers

While the value of OMs to consumers, carers and individual clinicians will typically be at the individual level, for team leaders and local service managers the same data, but at an

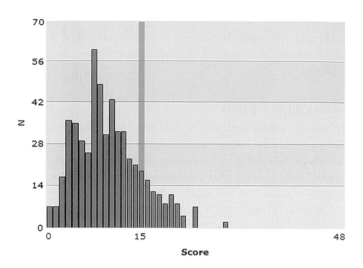

Figure 18.2 Chart display from Decision Support Tool (DST).

aggregated level, has a number of different uses, such as profiling the service and comparing with similar services, caseload management and promoting service quality.

(a) Profiling the service and comparing with similar services

Those responsible for services at a local level need to understand the population that is being served. They will typically rely on information that is routinely collected as part of registration of consumers with the service, such as demographic details and broad diagnostic categories. While these data have some value in their own right, they are limited in their capacity to capture service needs. Diagnosis is a fairly 'blunt' descriptor, with little discrimination of severity or acuity. Furthermore, diagnoses in new consumers, or at the beginning of episodes of care, are often deferred or provisional. OMs allow local managers to get a far stronger grasp and 'feel' for the kinds of problems that consumers in their services have. Where standard and quantitative measures are averaged across all consumers, a much clearer picture can be gained of the typical or modal presentation, as well as of the variation in presentations.

When similar services use the same instruments, the possibility arises for individual services to compare themselves against each other. Macdonald (2002) gives an example of this, comparing sector teams and wards within one hospital, and Trauer (2004) showed that the severity of patients seen by a psychiatric consultation-liaison team in a general hospital was similar to that of patients admitted to its acute psychiatric inpatient unit.

(b) Caseload management

One of the responsibilities of team leaders is to ensure that cases are allocated to service providers in an efficient and equitable way, having regard to the consumers' needs and the providers' capacities, skills and specialities. It is widely accepted that the cases constituting a caseload are likely to be unequal in terms of the time they will need, so some system of adjustment is required. Several such adjustment systems exist, but not all incorporate relevant consumer characteristics. King et al. (2004) included 'client needs and/or response difficulty' in their set of factors that should be included in a caseload management system, on the basis that this 'gives a quantitative value to the level of service required for each client.' (p. 458). Slade et al. (1999), studying the association between the HoNOS and the short form of the CAN, felt that the latter instrument was suitable for use as a caseload measure.

(c) Promotion of service quality

A recent British report noted: 'At the level of the individual clinician or clinical team, outcomes data will be valuable for performance management through quality improvement and clinical governance arrangements, revalidation, or to inform patient choice' (Office of Health Economics, 2008). One example of quality improvement is the report by Hoffmann et al. (1999), who described a project in which 'outcomes data were used to identify patterns in the responsiveness to treatment by diagnosis, monitor the effectiveness of performance improvement efforts in meeting goals, and illuminate factors outside of treatment approaches, such as population density of patients with particular diagnoses, that affected treatment outcomes' (p. 218). Another is Kersten et al. (1999), who, using clinical and functional measures based on both staff ratings and consumer self-reports in an adult community residential service, obtained data on consumers at intake and at 6-monthly intervals thereafter, as well as after discharge. Results were presented in team meetings, where staff displayed an interest in understanding the variations within and between consumers, and there were lively discussions about clinical practice, routines and standards of care.

There are numerous other reports of similar work and they share certain similarities. They are often time-limited and project-based, rather than ongoing and indefinite; the original idea for the project can be traced to the vision and drive of a small number of (sometimes just one) senior managers; the intervention is typically small-scale and local; and the project involves a 'whole of team' approach, not just a few key individuals.

Policy makers and funders

While uses of OMs with individual consumers may be considered 'low level', uses of the same data, but in aggregated form, by policy makers and funders may be thought of as 'high-level' applications. However, the validity of these high-level uses will be determined by whether the measures were obtained in a reliable and valid way in the first place, i.e. at the level of the clinician and the consumer.

In recent decades, new demands have been made of health services that planners and bureaucrats have had to respond to. Such demands have included calls for evidence of effectiveness, systems to ensure accountability and demonstrate 'value for money', and development of equitable and transparent bases for resourcing. These are challenging aspirations, and OMs can play a part in achieving them.

(a) Evidence of effectiveness of mental health services

Outcomes, in the sense of changes in measures of mental health status between assessments, hold the promise of providing evidence of beneficial effects in the average consumer of mental health services. Indeed, the key performance indicators (KPIs) for mental health in Australia (Information Strategy Committee, 2005) list consumer and carer outcomes as indicators of service effectiveness; significantly, however, both of these indicators have yet to be operationalized. The underlying principle is quite straightforward: when problems are measured at the beginning and end of episodes of care, the average difference represents overall effectiveness. Charlwood et al. (1999, pp. 33–4) proposed change in HoNOS score between admission and discharge as a candidate indicator for the severely mentally ill (SMI). The simplicity of this model, however, is deceptive. Various authors have pointed out dangers of incautious inference from pre–post studies not least because, in the absence of a 'control group' of untreated cases, it is difficult to know how much improvement may have occurred naturally (Salzer,

1996) and because of the large degree of uncertainty when there are only two points of assessment (Lambert et al., 2001). A large number of small positive changes can render an average difference statistically significant, when most of the actual changes may be well within the uncertainty of the measure used.

A different and possibly safer approach to demonstrating system effectiveness is to assign each treated case to a broad outcome category and count these. Such categories may be 'Progressing as expected', 'Progressing better than expected' and 'Progressing worse than expected', or 'Improved', 'Stayed the Same' and 'Worse'. There are technical issues in determining the thresholds between these categories (see Chapter 20 on change in this book). Using the classification approach, Hannan et al. (2005) found 7% of clients of a psychotherapy service deteriorated, and Parabiaghi et al. (2005) classified consumers in an Italian community mental health service into 91.6% stable, 5.6% improved and 1.8% deteriorated.

(b) Accountability and value for money

Funders in particular have a responsibility to ensure that scarce resources are deployed as efficiently as possible, and it is tempting to divide a measure of effectiveness, such as described in the previous section, by cost, to derive an index of efficiency. Some approaches to this will be considered later, but the very fact that OMs might be used in this way often creates negative reactions in the direct care staff, who have the principal responsibility for ensuring that the OMs are collected. Hodges and Wotring (2004, p. 400) wrote of the 'feelings of apprehension about being evaluated, which often accompany reporting of outcome data for accountability purposes', and Jacobs (2007, p. 16) noted that 'Clinicians in the USA are as resistant to routine outcome measures as their European counterparts for similar reasons – the driving force is seen to be the need for aggregate data for management and accountability purposes rather than direct clinical utility'. Speer (1998, p. 75) has noted that these concerns may also affect funders themselves: 'The downside of using provider ratings as outcome or response to treatment measures is the possible suspicion by policy makers that providers will be tempted to "gild the lily" when an evaluation of their own service program is involved'. He noted that measures completed by consumers are free of this contaminating effect.

Despite claims that OMs can be used to enhance accountability and promote efficiency, and the complementary reservations of clinicians and funders, there have been few reports of OM being actually used in this way.

(c) Equitable and rational basis for resourcing

Systems designed to allocated resources on the basis of consumer characteristics, or the outcomes of the inputs they receive, are often broadly termed casemix models. While numerous definitions of casemix exist, one suitable for present purposes, since it was used in a mental health context, is:

> The purpose of a casemix classification system is to classify episodes of care based on those factors which best predict the need for, and the cost of, care. In a casemix classification, episodes of care are grouped into classes based on two criteria. First each class should contain episodes with similar patterns of resource consumption. There is an implicit assumption that consumers who consume similar resources have similar needs. Second, each class should contain episodes that are clinically similar. (Gaines et al., 2003, p. 5)

The close association between outcomes and casemix is attested by the peak Australian agency responsible for outcomes, the Australian Mental Health Classification and Outcomes Network (AMHOCN), where 'Classification' refers, broadly, to casemix.

There have been two major casemix systems developed specifically for mental health, the Mental Health Classification and Service Costs (MH-CASC) project (Buckingham et al., 1998) in Australia and the Classification and Outcomes Study (CAOS) in New Zealand (Gaines et al., 2003, Trauer et al., 2004). Both incorporated OMs; this was because

> Although it is not unequivocal, the body of evidence suggests that severity of symptoms has an influence on mental health resource use. Studies that have directly examined the link have found severity to explain up to 24% of the variance in acute inpatient stays. The patterns of care literature indicates that severity is associated with greater use of all services, and particularly of higher Inpatient use and more intensive day and community treatment. Clinicians themselves rate severity as the greatest predictor of resource use, and this is evident in nursing classification instruments adopting severity as a factor which is predictive of high nursing dependency, and treatment guidelines pointing to specific differences in treatment depending on whether a person's symptoms are mild, moderate or severe. (Buckingham et al., 1998 pp. 37–8)

They noted that severity involves more than symptom severity or acuity; disability and level of personal functioning play a part in service costs as well. At the time of writing, there is little hard evidence of the performance of mental health casemix systems that rely to any great extent on OMs. However, there is interest and expressions of intent to use such systems, so this position may well change in the near future.

References

Bickman, L., Nurcombe, B., Townsend, C., et al. (1998). *Consumer Measurement Systems in Child and Adolescent Mental Health*. Canberra: Department of Health and Family Services.

Buckingham, W., Burgess, P., Solomon, S., Pirkis, J. and Eagar, K. (1998). *Developing a Casemix Classification for Mental Health Services*. Canberra: Department of Health and Ageing.

Callaly, T., Hyland, M., Coombs, T. and Trauer, T. (2006). Routine outcome measurement in public mental health – results of a clinician survey. *Australian Health Review*, **30**, 164–73.

Charlwood, P., Mason, A., Goldacre, M., Cleary, R. and Wilkinson, E. (1999). *Health Outcome Indicators: Severe Mental Illness. Report of a working group to the Department of Health*. Oxford: National Centre for Outcomes Development.

Coombs, T. and Meehan, T. (2003). Mental health outcomes in Australia: issues for mental health nurses. *International Journal of Mental Health Nursing*, **12**, 163–4.

Department of Human Services (2003). *Measuring Consumer Outcomes in Clinical Mental Health Services*. Melbourne.

Eisen, S. V. (1996). Behavior and Symptom Identification Scale (BASIS-32).In L. I. Sederer and B. Dickey, eds., *Outcomes Assessment in Clinical Practice*. Baltimore: Williams & Wilkins.

Gaines, P., Bower, A., Buckingham, W., et al. (2003). *New Zealand Mental Health Classification and Outcomes Study: Final Report*. Auckland: Health Research Council of New Zealand.

Goodman, R. (2001). Psychometric properties of the Strengths and Difficulties Questionnaire. *Journal of the American Academy of Child and Adolescent Psychiatry*, **40**, 1337–45.

Graham, C., Coombs, T., Buckingham, W., et al. (2001). *Consumer Perspectives of Future Directions for Outcome Self-Assessment*. Report of the Consumer Consultation Project, Wollongong.

Guthrie, D., McIntosh, M., Callaly, T., Trauer, T. and Coombs, T. (2008). Consumer attitudes towards the use of routine outcome measures in a public mental health service: a consumer-driven study. *International Journal of Mental Health Nursing*, **17**, 92–7.

Hannan, C., Lambert, M. J., Harmon, C., et al. (2005). A lab test and algorithms for identiying clients at risk for treatment failure. *Journal of Clinical Psychology*, **61**, 155–63.

Hansen, T., Hatling, T., Lidal, E. and Ruud, T. (2002). Discrepancies between patients and professionals in the assessment of patient needs: a quantitative study of Norwegian mental health care. *Journal of Advanced Nursing*, **39**, 554–62.

Hansson, L., Vinding, H. R., Mackeprang, T., et al (2001). Comparison of key worker and patient assessment of needs in schizophrenic patients living in the community: a Nordic multicentre study. *Acta Psychiatrica Scandinavica*, **103**, 45–51.

Hasler, G., Moergeli, H. and Schnyder, U. (2004). Outcome of psychiatric treatment: what is relevant for our patients? *Comprehensive Psychiatry*, **45**, 199–205.

Hodges, K. and Wotring, J. (2004). The role of monitoring outcomes in initiating implementation of evidence-based treatments at the state level. *Psychiatric Services*, **55**, 396–400.

Hoffmann, F. L., Leckman, E., Russo, N. and Knauf, L. (1999). In it for the long haul: the integration of outcomes assessment, clinical services, and management decision-making. *Evaluation and Program Planning*, **22**, 211–19.

Information Strategy Committee, AHMAC National Mental Health Working Group (2005). *Key Performance Indicators for Australian Public Mental Health Services*. Canberra.

Issakidis, C. and Teesson, M. (1999). Measurement of need for care: a trial of the Camberwell Assessment of Need and the Health of the National Outcome Scales. *Australian and New Zealand Journal of Psychiatry*, **33**, 754–9.

Jacobs, R. (2007). *Investigating Patient Outcome Measures in Mental Health: research report for the OHE Commission on NHS Productivity*. York: Centre for Health Economics, University of York.

Keppich-Arnold, S. (2005). Can HoNOS be used as a case load management tool? *Australian Mental Health Outcomes and Classification Network Newsletter*, **9**.

Kersten, E., Wilkinson, K. and Wright, S. (1999). Bringing staff on board: creating an outcomes project tied to continuous quality improvement in an adult community residential service. *Evaluation and Program Planning*, **22**, 232.

King, R., Meadows, G. and Le Bas, J. (2004). Compiling a caseload index for mental health case management. *Australian and New Zealand Journal of Psychiatry*, **38**, 455–62.

Lakeman, R. (2004). Standardized routine outcome measurement: pot holes in the road to recovery. *International Journal of Mental Health Nursing*, **13**, 210–15.

Lambert, E. W., Doucette, A. and Bickman, L. (2001). Measuring mental health outcomes with pre-post designs. *Journal of Behavioral Health Services & Research*, **28**, 273–86.

Macdonald, A. J. D. (2002). The usefulness of aggregate routine clinical outcomes data: the example of HoNOS65+. *Journal of Mental Health*, **11**, 645–56.

Mellsop, G. and Wilson, J. (2006). Outcome measures in mental health services: Humpty Dumpty is alive and well. *Australasian Psychiatry*, **14**, 137–40.

Miller, S. D., Duncan, B. L., Sorrell, R. and Brown, G. S. (2005). The partners for change outcome management system. *Journal of Clinical Psychology*, **61**, 199–208.

Office of Health Economics (2008). *NHS Outcomes, Performance and Productivity*.

Parabiaghi, A., Barbato, A., D'Avanzo, B., Erlicher, A. and Lora, A. (2005). Assessing reliable and clinically significant change on Health of the Nation Outcome Scales: method for displaying longitudinal data.

Australian and New Zealand Journal of Psychiatry, **39**, 719–25.

Phelan, M., Slade, M., Thornicroft, G., et al. (1995). The Camberwell Assessment of Need: the validity and reliability of an instrument to assess the needs of people with severe mental illness. *British Journal of Psychiatry*, **167**, 589–95.

Priebe, S., McCabe, R., Bullenkamp, J., et al. (2007). Structured patient-clinician communication and 1-year outcome in community mental healthcare. Cluster randomised controlled trial. *British Journal of Psychiatry*, **191**, 420–6.

Prowse, L. and Coombs, T. (2009). The use of the Health of the Nation Outcome Scales (HoNOS) to inform discharge and transfer decisions in community mental health services. *Australian Health Review*, **33**, 13–18.

Prowse, L. and Hunter, S. (2008). Using the LSP to inform programme decisions for individuals with Borderline Personality Disorder. *Australian and New Zealand Journal of Psychiatry*, **42**, A16.

Rosen, A., Hadzi-Pavlovic, D. and Parker, G. (1989). The Life Skills Profile: a measure assessing function and disability in schizophrenia. *Schizophrenia Bulletin*, **15**, 325–37.

Rosen, A., Hadzi-Pavlovic, D., Parker, G. and Trauer, T. (2006). *The Life Skills Profile: Background, Items and Scoring for the LSP–39, LSP–20 and the LSP–16*. Sydney, available at: http://www.blackdoginstitute.org.au/docs/LifeSkillsProfile.pdf.

Salzer, M. S. (1996). Interpreting outcome studies. *Journal of the American Academy of Child and Adolescent Psychiatry*, **35**, 1419.

Slade, M., Beck, A., Bindman, J., Thornicroft, G. and Wright, S. (1999). Routine clinical outcome measures for patients with severe mental illness: CANSAS and HoNOS. *British Journal of Psychiatry*, **174**, 404–8.

Slattery, T. and Anstey, S. (2008). Clinical utility of HoNOS in an inpatient setting. *Australian and New Zealand Journal of Psychiatry*, **42**, A6.

Speer, D. C. (1998). *Mental Health Outcome Evaluation*. San Diego, CA: Academic Press.

Stedman, T., Yellowlees, P., Mellsop, G., Clarke, R. and Drake, S. (1997). *Measuring Consumer Outcomes in Mental Health*. Canberra: Department of Health and Aged Care.

Stewart, M. (2009). Service user and significant other versions of the Health of the Nation Outcome Scales. *Australasian Psychiatry*, **17**, 156–63.

The Ohio Department of Mental Health (2008). *The Ohio Mental Health Consumer Outcomes System – Procedural Manual*, 10th edn. Columbus, OH.

Tobias, G. and Trauer, T. (2008). Routine outcome measurement and the perspectives of the different stakeholders: consumer, case manager, key worker. *Australian and New Zealand Journal of Psychiatry*, **42**, A15.

Trauer, T. (2004). Outcome measurement in a consultation-liaison mental health service. *Australasian Psychiatry*, **12**, 139–44.

Trauer, T. and Callaly, T. (2002). Concordance between mentally ill clients and their case managers using the Health of the Nation Outcome Scales (HoNOS). *Australasian Psychiatry*, **10**, 24–8.

Trauer, T., Eagar, K., Gaines, P. and Bower, A. (2004). *New Zealand Mental Health Consumers and their Outcomes*. Auckland: Health Research Council of New Zealand.

Trauer, T., Pedwell, G. and Gill, L. (2009). The effect of guidance in the use of routine outcome measures in clinical meetings. *Australian Health Review*, **33**, 144–51.

Wing, J. K., Beevor, A. S., Curtis, R. H., et al. (1998). Health of the Nation Outcome Scales (HoNOS). Research and development. *British Journal of Psychiatry*, **172**, 11–18.

Stakeholder perspectives in outcome measurement

Tom Trauer

In this chapter I examine stakeholders' views, perceptions and attitudes to OM. Despite the many actual and potential benefits of OM, as detailed in the previous chapter, there exists a wide range of feelings about OM, ranging from strongly positive to strongly negative. As Close-Goedjen and Saunders (2002) noted: 'OA [Outcomes Assessment] has not been universally embraced by health care providers' and they listed several reasons: 'Criticisms include concern that OA results in health care decisions and procedures that do not reflect the unique qualities and needs of the individual patient, thus undermining the clinician's professional autonomy and clinical judgement. Clinicians complain that OA is too time consuming, intrudes on the therapeutic relationship, and is potentially harmful to the patient. In short, OA is often perceived to lack both value and practical application' (p. 100). We shall review some of this evidence, and attempt to explain its causes and effects. The material will be structured into three broad categories of stakeholders: clinicians, other providers, and consumers and carers.

Clinicians

Since the advent of routine OM in the mid-1990s, there has been a fairly steady stream of writing regarding clinicians' feelings about OM. Perhaps unsurprisingly, the literature is somewhat polarized.

Close-Goedjen and Saunders (2002) investigated the provision of technical support, in the form of scored and profiled results of an outcomes instrument, on the attitudes (general value, clinical relevance, ease of use) and behaviours (frequency of administration, analysis and use) of mental health clinicians. They found that both attitudes and behaviours improved while the support was provided. Once the support was withdrawn, however, attitudes remained elevated, but behaviours fell back to pre-support levels. They concluded that 'clinicians are not opposed to OA per se, but rather were opposed and resistant to the potential additional paperwork and administrative requirements that OA protocols often represent. . . . This suggests that, when clinicians are given an opportunity to utilize outcome measures without additional burdens on their time or workload, they are more able to appreciate their potential' (p. 107).

Huffman et al. (2004) administered questionnaires to staff in two child and adolescent facilities. While the respondents viewed outcome measurement as very important, and useful at initial assessment, they perceived only a small to moderate effect of outcomes data on their clinical practice. The authors also found correlational evidence that the perception of outcomes evaluation as burdensome was inversely related to the perception of outcomes evaluation as important. Psychiatrists were significantly less positive to OM than psychologists with regard to overall importance and research utility, which the authors speculated could be due to their medical training 'in which the use of individual interviews and unstructured progress monitoring are emphasized' (p. 186). Around the same time Merry et al. (2004) sought the views of families, consumers and clinicians of child and adolescent routine outcome measures in New Zealand. There was generally strong support for OM from all the groups. Clinicians' concerns revolved around workload burden, the possibility that OMs might be used to monitor their performance adversely and fears that OMs could be used to limit access to services. Also, Hatfield and Ogles (2004) reported that cognitively and behaviourally oriented psychologists were more likely to use OMs than those who were insight-oriented or eclectic.

Garland et al. (2003) also studied clinicians in child and adolescent services. Using focus groups and semi-structured interviews, they discovered great variability in their attitudes to empirical methods of treatment evaluation, with roughly equal numbers thinking it was or was not possible. Over 90% reported that they had never used the scores from the mandated standardized instruments in their clinical practice, yet over 60% commented on the usefulness of administering them to youths and their parents, especially in the intake process. While these clinicians were overwhelmingly of the view that OMs were not useful, they drew a clear distinction between the use of scores from OMs (not useful) and the process of using OMs with youths and parents (useful). Barriers to the wider use of OMs fell into three categories. First, there were feasibility issues, which included time burden, the fact that the measures were difficult for the service recipients to understand and the fact that negative feedback from service recipients was much more common than positive feedback. Second, there were doubts about the validity of standardized outcome measures, with over half believing that they were neither appropriate nor valid for their particular patient population. Third, many staff felt that the scores were difficult to understand, and even most of those who did not indicated that they didn't find the scores helpful in practice. What then did these clinicians want? Mostly, they wanted easier and briefer measures, reports that were easier to understand, with, for example, graphical and narrative summaries, and more information and training on how to use the results in practice. Abrahamson (1999) also discerned three main sources of resistance and concern among clinicians, these being performance measurement issues, logistical considerations and conceptual appropriateness of the measures.

In a study in rural Western Australia, Aoun et al. (2002) observed a similar wide spread of opinion. They found 44% of clinical staff thought outcome ratings were a waste of time, an equal proportion thought they were useful for tracking clients, and the remainder were unsure. Despite this, 78% indicated that they were in favour of OM. Unlike in certain other studies, the complaint of time burden was not observed, with 90% saying they found the time spent in undertaking measurement to be reasonable. Their findings revealed a 'need to provide staff with reasons and incentives for incorporating outcome measurement into routine practice, . . . as is provision of thorough and on-going training and support for participants in both time and resources' (p. 306).

In another Australian study, Crocker and Rissel (1998) sent questionnaires to community mental health clinicians. The responses identified some pessimism about what focusing on outcomes would achieve for them or their clients. It was felt that better uptake might be achieved by training in the practical applications of OMs, greater involvement with and ownership of the process, and recognition of OM achievements.

In the same year, Walter et al. (1998) reported a survey of staff in an urban Mental Health Service that had taken part in a time-limited Commonwealth-funded project which had required them to rate patient outcome. 'The major concern expressed by respondents was that rating outcome was too time-consuming. More than half were not in favour of measuring outcome routinely even if it meant providing a better service to patients' (abstract). However, a report from the same service a few years later (Cleary et al., 2002) described a workshop for mental health nurses in which 92% of attenders believed that measuring outcomes could improve patient care.

Callaly and Hallebone (2001) sought the views of clinicians, managers, consumers and carers in an area service that had recently initiated routine OM. 'A recurring theme for clinicians and managers was that of respect for their professionalism' (p. 46) in that the requirement to complete measures could be taken as meaning that clinicians were not already discussing issues with consumers and including them in their planning. Almost every staff member interviewed was suspicious of management and government rhetoric about their motivation in introducing OM; they were comfortable with using them to increase accountability, but had reservations about using them in funding formulas for mental health. They also noted a number of positive uses of OMs, including encouraging clinicians to think more critically about consumers' difficulties, encouraging listening, engagement and collaboration with consumers, and providing a common language for dialogue.

Writing from a specifically mental health nursing perspective, Coombs and Meehan (2003) noted that the workload of ROM falls mainly on nursing staff, and it provides them with an opportunity to take the lead in service monitoring and evaluation. This elicited a dissenting response from Lakeman (2004), who saw ROM as failing to capture the subtlety of individual differences, contributing to low quality of research, not actually delivering improved outcomes, and distracting from the more fundamental task for nurses, namely focusing on the personal recovery of those they care for. Browne (2006) echoed Lakeman's complaint that ROMs do not reflect a recovery philosophy. In the same year Meehan et al. (2006) summarized 34 focus groups held with 324 staff, over half of whom were mental health nurses. 'While the majority of participants endorsed the collection and utilization of outcomes data, many raised questions about the merits of the initiative. Ambivalence, competing work demands, lack of support from senior medical staff, questionable evidence to support the use of outcome measures, and fear of how outcomes data might be used emerged as key issues. At 8 months after implementation a significant number of clinical staff remained ambivalent about the benefits of outcome measurement and had not engaged in the process.'

The other major group that have expressed views about ROM are psychiatrists, and their public expressions have been predominantly negative. Perhaps the first specific comments were by Stein (1999), in the editorial of a special issue of the *British Journal of Psychiatry* devoted to the Health of the Nation Outcome Scales (HoNOS). In a generally sceptical review, he expected that the HoNOS was unlikely to enter routine practice in the National Health Service (NHS), although it could come to play a role in mental health service research. In the same issue, Sharma et al. (1999), writing from the perspective of using the HoNOS in psychiatry in general practice, concluded that while the instrument may be feasible, it was of limited value in the day-to-day clinical management of patients, and its widespread adoption into clinical practice was premature. A few years later, in the same journal, Gilbody et al. (2002), in a paper entitled 'Psychiatrists in the UK do not use outcome measures', reported a survey of psychiatrists in the NHS. Most did not use OMs routinely, and many of the comments were negative ('simplistic', 'pseudo-scientific gloss'). Concerns were expressed about the usefulness of OMs and their detraction from the therapeutic relationship (see also Bewick et al., 2006). As to the HoNOS, negative comments (time burden, psychometric concerns) outnumbered positive comments. Courtenay (2002) responded by pointing out that there was already considerable reliance on well-validated tools in psychiatry. More recently, Zimmerman and McGlinchey (2008) conducted a study similar to that of Gilbody et al. in the United States. Fewer than 20% of psychiatrists routinely use scales to monitor outcome when treating depression. The main reasons for non-use were the belief that scales would not be clinically helpful, that scales take too much time to use and that they were not trained in the use of such measures.

There are a number of studies of clinician attitudes in Australia that were conducted in or after 2003, which is the year that routine OM became mandatory throughout the country. These studies therefore have somewhat different significance to some of the above, since the clinicians were working in an environment where they were expected to comply with mandatory nation-wide OM collection protocols.

Callaly et al. (2006) conducted focus groups with clinical staff, who were equally divided on the question of the value of OM to their clinical work, thought that the consumer self-rated measure was more valuable than the clinician-rated measures, and thought that the government's interest in OM was to control expenditure and develop new models of funding. The staff identified training and useful forms of feedback as areas that could be developed further. Patterson et al. (2006) identified low compliance with mandatory collection protocols as a kind of proxy for opinions of low value or utility. In the state-level system that they studied, OMs were embedded in a much wider set of information that was required to be collected, and it is possible that the antipathy expressed to OMs was partly due to the cumbersome system within which they were embedded.

Prabhu and Oakley Browne (2008) described the use and uptake of OM in an out-reach rehabilitation service that operated on a strong collaborative recovery model. The staff group were very positive toward the HoNOS, which they found objective and providing a baseline against which to judge improvement. Staff selection may have accounted for this finding because 'A positive attitude towards objective assessments and structured interventions were a strong prerequisite in obtaining positions within this team'. They also pointed out that 'The group of clinicians in the team were not representative of the mental health workforce across other clinical services' (p. 198).

Trauer et al. (2009b) studied clinicians' attitudes before, after and at follow-up of an intervention aimed at assisting them to understand and interpret the OMs that they collected. Attitudes became more positive while the intervention lasted and, unlike Close-Goedjen and Saunders (2002), most of these gains were maintained at follow-up. Despite these average trends, there were significant differences between individual clinicians and between clinical teams. In another study, Trauer et al. (2009a) administered an attitude survey to over 200 staff in two adult area mental health services, an overall return rate of 77%. Summary attitude scores showed that staff in administrative positions judged the highest value for OM, and clinical staff in community settings the lowest. Comparing staff trained in OM with the untrained, the trained found OMs easier to use than untrained, but there was no difference in judgements of overall value. Asked to rate the usefulness of the actual instruments in use in those services, the whole range of opinion, from very positive to very negative, was observed. Although the average was more positive than negative, about 10% thought all the instruments had utility for any purpose, and a similar percentage thought all the instruments lacked utility for any purpose. This is similar to the finding by Callaly et al. (2006) of equally divided opinion.

Other providers

In this section we will review the perspective of those who are neither direct services providers, like clinicians, nor recipients of services, like consumers and carers. This group therefore comprises managers, administrators, policy makers and funders. The potential benefits of

OMs to these groups were summarized in the previous chapter as providing evidence of effectiveness of services and assisting with decisions about value for money and equitable resourcing. Typically, these 'organizational' uses involve aggregates or averages of individual OM assessments, partly because they are more suited to 'big picture' questions, but also because the original measures will be subject to privacy, confidentiality and 'need to know' considerations.

One of the earliest indications of the nexus between outcomes and management was by Ellwood (1988), who used the term 'outcomes management', a central component of which was to be a 'national data base containing information and analysis on clinical, financial and health outcomes that estimates as best we can the relation between (medical) interventions and health outcomes; and an opportunity for each decision-maker to have access to the analyses that are relevant to the choices they must make'. Epstein (1990) identified three elements in the origin of the 'outcomes movement': cost containment, a renewed sense of competition and concerns over equitable distribution.

Early evidence of what senior management and medical staff thought of OM was reported by Linder (1991), who conducted interviews with such staff at 31 hospitals. Three patterns of usage emerged. Hospitals embracing the *status quo* used OM to insulate themselves from change. Other hospitals exerted *administrative control* of medical quality by carefully monitoring physicians with outcomes information. The third group of hospitals managed quality and cost through informed and open discussion of difficult medical issues with the *professional network*. Status quo hospitals were characterized by disdain for OM, allocation of junior or ineffective staff to OM roles, little involvement beyond a perfunctory attempt at compliance, discrediting of scoring systems and ensuring a strict separation between measurement information and clinical decision-making. Nevertheless, staff at these hospitals were 'mildly pleased' with their use of OM, because they were able to demonstrate that their 'quality' was comfortably within national norms of practice. Senior medical staff were the dominant group in these hospitals. In administrative control hospitals, administrators and nurses were the dominant groups. OM was seen as assisting financial outcomes in a competitive environment. As far as possible, treatment was standardized, by use of protocols and checklists. Executives in these hospitals valued OM for its capacity to reduce utilization, but complained that it was not sufficiently technically sophisticated. It was in the professional network hospitals where OM appeared to flourish. Administrative and medical staff combined to maximize quality, through continuous assessment and improvement activities. Executives at these hospitals were more likely to say 'Our physicians are hungry for data. All we have to do is let them see how they compare with others, and they begin to change' (p. 28). The ideal information products in these hospitals consisted of tailored studies that included both clinical and cost information from the database. Despite these varying stances in relation to OM, only four of the 31 hospitals claimed that quality of care had improved as a result of using OM (p. 29).

Studies that have been able to directly compare the attitudes to OM of different categories of staff (e.g. Trauer et al., 2009a) have typically found that those in management positions are on average more favourable than those in direct care positions. Ciarlo (1982) suggests that at least one reason may be the drive for accountability through demonstrated effective performance. He cited earlier moves to regard 'improved mental status of individuals . . . as measurable program products' (p. 32). Another management incentive for OM is cost containment, which has been seen as the main driver of OM in the USA (Jacobs, 2007, p. 15).

Consumers and carers

The literature on consumer and carer attitudes to OM is somewhat limited, not because they are apathetic to OM, but because they are less likely to have the connections, skills and opportunities to make their views known via academic or professional outlets. Nevertheless, there are a number of valuable resources, many written by consumers or consumer-academics in conjunction with service providers or clinicians.

Stedman et al. (1997, 2000) reported the field trials of instruments recommended by Andrews et al. (1994) for national use in Australia with adult consumers. As part of their project they conducted focus groups with consumers to seek their views about the instruments. While generally endorsing the principle of OM, and being mostly favourable to the specific instruments, consumers raised issues about the language and scoring of the forms, and about omitted domains such as wellness and consumers' individuality. Qualitative feedback indicated that process and context issues, such as how the responses are obtained and how they are then used, may be as important to the success of OM as the choice of instrument. At around the same time, Bickman et al. (1998) produced a similar report in relation to child and adolescent services. From their wide-ranging consultations, most stakeholders felt that an outcomes system was important and, provided the system is not too burdensome, resistance from clients or parents would not be a problem. Reservations included concern that the information could be abused through attempts to evaluate the cost-effectiveness of services.

Graham et al. (2001) reported the results and recommendations of consultations with consumers about the introduction of OM in the Australian state of Victoria. They summarized previous work thus:

- *Outcomes for consumers are about more than relief from symptoms*
  Well-being, Personhood, Empowerment, Recovery and Minimizing the detrimental effects of treatment and care regimes are particularly important outcomes for consumers.

- *Consumers want the link between health outcome and service quality to be recognized in self-assessment measures*
  'Put simply, the question is whether it is meaningful to consumers to gather information about their health outcome without also asking whether they regard the service being provided to them as meeting their needs'. (p. 15).

- *Consumers rate their outcomes differently from clinicians*
  This does not mean that either is right or wrong – instead, it means that both parties approach the question from different perspectives and that these need to be brought together for a full understanding.

- *No single measure is universally accepted as the best measure*
  They noted that the work involved in the development of a comprehensive new instrument is substantial and there is no guarantee that such a new instrument would not also be seen to have faults.

- *The process of measurement is as important as the outcome measure*
  Process refers to *how* rather than *what* – e.g. how consumers are approached for information, how it is used by clinicians, how it influences treatment planning, how privacy is protected and so forth. The process should include explanation of the purpose, confirming the right to refuse, and offers of assistance where required.

- *Comprehensiveness needs to be balanced by brevity*

An overly long instrument was thought to be impractical for routine use.

In the early 2000s, New Zealand undertook preliminary work toward the development of a self-assessed measure of consumer outcome, reported by Gordon et al. (2004). The consultations revealed that consumers were positively disposed to having a tool that would support them in reflecting on and monitoring their mental well-being. Most expressed a desire that such a tool should have direct potential benefits to the consumer and that it should afford them space to write free text.

Guthrie et al. (2008) explored the views of 50 case-managed adult consumers. Forty had been offered a consumer self-report measure, but of those fewer than half said their case manager had explained what it would be used for, or had discussed their responses with them. Nevertheless, three-quarters thought that their completion of the measure had helped their case manager to understand them better and two-thirds believed that completing the measure had led to them receiving better care. Very few were aware that their case manager was routinely completing other measures on them. The results suggested that consumers see the benefit of routine OM and believe it leads to improved care, but that more information about OM, including the clinician-rated measures, needs to be provided to consumers if they are to be engaged constructively in this exercise.

About the same time as the Guthrie et al. (2008) paper, Black et al. (2009) reported a study of the knowledge and attitudes of consumers and carers in the same region. A mailed survey revealed that only 27% of consumer responders and 4% of carers had heard of routine OM before reading the enclosed brochures. In a setting where OM had been mandatory for several years, not all (84%) of clinicians knew about it. These findings, combined with subsequent workshops, led the authors to conclude that 'the major barrier to completion of the measures is not the consumers' willingness to engage, but the continued resistance of clinicians to embrace the measures in their clinical practice' (p. 98). For most consumers, the most important factor in their treatment was the relationship they had with their clinician, and they saw routine OM as one way of valuing their input to the treatment process, and thereby strengthening this relationship.

Summary and conclusions

The common finding among clinicians is of wide variation in views, frequently equally split between for and against OM. We may infer from this that as well as definite views, there is also a good deal of ambivalence. While most clinicians surveyed are prepared to endorse the *idea* of OM, they list multiple barriers, most commonly time constraints, devaluing of their clinical judgement, detrimental effects on the therapeutic relationship, psychometric concerns, worries about uses of OM by 'management' that would restrict their freedom of action, and lack of ongoing institutional support. Milne et al. (2001) speculated that the non-users of OM used their negative evaluation to justify their non-compliance. A succinct summary has been provided by Jacobs (2007): 'Probably the most crucial barrier to the introduction of outcome measures is that clinicians are unable to see the clinical benefits, partly because they have not been given a clear rationale for their use, partly because they are simply told to complete scores, but primarily because they never receive any feedback on them. Many see it as a paper-filling exercise for managers' (p. 8) and 'Many clinicians had concerns over outcome measurement being used for performance management. The fear was that outcome measures would be used to distinguish good clinicians from poor ones. Any kind of league-tabling approach will make clinicians very afraid' (p. 66). A perceived lack of everyday utility was a recurring theme.

This is not restricted to mental health; Meadows et al. (1998) studied the attitudes of general practitioners and clinic nurses to the use of health outcome questionnaires with diabetic patients in routine outpatient care. While the majority expressed support for the idea of health outcome measurement, nearly half were unclear about how they would actually use such data. In addition to affecting compliance and return rates, negative attitudes may even affect the accuracy of ratings; Söderberg et al. (2005) found that attitude and motivation affected the reliability of ratings that clinicians made. Given the large role of measurement error in the assessment of change in the individual, they concluded that a positive outlook toward rating instruments would minimize errors and maximize reliability.

In contrast, most consumer and carer opinion is strongly positive, for the reason that OM affords them a more effective voice in their care. However, consumer and carer support is not unqualified; they want reassurance on issues such as confidentiality, and that their responses will actually be used for their benefit. Like the clinicians, they were generally unimpressed by potential uses for organizational purposes, such as quality assurance, performance management, cost containment and the like. They often wanted a wider coverage of issues, beyond the 'negatives' of symptoms and dysfunction, extending to such 'positives' as empowerment, quality of life and recovery. We cannot be sure how representative those consumers and carers who participated in the focus groups etc. were, since they were often largely self-selected. As Frese et al. (2001) have pointed out, enthusiasm for the more abstract health aspirations may be more prevalent among more recovered consumers, with those who are less advanced on the road to recovery being more focused on basic and practical objectives.

Despite caution about the representativeness of attitudinal findings, the picture appears to be of variable support and ambivalence to OM among direct service providers, contrasting with much stronger support for OM among consumers and carers, along with hopes of extending the range of coverage of OMs beyond the narrow interests of clinicians, to incorporate some of the concepts of more immediate concern to service recipients. These two broad groups of stakeholders are suspicious or fearful of some of the uses to which OM might be put by managers, administrators and funders.

References

Abrahamson, D. J. (1999). Outcomes, guidelines, and manuals: on leading horses to water. *Clinical Psychology: Science and Practice*, **6**, 467–71.

Andrews, G., Peters, L. and Teesson, M. (1994). *The Measurement of Consumer Outcome in Mental Health: a Report to the National Mental Health Information Strategy Committee*. Sydney: Clinical Research Unit for Anxiety Disorders.

Aoun, S., Pennebaker, D. and Janca, A. (2002). Outcome measurement in rural mental health: a field trial of rooming-in models. *Australian Journal of Rural Health*, **10**, 302–7.

Bewick, B. M., Trusler, K., Mullin, T., Grant, S. and Mothersole, G. (2006). Routine outcome measurement completion rates of the CORE-OM in primary care psychological therapies and counselling. *Counselling and Psychotherapy Research*, **6**, 33–40.

Bickman, L., Nurcombe, B., Townsend, C., et al. (1998). *Consumer Measurement Systems in Child and Adolescent Mental Health*. Canberra: Department of Health and Family Services.

Black, J., Lewis, T., McIntosh, P., et al. (2009). It's not that bad: the views of consumers and carers about routine outcome measurement in mental health. *Australian Health Review*, **33**, 93–9.

Browne, G. (2006). Outcome measures: do they fit with a recovery model? *International Journal of Mental Health Nursing*, **15**, 153–4.

Callaly, T. and Hallebone, E. L. (2001). Introducing the routine use of outcomes measurement to mental health services. *Australian Health Review*, **24**, 43–50.

Callaly, T., Hyland, M., Coombs, T. and Trauer, T. (2006). Routine outcome measurement in public mental health – results of a clinician survey. *Australian Health Review*, **30**, 164–73.

Ciarlo, J. A. (1982). Accountability revisited: the arrival of client outcome evaluation. *Evaluation and Program Planning*, **5**, 31–6.

Cleary, M., Jordan, R. and Happell, B. (2002). Measuring outcomes in the workplace: The impact of an education program. *International Journal of Mental Health Nursing*, **11**, 269–75.

Close-Goedjen, J. L. and Saunders, S. M. (2002). The effect of technical support on clinician attitudes toward an outcome assessment instrument. *Journal of Behavioral Health Services & Research*, **29**, 99–108.

Coombs, T. and Meehan, T. (2003). Mental health outcomes in Australia: issues for mental health nurses. *International Journal of Mental Health Nursing*, **12**, 163–4.

Courtenay, K. P. (2002). Use of outcome measures by psychiatrists. *British Journal of Psychiatry*, **180**, 551.

Crocker, T. and Rissel, C. (1998). Knowledge of and attitudes to the health outcomes approach among community mental health professionals. *Australian Health Review*, **21**, 111–26.

Ellwood, P. M. (1988). Shattuck Lecture: Outcomes Management – a technology of experience. *New England Journal of Medicine*, **318**, 1549–56.

Epstein, A. M. (1990). The outcomes movement – will it get us where we want to go? *New England Journal of Medicine*, **323**, 266–70.

Frese, F. J., Stanley, J., Kress, K. and Vogel-Scibilia, S. (2001). Integrating evidence-based practices and the recovery model. *Psychiatric Services*, **52**, 1462–8.

Garland, A. F., Kruse, M. and Aarons, G. A. (2003). Clinicians and outcome measurement: what's the use? *Journal of Behavioral Health Services & Research*, **30**, 393–405.

Gilbody, S. M., House, A. O. and Sheldon, T. A. (2002). Psychiatrists in the UK do not use outcome measures. *British Journal of Psychiatry*, **180**, 101–3.

Gordon, S., Ellis, P., Haggerty, C., et al. (2004). *Preliminary Work towards the Development of a Self-assessed Measure of Consumer Outcome*. Auckland: Health Research Council of New Zealand.

Graham, C., Coombs, T., Buckingham, W., et al. (2001). *Consumer Perspectives of Future Directions for Outcome Self-Assessment*. Report of the Consumer Consultation Project, Wollongong.

Guthrie, D., McIntosh, M., Callaly, T., Trauer, T. and Coombs, T. (2008). Consumer attitudes towards the use of routine outcome measures in a public mental health service: a consumer-driven study. *International Journal of Mental Health Nursing*, **17**, 92–7.

Hatfield, D. R. and Ogles, B. M. (2004). The use of outcome measures by psychologists in clinical practice. *Professional Psychology: Research and Practice*, **35**, 485–91.

Huffman, L. C., Martin, J., Botcheva, L., Williams, S. E. and Dyer-Friedman, J. P. (2004). Practitioners' attitudes toward the use of treatment progress and outcomes data in child mental health services. *Evaluation & the Health Professions*, **27**, 165–88.

Jacobs, R. (2007). *Investigating Patient Outcome Measures in Mental Health: research report for the OHE Commission on NHS Productivity*. York: Centre for Health Economics, University of York.

Lakeman, R. (2004). Standardized routine outcome measurement: pot holes in the road to recovery. *International Journal of Mental Health Nursing*, **13**, 210–15.

Linder, J. C. (1991). Outcomes measurement: compliance tool or strategic initiative? *Health Care Management Review*, **16**, 21–33.

Meadows, K. A., Rogers, D. and Greene, T. (1998). Attitudes to the use of health outcome questionnaires in the routine care of patients with diabetes: a survey of general practitioners and practice nurses.

British Journal of General Practice, **48**, 1555–9.

Meehan, T., McCombes, S., Hatzipetrou, L. and Catchpoole, R. (2006). Introduction of routine outcome measures: staff reactions and issues for consideration. *Journal of Psychiatric and Mental Health Nursing*, **13**, 581–7.

Merry, S., Stasiak, K., Parkin, A., et al. (2004). *Child and youth outcome measures: Examining current use and acceptability of measures in mental health services and recommending future directions*, Auckland, available at: http://www.hrc.govt.nz.

Milne, D., Reichelt, K. and Wood, E. (2001). Implementing HoNOS: an eight stage approach. *Clinical Psychology and Psychotherapy*, **8**, 106–16.

Patterson, P., Matthey, S. and Baker, M. (2006). Using mental health outcome measures in everyday clinical practice. *Australasian Psychiatry*, **14**, 133–6.

Prabhu, R. and Oakley Browne, M. (2008). The use of the Health of the Nation Outcome Scale in an outreach rehabilitation program. *Australasian Psychiatry*, **16**, 195–9.

Sharma, V. K., Wilkinson, G. and Fear, S. (1999). Health of the Nation Outcome Scales: a case study in general psychiatry. *British Journal of Psychiatry*, **174**, 395–8.

Söderberg, P., Tungström, S. and Armelius, B. Å. (2005). Reliability of global assessment of functioning ratings made by clinical psychiatric staff. *Psychiatric Services*, **56**, 434–8.

Stedman, T., Yellowlees, P., Mellsop, G., Clarke, R. and Drake, S. (1997). *Measuring Consumer Outcomes in Mental Health*. Canberra: Department of Health and Aged Care.

Stedman, T., Yellowlees, P., Drake, S., et al. (2000). The perceived utility of six selected measures of consumer outcomes proposed for routine use in Australian mental health services. *Australian and New Zealand Journal of Psychiatry*, **34**, 842–9.

Stein, G. S. (1999). Usefulness of the Health of the Nation Outcome Scales. *British Journal of Psychiatry*, **174**, 375–7.

Trauer, T., Callaly, T. and Herrman, H. (2009a). Attitudes of mental health staff to routine outcome measurement. *Journal of Mental Health*, **18**, 288–96.

Trauer, T., Pedwell, G. and Gill, L. (2009b). The effect of guidance in the use of routine outcome measures in clinical meetings. *Australian Health Review*, **33**, 144–51.

Walter, G., Cleary, M. and Rey, J. M. (1998). Attitudes of mental health personnel toward rating outcome. *Journal of Quality in Clinical Practice*, **18**, 109–15.

Zimmerman, M. and McGlinchey, J. B. (2008). Why don't psychiatrists use scales to measure outcome when treating depressed patients? *Journal of Clinical Psychiatry*, **69**, 1917–19.

Assessment of change in outcome measurement

Tom Trauer

A central feature of the outcome measurement (OM) philosophy is the ability of OMs obtained at points in time to detect and measure change between those points. It has been suggested that single assessments merely represent measures of current status, and that they only become actual measures of outcome once there are two or more of them, allowing any change in status, or lack of change, to be captured.

The present consideration of this topic is predicated on the idea that OMs are capable of delivering information regarding change at two levels: one is at the level of the individual consumer and the other is at the level of the group. It is likely that the former level will be of primary interest and relevance to clinicians and other direct care providers, and to carers and consumers themselves, while the aggregate level will hold more for team leaders, managers, funders and those responsible for policy. This distinction should not be overstated; many people will be interested in findings at both levels. Also, the two levels are intimately connected, since the aggregate level data are constructed from assessments conducted at the individual level. Group-level results can inform interpretation at the individual level, and vice versa (Cella et al., 2002). However, generally speaking, different methods are required, not least because the confidence provided by the usually large numbers in group studies are lacking in the individual case (op. cit., p. 389).

We shall review some of the approaches that have been taken to assessing change at both the individual and group level. It will be apparent that numerous methods exist. Despite differences in approach, there is an overwhelming consensus on the inappropriateness of using statistical significance to evaluate change. The reasons for this are (a) statistical significance is primarily for evaluating between-group rather than within-individual differences, (b) statistical significance is concerned with the likelihood rather than the magnitude of change and (c) even very small differences, such as would be clinically meaningless, can achieve statistical significance if based on very large numbers.

Assessment of change in the individual

(a) Reliable change

The concept of reliable change arises from the fact that all measurement in science and clinical practice is subject to what statisticians call 'error'. The term error is used in the special sense of random inaccuracy in measurement, and not the everyday sense of 'mistake'. (Inaccuracy that is not random, but is consistent and systematic, is called bias.) All measurement, whether by laboratory equipment or by questionnaires, will be prone to some degree of error.

Random error can be illustrated by a simple example. You step on the bathroom scales and note the weight displayed. You then step off the scales and immediately step back on. You may see that the weight displayed is now slightly different from the first. You do not conclude that your weight has actually changed in the few seconds between weighings; rather, you conclude that the bathroom scales are somewhat erratic. The point of this example is that the allowance we make for the bathroom scales has a direct parallel with OMs. They too will be somewhat erratic, and this must be taken into account when making single assessments and when assessing change.

The notion of (in)accuracy of measurement leads directly to the concept of (un)reliability. There are several formal definitions of reliability, but for present purposes it may be thought of as the accuracy with which something is measured. Estimates of the reliability can be derived in a number of ways: retesting after a brief interval (test–retest), getting two or more measurements/ratings from different raters (inter-rater) and seeing to what extent the components of a measure (like the questions in a questionnaire) yield the same values (internal consistency). In each of these methods, multiple measurements are made of a single, presumably invariant, quantity. The reliability of the instrument is then derived from how close the measurements agree with each other. Estimates of reliability can range between zero (totally unreliable) and one (totally reliable). What constitutes a satisfactory level of reliability? Nunnally and Bernstein (1994, pp. 264–5) suggest that a 'modest' 0.70 may be acceptable for preliminary and basic research, while 0.80 and above is required when measurements will be used to make decisions about individuals.

In assessing change, when both the first and subsequent scores are measured with imperfect reliability, there will be some differences that are simply the result of that unreliability. The first major work to identify the concept of reliable change was that of Jacobson et al. (1984), subsequently refined by Christensen and Mendoza (1986). The essence of this approach is to identify how large a difference between two scores from the same person must be in order to be very unlikely to be the result of unreliability, i.e. how large must a difference be to be beyond the margin of measurement error. This difference is known as the Reliable Change Index (RCI). To calculate an RCI, one combines the reliability (r) and the standard deviation of the measure (SD) to produce the Standard Error of Measurement (SEm) using the formula $SEm = SD\sqrt{1-r}$, from which is derived the Standard Error of Difference (SEdiff) from the formula $SEdiff = \sqrt{2}\ SEm$. For an RCI with 95% confidence that the difference is beyond measurement error, RCI = 1.96 × SEdiff; the RCI for 90% confidence would be 1.64 × SEdiff.

Using a study group of nearly 5,000 consumers who had been assessed at least twice with the Health of the Nation Outcome Scales (HoNOS, Wing et al., 1998), Parabiaghi et al. (2005) observed a reliability of 0.73 (internal consistency) and an SD of the total score of 5.6. Using the above procedure, they calculated an RCI of 8, meaning that changes between assessments of 8 or greater were 95% likely to be reliable. This in turn allowed them to say that 91.6% of the group were stable, 5.6% improved reliably and 1.8% worsened reliably. Trauer, in a smaller study, (2004, Analysis of outcome measurement data from the four Victorian 'Round One' agencies; unpublished report), examined change in HoNOS total scores in consumers assessed at review in the community. With an estimate of reliability of 0.68 and an SD of 5.9, he obtained an RCI of 9.2. RCIs were larger when two different clinicians conducted the two assessments, and smaller when they were conducted by the same clinician. That is, the fact that a different clinician undertook the two ratings constituted a source of difference that was unrelated to the 'real' change.

(b) Clinically significant change

The idea of clinically significant change is based on the expectation that not only can scores change beyond the margin of measurement error, they can also change from abnormal or pathological levels to normal or healthy levels (and vice versa). For example, a reduction in Body Mass Index (BMI) in an obese person from 40 to 35 may well be large enough to be reliable, and may exceed an RCI, but it remains in the 'too high' range, and in that sense is not as clinically significant as if it had fallen to below 30, the criterion for obesity. In this strictly quantitative sense, a clinically significant change is one where the re-test score crosses a threshold between scores typical of the 'sick' and scores typical of the 'well'. This requires access to the distribution of OM scores of sick and well populations, such as is displayed schematically in Figure 20.1.

This figure shows the scores of a large non-depressed group and a smaller depressed group on a notional depression measure. A score of 20 best separates the two groups. In this context, a reduction from a first score of 25 to a second score of 15 would be deemed a 'clinically significant' improvement, while a rise from a first score of 15 to a second score of 25 would be a clinically significant deterioration. Note that even large improvements, as for example from 45 to 25, would not be deemed clinically significant because they remained above the threshold for clinical significance, i.e. the second score, while clearly better than the first, is still typical of depressed persons.

There are two potential limitations of this conceptualization of clinically significant change. One is that it requires data from a normative, or 'normal', sample. Certain instruments used in OM, such as the HoNOS and the Life Skills Profile (LSP, Rosen et al., 1989), were not designed to be used with persons without mental health problems, and normative data do not exist. The other limitation is that for chronic, intractable or incurable conditions, the 'return to normal' criterion may be unrealistic (Wise, 2004).

(c) Reliable and clinically significant change

Several studies have simultaneously examined reliable and significant change using OMs. Evans et al. (1998) studied 40 clients receiving short-term psychological intervention at a university student counselling service, using the CORE measure (Evans et al., 2000). Using the methods described above, they were able to classify the clients into those who showed reliable and significant change at follow-up, those who showed either reliable or significant change but not both, and those who showed neither. Piersma and Smith (1991) also used the reliable and significant change approach with a group of depressed psychiatric inpatients. They found that 36% of their group met both criteria, and noted: 'One purpose in this study

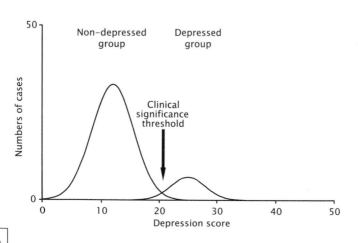

Figure 20.1 Schematic representation of scores of depressed and non-depressed individuals on a depression scale.

was to illustrate how reporting results to emphasize individual improvement can highlight variability among patients, particularly when compared with the usual method of reporting findings, that is, group means and statistical significance tests' (p. 231). Audin et al. (2001), like Parabiaghi et al. (2005), derived reliable and significant change criteria for the HoNOS, and classified consumers into nine categories according to the reliability of their change (reliable deterioration, no reliable change, reliable improvement) and the clinical significance of their change (clinical deterioration, no clinical change, clinical improvement).

While the reliable and clinically significant change methodology described above remains the most commonly reported approach (Ogles et al., 2001), limitations, such as the effect of regression to the mean, have been described (Speer, 1992). Numerous other methods exist, including the 'Minimally Important Difference' and 'Minimally Detectable Difference' (Norman et al., 2003) and Effect Size (Burgess et al., 2006). There are now a number of studies that compare and contrast the different approaches (e.g. Wyrwich et al., 2005, Eisen et al., 2007).

(d) Longitudinal models

The reliable and clinically significant approach described above is suitable when there are just two assessments, typically one at the start and the other at the end of treatment. Other more sophisticated and powerful methods that look at overall trajectory of change are available when there are more than two assessments (see also the chapter by Michael Lambert (Chapter 6) in this book).

Lambert et al. (2001) have noted that one of the limitations of the classical pre–post design is the excessively large intervals of uncertainty for individual outcomes, that is, 'The real issue is that two observations per client do not provide enough information to answer the questions that outcome evaluators must ask' (p. 276), and that 'When data are "soft" in the sense of having low reliability or large variability . . . Multiple repeated measurements add precision' (p. 277). They noted that three serial assessments are much more powerful than the minimum two, and that the value of additional observations is very small after six or seven observations.

A study employing this longitudinal approach was reported by Monzani et al. (2008), who assessed consumers receiving different 'packages of care' up to three times in a year using the Italian translation of the HoNOS (Lora et al., 2001). The analytic method used (longitudinal random effects modelling) allowed a comparison of the average reduction in HoNOS scores between care packages, controlling for a number of baseline variables, using all the available assessment data, i.e. two or three assessments in the year. These authors noted the flexibility and power of the random effects model, in particular its ability to handle complex, clustered, unbalanced and incomplete assessment data collected from routine practice. These methods, also known as multilevel methods, have been shown to be effective in quality of life research (Beacon and Thompson, 1996), compared favourably with standard pre–post methods in assessing individual change (Speer and Greenbaum, 1995) and were used by Ecob et al. (2004) to understand the respective contributions of consumer and clinician factors in HoNOS scores.

(e) Change according to whom?

It is well established that measures obtained from clinicians and consumers are only weakly correlated at best (e.g. Stedman et al., 1997, Trauer and Callaly, 2002). This is because they have differing perceptions of the nature and severity of problems, but also because certain areas of life that are of significance to many consumers, for example existential or spiritual concerns, are not reflected in many of the predominantly illness-oriented instruments employed by clinicians (Hasler et al., 2004). Thus, the low correspondence between changes on clinician and consumer scales may be due in part to their different content. It follows, therefore, that changes, estimated by whatever method, in measures based on clinician ratings may have little relation to changes based on consumer self-assessments. Two conclusions arise from this: first, always attempt to get change information from more than one source, and second, where possible, have those sources use the same instrument, or instruments that are closely linked. Examples of these are the Camberwell Assessment of Need (Phelan et al., 1995) for adults, which has forms for both clinician and consumer, and the Strengths and Difficulties Questionnaire (Goodman, 2001) for children and adolescents, which has forms for the young person as well as parents and teachers.

(f) Issues in communicating individual change information

Given the diverse ways in which individual change may be measured, and their complexities, the challenge is to find ways to present the results to interested parties, not least to the consumer whose change has been assessed. The relevant issues may be grouped into those of presentation and those of interpretation. Many consumers, as well as some staff, find numerical presentations difficult and even threatening, There is evidence that staff are most comfortable with graphical presentations (Trauer et al., 2009), and this could be true for consumers and carers as well. Interpretation involves assisting those who use OM change results to understand correctly what they mean. The concept of reliable change protects against over-interpreting small changes. Anecdotally, it has been noticed that clinicians experience less difficulty in communicating improvement than deterioration. Also, depending on the clinician's or the consumer's expectations, 'no change' may be regarded as a 'good outcome' (i.e. stability) or a disappointing result. It is possible that some of the concerns that clinicians have in discussing OM results with their consumers are based on anxieties about communicating 'poor' outcomes.

Assessment of change in groups

As mentioned at the beginning of the chapter, changes at the individual level can be aggregated to yield information at the group or collective level. The most common and generic reason for using OMs in this way is to demonstrate the effectiveness of services. This is implicit in the policy statement that initiated OM in Australia, which urged 'that specific and quantifiable measures be developed to assess the impact of services on consumer outcomes' (Australian Health Ministers, 1992, p. 30).

Many studies, e.g. Dalton (2005), have reported comparisons of 'before and after' average scores on routinely administered OMs and demonstrated significant average changes in a beneficial direction. Almost all of these studies are undertaken as service evaluation projects, and not as controlled experiments, and, while valuable in many respects, one limitation is that there is usually no way to ascertain how much of the observed change could be attributed to the service. In the absence of rigorous methodologies, resort may be made to statistical adjustments.

(a) Comparison of services adjusting for consumer and episode characteristics

This section describes one approach to the comparison of services using change scores on OMs. Referred to in the chapter by Graham Mellsop and Mark Smith (Chapter 3), the

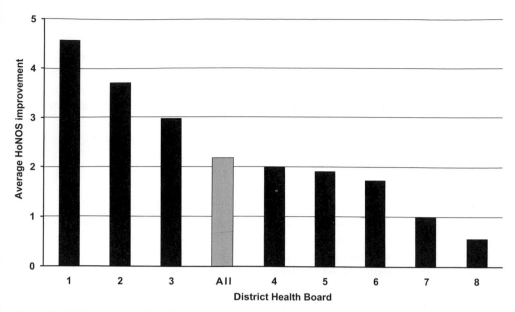

Figure 20.2 Mean change in HoNOS total score in eight New Zealand DHBs.

Classification and Outcomes Study (CAOS) in New Zealand (Gaines et al., 2003, Trauer et al., 2004) obtained 5,567 pairs of HoNOS assessments from 4,990 consumers in the eight participating District Health Boards (DHBs).

Figure 20.2 shows the mean change in HoNOS total score in the eight DHBs, with the overall average of 2.2. Note the great difference between the mean improvement of 4.6 in one service and the mean of 0.5 in another. One explanation might be that DHB 1 provides more effective mental health care, but another is that the mix of consumers is different, with DHB 8 having more 'difficult' cases.

One way to take differences in the characteristics of consumers' episodes into account is by using a casemix approach, defined in the CAOS study as:

> The purpose of a casemix classification system is to classify episodes of care based on those factors which best predict the need for, and the cost of, care. In a casemix classification, episodes of care are grouped into classes based on two criteria. First each class should contain episodes with similar patterns of resource consumption. There is an implicit assumption that consumers who consume similar resources have similar needs. Second, each class should contain episodes that are clinically similar. (Gaines et al., 2003, p. 5)

For adults, the CAOS study, which was itself based on an earlier Australian mental health casemix study (MH-CASC, Buckingham et al., 1998), derived 29 classes, 16 for inpatient episodes and 13 for community episodes. These classes were based on combinations of the following variables:

- age group
- legal status: voluntary or involuntary

- ethnicity: Maori/Pacific Islander/All Others
- whether the episode was for the purpose of Assessment Only
- start of episode scores on HoNOS items 4 (cognitive impairment), 5 (physical problems) and 6 (hallucinations and/or delusions)
- Focus of Care: a classification of the main objective of the completed episode, one of Acute/Functional Gain/Intensive Extended/Maintenance (Buckingham et al., 1998, pp. 62–3).

The classification showed that the most expensive classes of adult episodes were involuntary inpatient episodes of the three ethnicity groups, with average costs 9 to 11 times the average cost of all episodes, while the least costly were Assessment Only episodes in the community, which cost just 9%.

The 5,567 HoNOS change scores were grouped into the casemix classes that their episodes belonged to. This showed, at one extreme, that the classes that showed the greatest improvement were involuntary inpatient episodes that had an Acute Focus of Care, and had moderate to severe admission ratings on the hallucinations and/or delusions HoNOS item. For these classes, the admission HoNOS total scores at episode start were around 17 to 19, and at episode end around 7, an improvement of 10 to 12 points. At the other extreme, the least change was seen in voluntary community episodes with Intensive Extended Focus of Care; for these the HoNOS total score at both start and end of episodes was 13.9, showing zero overall change.

The next step was, for each episode, to subtract the average change for the casemix class that it belonged to from the actual change. For example, a voluntary community episode with an Intensive Extended Focus of Care with a HoNOS improvement of 5 points would have the change score of that casemix class, zero, subtracted. The resultant +5 means that this episode showed 5 more points of improvement than expected.

The final step was to average these actual minus expected change scores within each DHB. This is shown in Figure 20.3.

The dark bars in Figure 20.3 are the same as in Figure 20.2 and the lighter bars are the mean improvements expected based on the casemix classes. DHB 8, which achieved the lowest mean improvement of 0.5, could have been expected to achieve 1.3 on the basis of its casemix. DHB 1, which achieved the highest raw improvement (4.6), slightly exceeded its casemix-based expectation of 4.5. The difference between the mean achieved and the mean expected has been termed the Casemix Adjusted Relative Mean Improvement, or CARMI (Trauer et al., 2004, p. 92). On the basis of CARMI, the best performing service was DHB 3, which achieved an average improvement of nearly 3 despite a casemix-based expectation of 1.9, giving a CARMI of +1.1.

Trauer et al. (2004, Ch. 10) present similar analyses for the Life Skills Profile (LSP-16, Rosen et al., 1989, Buckingham et al., 1998), HoNOSCA (Gowers et al., 1999) and the CGAS (Schaffer et al., 1983). They concluded that 'The CARMI is a way that the outcomes achieved by different mental health services can be fairly compared for benchmarking and quality improvement purposes because it takes into account the unique mix of consumers at each DHB' (p. 105).

(b) Key Performance Indicators

Performance indicators are service descriptors that allow services to be evaluated and compared in terms of their performance and the quality of care they deliver. Key Performance

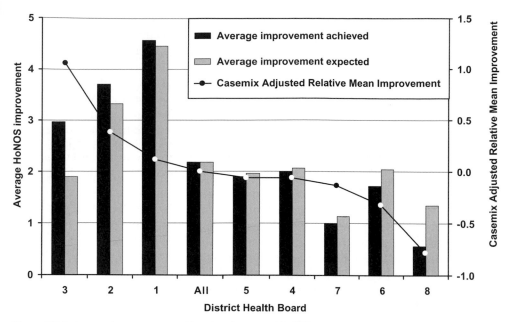

Figure 20.3 Average improvements achieved and expected, by DHB.

Indicators (KPIs) are an agreed and standard set of descriptors derived from nationally collected data. Ideally, an outcomes indicator should meet a number of criteria; McGlynn (1998) proposed seven: (1) whether the outcome is a health outcome; (2) the extent to which expectations for performance can be defined; (3) the role medical care plays in achieving the outcome; (4) the relative complexity of events that produce the outcome; (5) the degree to which attribution can reasonably be made; (6) the suitability of risk adjustment for limiting external sources of variation; and (7) the likelihood that the measure provides perverse behavioural incentives.

In 2005, the Australian government issued a framework for mental health KPIs, as part of overall performance monitoring (Information Strategy Committee, 2005). Nine domains were identified; services should be: Effective, Appropriate, Efficient, Accessible, Continuous, Responsive, Capable, Safe and Sustainable. Within each domain lay one or more subdomains. Each subdomain then required operationalizing into a KPI, which means specifying the data requirements and formula for its computation. In all, the nine domains encompassed 20 subdomains, not all of which had corresponding indicators at that time. The Effective domain comprised Consumer outcomes, Carer outcomes and Community tenure, and only the last of these had an indicator that could be computed from currently available data.

The Consumer outcomes KPI is intended to measure the impact of health care on the consumer's clinical status and functioning (and for Carer outcomes, impact on quality of life). Clearly identified as an area requiring further development, an example of what the Consumer outcomes KPI might look like was the percentage of consumers showing improvement on the HoNOS (clinical status) or LSP (functioning).

Since that time, further conceptual work has been undertaken to develop a Consumer outcomes KPI. Burgess and Pirkis (2008) identified the task as assessing clinically significant change. They compared and contrasted four methods: Classify and Count and the three main methods identified by Eisen et al. (2007): Effect Size (ES), Reliable Change Index (RCI) and Standard Error of Measurement (SEM). The Classify and Count method refers to the approach applied by Lelliott (1999) to the HoNOS whereby an assessment with a score of four on at least one item or a score of three on at least two was classified as severe. At reassessment one could count the number of cases that changed from meeting or no longer meeting this criterion. The ES approach was developed by Cohen (1988) to assess the magnitude of a treatment effect in an experiment; in its most common form, it is the difference between pre-treatment and post-treatment mean scores divided by the standard deviation of the pre-treatment scores. The RCI was described earlier in this chapter, and is closely related to the SEM in that they both explicitly incorporate the reliability of the measure (Cella et al., 2002).

Burgess and Pirkis assessed these different approaches against a number of desirable properties for a service-based KPI of effectiveness, and recommended the Classify and Count and the ES as suitable for further trialling. As an example of the ES approach, Burgess et al. (2006), analysing aggregated Australian adult data, showed that changes in HoNOS total scores between start and end of episodes of care amounted to ESs of about 1.0 in acute inpatient settings, and about 0.5 in community settings. Given Cohen's (1988) rule of thumb that an ES of ≥ 0.8 is large and 0.5 is medium, they concluded that, on the whole, consumers of the country's public mental health services do improve.

At the time of writing, there is general consensus in Australia that a KPI will express the percentage of cases meeting some improvement criterion, appropriately adjusted for factors beyond the control of the service, but debate continues as to whether the improvement criterion is based on the more population-based ES or the RCI, which is more individual-based and acknowledges the reliability of the instrument from which the KPI is calculated.

(c) Benchmarking

One useful definition of benchmarking as applied to health services is that of Bullivant (1994), who described it as 'the systematic process of searching for and implementing a standard of best practice within an individual service or similar groups of services'. Typically, this process is seen as a cycle, whereby standards are set, data are collected, comparisons made, differences discussed and interpreted, and services modify their practices, after which further rounds of data collections etc. may be undertaken. Benchmarking is closely related to KPIs, which are often used as the standards representing best practice.

One of the most developed uses of changes on outcome measures for benchmarking comes from the CORE-OM (Clinical Outcome in Routine Evaluation – Outcome Measure) system, whose 'core' is a 34-item self-completed form covering subjective well-being, personal functioning, problems and symptoms, and risk to self or others (Barkham et al., 1998). Designed primarily as a tool for assessing outcome in counselling and psychotherapy services, Mullin et al. (2006) used CORE-OM to construct recovery and improvement benchmarks from over 11,000 intake and end of therapy assessments with over 500 practitioners in 32 NHS (National Health Service) trusts. Using cut-off criteria for reliable and clinically significant change from Evans et al. (2002), they classified clients into four categories: recovery, improvement, no reliable change and reliable deterioration. Services as well as practitioners could be grouped according to how many of their clients fell into the four outcome categories. With their results they were able to show, among other things, that between 5 and 6 clients out of every 10 in the average service met the criterion of recovery, and a rate of below 5 would place a service in the bottom quarter of services. Success rates could also be computed for practitioners separately for their severely and non-severely distressed clients. They conclude with:

> benchmarks are not, in themselves, good or bad. They act as a mirror of the service, reflecting it against other services and practitioners. That is, they provide signals as to possible areas of variation within a service that might need attention. Hence, the overriding point to be made here is that the information yielded by the benchmark data needs to lead to a line of inquiry at multiple levels - the individual practitioner, the manager, and the service. Inasmuch as benchmarks can initiate this reflective practice, then they have something of the quality of clinical supervision by ensuring the delivery of quality services to clients. (p. 75)

Conclusions

This chapter has surveyed some of the more commonly used approaches to assessing change from outcome measures. It is a large and sometimes confusing area, and our coverage is by no means comprehensive. While there appears to be no general consensus as to which method or methods are best for a particular situation, a number of principles appear to be reasonably well endorsed.

First, most authorities agree that statistical significance testing is not helpful when it comes to judging whether change has occurred and, if so, how much. A statistically significant difference means only that it is most unlikely that the true change is exactly zero; while this may be a relevant question in an experiment or research project, it doesn't answer the kinds of questions that most users have of routinely collected measures in a service delivery context. Second, different methods, albeit related to a degree, are usually required for judgements of change in individuals compared to judgements of change in groups. Real and valid changes at the group level will generally not apply to all the members of the group, a misunderstanding that goes by the name of the Ecological Fallacy.

A third principle is that detection and quantification of change are much more powerful if there are more than just two (e.g. before and after) assessments. Nevertheless, the most widely used methods have been Reliable Change, with or without Significant Change. However, the development and increasing availability of powerful and sophisticated analytic methods that allow the characterization of change trajectories hold the promise of more useful reports.

Despite significant advances in methods to assess change, several challenging issues, which are comparatively under-researched, remain. One of these is how to combine and reconcile the often differing perspectives of change held by different stakeholders. Another is to ensure that the methods are not overly complicated, so that they can be used easily but validly at the clinical interface. This has implications for the training of clinical staff. Quite apart from correctly appreciating what differences in scores mean, many clinicians will need to develop or upgrade their skills in communicating these to consumers and carers in a positive and constructive fashion – a task that may be more difficult when the assessments are not progressing as hoped.

References

Audin, K., Margison, F., Clark, J. M. and Barkham, M. (2001). Value of HoNOS in assessing patient change in NHS psychotherapy and psychological treatment services. *British Journal of Psychiatry*, **178**, 561–6.

Australian Health Ministers (1992). *National Mental Health Policy*. Canberra: Australian Government Publishing Service.

Barkham, M., Evans, C., Margison, F., et al. (1998). The rationale for developing and implementing core outcome batteries for routine use in service settings and psychotherapy outcome research. *Journal of Mental Health*, **7**, 35–47.

Beacon, H. J. and Thompson, S. G. (1996). Multi-level models for repeated measurement data: application to quality of life data in clinical trials. *Statistics in Medicine*, **15**, 2717–32.

Buckingham, W., Burgess, P., Solomon, S., Pirkis, J. and Eagar, K. (1998). *Developing a Casemix Classification for Mental Health Services*. Canberra: Department of Health and Ageing.

Bullivant, J. R. N. (1994). *Benchmarking for Continuous Improvement in the Public Sector*. London: Longman.

Burgess, P. and Pirkis, J. (2008). *Key Performance Indicators for Australian Public Mental Health Services – Potential Contributions of MH-NOCC Data: Developing Indicators of Effectiveness Version 2.0*. Brisbane, Queensland.

Burgess, P., Pirkis, J. and Coombs, T. (2006). Do adults in contact with Australia's public sector mental health services get better? *Australia and New Zealand Health Policy*, **3**, 9.

Cella, D., Bullinger, M., Scott, C., Barofsky, I. and The Clinical Significance Consensus Meeting Group (2002). Group vs individual approaches to understanding the clinical significance of differences or changes in quality of life. *Mayo Clinic Proceedings*, 77, 384–92.

Christensen, L. and Mendoza, J. L. (1986). A method of assessing change in a single subject: an alteration of the RC index. *Behaviour Therapy*, **17**, 305–08.

Cohen, J. (1988). *Statistical Power Analysis for the Behavioral Sciences*, 2nd edn. Hillsdale, NJ: Lawrence Erlbaum.

Dalton, R. (2005). Client progress in a community team for mentally disordered offenders. *The British Journal of Forensic Practice*, **7**, 18–22.

Ecob, R., Croudace, T. J., White, I. R., et al. (2004). Multilevel investigation of variation in HoNOS ratings by mental health professionals: a naturalistic study of

consecutive referrals. *International Journal of Methods in Psychiatric Research*, **13**, 152–64.

Eisen, S. V., Ranganathan, G., Seal, P. and Spiro, A. I. (2007). Measuring clinically meaningful change following mental health treatment. *Journal of Behavioral Health Services & Research*, **34**, 272–89.

Evans, C., Margison, F. and Barkham, M. (1998). The contribution of reliable and clinically significant change methods to evidence-based mental health. *Evidence-based Mental Health*, **1**, 70–2.

Evans, C., Mellor-Clark, J., Margison, F., et al. (2000). CORE: clinical outcomes in routine evaluation. *Journal of Mental Health*, **9**, 247–55.

Evans, C., Connell, J., Barkham, M., et al. (2002). Towards a standardised brief outcome measure: psychometric properties and utility. *British Journal of Psychiatry*, **180**, 51–60.

Gaines, P., Bower, A., Buckingham, W., et al. (2003). *New Zealand Mental Health Classification and Outcomes Study: Final Report*. Auckland: Health Research Council of New Zealand.

Goodman, R. (2001). Psychometric properties of the Strengths and Difficulties Questionnaire. *Journal of the American Academy of Child and Adolescent Psychiatry*, **40**, 1337–45.

Gowers, S. G., Harrington, R. C., Whitton, A., et al. (1999). Brief scale for measuring the outcomes of emotional and behavioural disorders in children. Health of the Nation Outcome Scales for Children and Adolescents (HoNOSCA). *British Journal of Psychiatry*, **174**, 413–16.

Hasler, G., Moergeli, H. and Schnyder, U. (2004). Outcome of psychiatric treatment: what is relevant for our patients? *Comprehensive Psychiatry*, **45**, 199–205.

Information Strategy Committee, AHMAC National Mental Health Working Group (2005). *Key performance indicators for Australian public mental health services*, November 2004. Commonwealth of Australia.

Jacobson, N. S., Follette, W. C. and Revensdorf, D. (1984). Psychotherapy outcome research:

Methods for reporting variability and evaluating clinical significance. *Behaviour Therapy*, **15**, 336–52.

Lambert, E. W., Doucette, A. and Bickman, L. (2001). Measuring mental health outcomes with pre-post designs. *Journal of Behavioral Health Services & Research*, **28**, 273–86.

Lelliott, P. (1999). Definition of severe mental illness. In P. Charlwood, A. Mason, M. Goldacre, R. Cleary and E. Wilkinson, eds., *Health Outcome Indicators: Severe Mental Illness. Report of a Working Group to the Department of Health*. Oxford: National Centre for Health Outcomes Development.

Lora, A., Bai, G., Bianchi, S., et al. (2001). The Italian version of HoNOS (Health of the Nation Outcome Scales), a scale for evaluating the outcome and the severity in mental health services. *Epidemiologia e Psichiatria Sociale*, **10**, 198–204.

McGlynn, E. A. (1998). The outcomes utility index: will outcomes data tell us what we want to know? *International Journal for Quality in Health Care*, **10**, 485–90.

Monzani, E., Erlicher, A., Lora, A., Lovaglio, P. and Vittadini, G. (2008). Does community care work? A model to evaluate the effectiveness of mental health services. *International Journal of Mental Health Systems*, **2**, 10.

Mullin, T., Barkham, M., Mothersole, G., Bewick, B. M. and Kinder, A. (2006). Recovery and improvement benchmarks for counselling and the psychological therapies in routine primary care. *Counselling and Psychotherapy Research*, **6**, 68–80.

Norman, G. R., Sloan, J. A. and Wyrwich, K. W. (2003). Interpretation of changes in health-related quality of life: the remarkable universality of half a standard deviation. *Medical Care*, **41**, 582–92.

Nunnally, J. C. and Bernstein, I. H. (1994). *Psychometric Theory*, 3rd edn. New York: McGraw-Hill.

Ogles, B. M., Lunnen, K. M. and Bonesteel, K. (2001). Clinical significance: history, application, and current practice. *Clinical Psychology Review*, **21**, 421–46.

Parabiaghi, A., Barbato, A., D'Avanzo, B., Erlicher, A. and Lora, A. (2005). Assessing reliable and clinically significant change on Health of the Nation Outcome Scales: method for displaying longitudinal data. *Australian and New Zealand Journal of Psychiatry*, **39**, 719–25.

Phelan, M., Slade, M., Thornicroft, G., et al. (1995). The Camberwell Assessment of Need: the validity and reliability of an instrument to assess the needs of people with severe mental illness. *British Journal of Psychiatry*, **167**, 589–95.

Piersma, H. L. and Smith, A. Y. (1991). Individual variability in self-reported improvement for depressed psychiatric inpatients on the MCMI-II. *Journal of Clinical Psychology*, **47**, 227–32.

Rosen, A., Hadzi-Pavlovic, D. and Parker, G. (1989). The Life Skills Profile: a measure assessing function and disability in schizophrenia. *Schizophrenia Bulletin*, **15**, 325–37.

Schaffer, D., Gould, M. S., Brasic, J., et al. (1983). A children's global assessment scale (CGAS). *Archives of General Psychiatry*, **40**, 1228–31.

Speer, D., C. (1992). Clinically significant change: Jacobson and Truax (1991) revisited. *Journal of Consulting and Clinical Psychology*, **60**, 402–8.

Speer, D. C. and Greenbaum, P. E. (1995). Five methods for computing significant individual client change and improvement rates: support for an individual growth curve approach. *Journal of Consulting and Clinical Psychology*, **63**, 1044–8.

Stedman, T., Yellowlees, P., Mellsop, G., Clarke, R. and Drake, S. (1997). *Measuring Consumer Outcomes in Mental Health*. Canberra: Department of Health and Aged Care.

Trauer, T. and Callaly, T. (2002). Concordance between mentally ill clients and their case managers using the Health of the Nation Outcome Scales (HoNOS). *Australasian Psychiatry*, **10**, 24–8.

Trauer, T., Eagar, K., Gaines, P. and Bower, A. (2004). *New Zealand Mental Health Consumers and their Outcomes*. Auckland: Health Research Council of New Zealand.

Trauer, T., Pedwell, G. and Gill, L. (2009). The effect of guidance in the use of routine outcome measures in clinical meetings. *Australian Health Review*, **33**, 144–51.

Wing, J. K., Beevor, A. S., Curtis, R. H., et al. (1998). Health of the Nation Outcome Scales (HoNOS). Research and development. *British Journal of Psychiatry*, **172**, 11–18.

Wise, E. A. (2004). Methods for analyzing psychotherapy outcomes: a review of clinical significance, reliable change, and recommendations for future directions. *Journal of Personality Assessment*, **82**, 50–9.

Wyrwich, K. W., Bullinger, M., Aaronson, N., et al. and The Clinical Significance Consensus Meeting Group (2005). Estimating clinically significant differences in quality of life outcomes. *Quality of Life Research*, **14**, 285–95.

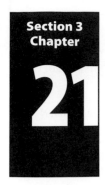

Section 3
Chapter

21

Current Issues in Outcome Measurement

Routine outcome measurement: perspectives on skills and training

Tom Trauer and Tim Coombs

In order to gain the most value from routine outcome measures (ROM), clinicians and others involved in the delivery of services need to acquire certain knowledge and skills. This chapter will review a number of issues in relation to knowledge, skills and training that have arisen over the course of the implementation of ROM in Australian public-sector mental health services. The extent to which the Australian experience is relevant and informative to services in other countries will depend on the similarities of their mental health systems, how ROM fits with these, and the specifics of the instruments and protocols they use. The coverage will start with a brief overview of the mental health workforce and some of its characteristics that are particularly relevant to training. This will be followed by an account of salient events in ROM training in Australia; the way ROM itself operates in that country is covered in the chapter by Jane Pirkis and Tom Callaly (Chapter 2). The training and related activities, which date back to the late 1990s, have provided a good deal of experience, including what some of the critical issues are. Several of the most important of these will be discussed, namely: what format training should take, whether training should be different for different users of ROM, how necessary training is, what the content of training should be, and the role of information technology infrastructure.

The mental health workforce

The mental health workforces in most developed countries have similar compositions. Typically, they comprise a variety of disciplines including medical staff, nurses, psychologists, social workers, occupational therapists and possibly several other disciplines. To support those who deliver services there are a number of administrative personnel who may have responsibility for such processes as data entry and the production of periodic reports. This workforce is not static but in a constant state of flux. The workforce has tended to become more diverse, with the creation of new roles and responsibilities, such as nurse practitioners, specialist support workers, helpers and mentors, and paid consumer and carer consultants. Also, the workforce is subject to a high level of turnover; Woltmann et al. (2008) reviewed evidence that it was between 25% and 50% per year in the United States. Further complicating the picture is that clinical staff are distributed across a variety of settings such as inpatient, community, residential, drug and alcohol and justice/corrections, and to these may be added the non-clinical staff who work in non-government organizations (NGOs) working with the mentally ill. In Australia, there are significant skill shortages (Gough and Happell, 2007), difficulty in the recruitment and retention of staff, workplace violence and aggression (Happell, 2008b) and an increasingly ageing workforce with a lack of training and support, poor working conditions and poorly defined career paths (Productivity Commission, 2005). To overcome some of these issues there has been an increasing reliance on overseas-trained staff to provide clinical services. These factors have posed significant challenges for the development of training materials and delivery of the right kind of training to the right recipients.

The development of ROM training in Australia

The first large-scale attempt to introduce ROM into public mental health services began in 2000 when a team undertook a project to develop training materials and deliver training to clinical staff in four adult mental health services in the state of Victoria. The team's approach was based on a set of principles:

- training should be flexible and tailored to local needs
- flexible modes of delivery, using various training methods
- local ownership of the implementation
- establishment of a self-sustaining training system
- the data collected should be of sufficient quality to convert to useful information
- consumers should be supported to be involved in the training.

To meet its objectives the team developed a number of resources. A training manual (Eagar et al., 2000), which set out the national and state context of ROM at the time, explained the concept of outcome, described the instruments to be used and set out a collection protocol, the set of rules that governed which instruments were to be applied with which consumers on which occasions. The manual's appendices presented materials for use in training, such as model course outlines for training sessions of varying lengths, teaching aids and sample evaluation forms.

Another resource was a set of training video vignettes – carefully scripted fictitious clinical cases with the roles of consumers, clinicians, family members and others played by actors, portraying scenarios in inpatient and community and metropolitan and country settings. The 'cases' portrayed were relatively severe, in order to provide practice in judging the severity of problems, and thereby arriving at the correct rating. These vignettes were structured so that not only would trainees have the necessary information to make practice ratings on the consumer at a single point in time, but some vignettes saw the same consumer at different points in time. This allowed trainees to make practice ratings at different stages in an episode of care. In this way, trainees not only practised rating the measures but also had the opportunity to see how the measures can be used to monitor change over time. The vignettes were accompanied by extracts from 'case notes' and recommended (i.e. 'correct') ratings of the vignettes on the instruments. These recommended ratings were for trainers to use in discussion, and to rectify misconceptions and reinforce the rating rules.

The project left a legacy of reports and materials that were used in subsequent training activities. One report (Graham et al., 2001) outlined the results of extensive consultations with consumers to understand their perspectives on self-assessment. Another (Eagar et al., 2001b) described the various printed outcomes reports that were developed, such as individual and aggregate, and for assessments made at one point in time and change over time. The final project report (Eagar et al., 2001a) documented what had been learned and made several recommendations, such as the need to provide ongoing support to agencies and the critical nature of information technology.

The project is further described in Trauer et al. (2002). They concluded that:

> A critical success factor in the successful introduction of outcome measurement within a service is that both senior and middle managers embrace and enthusiastically support its implementation. This ensures that staff are released for training and that the measures become embedded in the ongoing activity of the organisation. This type of leadership is essential from psychiatrists within the service since the involvement of this group is important to the clinical credibility to the routine use of outcome measurement. Regrettably, very few psychiatrists participated in the training we conducted. (p. 129)

At the same time, the project was evaluated by Coombs et al. (2002). They reported that, while most participants rated the training positively, 45% in one agency and 64% in another felt they needed more training, which was probably a result of their receiving much shorter training sessions than the other two agencies. In general, it was possible to show that, even after relatively short training sessions, staff can demonstrate sufficient knowledge and skill in the application of the main instruments to begin data collection using these measures. Following this early work, the different states and territories then began the process of training their own workforces.

We turn now to a consideration of some of the key issues identified in Australia, along with relevant experience from other countries, some of which is covered separately in other chapters.

'Train the Trainer' or 'Train the Troops'?

Different approaches to the process of training and implementation were adopted in different states and territories. The Victorian project had trialled two training formats: one, called 'Train the Troops', involved direct training of clinical staff by central trainers, while the other, called 'Train the Trainers', had the central trainers delivering training to locally nominated trainers, who then returned to their services and trained the clinical staff, and continued to be local resources. One state (Queensland) adopted a 'Train the Troops' approach; they created a team of four trainers who were responsible for directly training the clinical workforce across the whole state. Over a 12-month period they delivered a consistent training package to about 3,000 staff. In contrast, another state (New South Wales) adopted a 'Train the Trainer' approach; a series of 2-day workshops were attended by about 500 staff with the expectation that they would return to their host organizations and undertake training.

Both of these models had advantages and disadvantages, largely complementary. The advantage of a small team of trainers is that the workforce receives consistent training messages, but the disadvantage is the burden on team members in travelling to deliver the training, and the large disruptive effect of the loss of even a single team member. The 'Train the Trainer' approach had its own problems. New South Wales encountered inconsistencies in the training delivered by the designated trainers when they returned to their services. For example, some trainers characterized ROM as essentially a quality-improvement activity (a key training message in the 'Train the Trainer' workshops), while others highlighted the possibility of ROM being used to fund mental health services, a message that was not promoted in the workshops they had attended. Additional activities, such as forums, training and retraining, were required to correct these distortions.

Other states adopted hybrid models combining small centralized training teams as well as 'Train the Trainer' activities. One of the criticisms of the New South Wales training was the inadequate development of training and educational skills (as distinct from knowledge about ROM) in those who were expected to become trainers following attendance at the 'Train the Trainer' workshops. To combat these concerns, South Australia specifically invested in the development of training skills in those attending their 'Train the Trainer' sessions, awarding them a nationally recognized trainer qualification. The experience in that state revealed another potential limitation of the 'Train the Trainer' approach. Some of the trainers they produced were not subsequently utilized as ROM trainers when they returned to their host organizations and never had the chance to use the skills that had been developed, while others used the qualification they had acquired to gain positions as educators but, in those new roles, were engaged in duties other than ROM training.

Since these events, much of the training around the nation has been coordinated by the Training and Service Development function of the Australian Mental Health Outcomes and Classification Network (AMHOCN), which was set up in late 2003. From its central position, it has been able to bring some uniformity and consistency of message to training around the country, not least by its further development of training materials and support of local training initiatives. It has also introduced online training in order to (a) overcome some of the practical obstacles, such as releasing staff for training and time pressures, and (b) make training more accessible to staff in rural and remote locations. While bringing certain benefits, online training also has certain limitations: currently it only provides basic training in the administration of the measures, and there is the danger that staff may regard themselves as fully trained after only a brief and limited exposure to the measures.

Different training for different staff?

In Australia, whenever ROM training was delivered at the local agency (whether by central trainers or by local staff who had themselves been recently trained), little consideration was given to the composition of the group to be trained. The expectation has generally been that all clinical staff who would be engaged in ROM would attend the same session. In this way, the same training package would be delivered to, and the same skills acquired by, all clinicians in an agency, and consistency would be maintained. There is some evidence that ratings on the Health of the Nation Outcome Scales (HoNOS, Wing et al., 1998) can vary according to the profession of the rater: Ecob et al. (2004) found that 'As HoNOS total and subscale scores show much larger variation by assessor than by referral source, investigations of HoNOS scores must take assessors into account' and this led them to recommend that 'Services should implement and evaluate interdisciplinary training to improve consistency in use of rating thresholds' (abstract).

The default expectation that training would be multidisciplinary was not always realized. One common occurrence was that the medical staff did not attend, even when sessions had been well advertised in advance. In some cases this was because medical staff were unsure whether they were expected to complete outcome measures, or whether those instruments were to be completed only by nurses or non-medical case managers. In other cases it appeared that medical staff were unused to participating in mixed training events, and were more comfortable in exclusively medical educational forums. Since ROM training was always delivered by clinicians from non-medical backgrounds, it may even have been that some doctors were uncomfortable in receiving training from staff that they would otherwise expect to be subordinate or junior to them. Their non-attendance may have been related to their generally lower enthusiasm for ROM (reviewed in the chapter on stakeholder perspectives (Chapter 19) in this book). Pring (1998), a psychiatrist writing for his colleagues, observed: 'I am concerned about the fact that few psychiatrists seem to be interested in undergoing the training to regularly use the HoNOS instrument', and the Office of Health Economics in the UK (2008) noted that 'To sustain the routine use of outcome measures there needs to be training in their use for all clinicians including new doctors' (p. 7) and also that it should be part of medical education for new doctors (p. 62).

We have no evidence as to the relative contribution of the possible causes, but the end result was that far fewer of the medical staff received training. This is likely to have had a detrimental effect on the use of ROM in the workplace, since it meant that they were less able to contribute to discussion and interpretation of measures performed by other staff, and the lack of involvement of some of the most senior professionals in the team detracted from the perceived importance of ROM.

Another group who were potentially problematic were the non-clinical staff, such as team leaders and service managers, who may have had clinical roles in their past, but were currently engaged in non-clinical duties. From one point of view it was good that these people could see what the clinical staff were being expected to do, but on the other it was sometimes difficult for them to participate to the full, especially when it came to making ratings of the clinical vignettes.

How important is training anyway?

Many services would not contemplate requiring its clinical staff to begin using instruments to assess consumers' problems without at least some degree of initial training. In relation to the HoNOS, James (James and Mitchell, 2004), who conducted much of the HoNOS training in the United Kingdom, wrote: 'It is not uncommon for clinical staff to receive a HoNOS pack with directions to start using it immediately. Whilst this might allow a service provider to rightly claim that they are using outcome measurement, such a strategy is fraught with dangers, the most obvious of which is that, without adequate training and ongoing supervision, the HoNOS data collected would not stand up to questions of validity and reliability' (p. 44) and 'In addition, it is thought that a brief one-off training course is not sufficient to guarantee comparability between individual raters or between groups of raters and that practice and ongoing supervision are required to maintain reliability and data quality' (p. 45). Other authors have similarly pressed the necessity for training.

However, other studies have questioned the effect of training. Brooks (2000) found that while inter-rater reliability of the HoNOS did improve following training, it remained at unsatisfactory levels. Rock and Preston (2001) tested the inter-rater reliability (IRR) of groups of mental health nurses and two groups of non-clinicians, one with prior exposure to mental health consumers and the other without, in the rating of standard text-based training vignettes. They found no significant difference between IRR scores post-training compared with the pre-training scores. There was also no significant difference between nurses and the non-clinicians who had prior exposure to mental health consumers. However, unlike the study by Brooks, all their groups achieved adequate reliability coefficients. They proposed two possible interpretations. First, the HoNOS is so well designed that only familiarity with mental consumers is sufficient to achieve adequate reliability even without training, and/or using written vignettes does not provide a valid measure of reliability for the HoNOS.

Despite these two reports, the consensus of opinion appears to be that training is required. Indeed, there are several reports of trained staff wanting additional training (Garland et al., 2003, Callaly et al., 2006). In most cases, training involves more than simply ensuring that clinicians can complete the assessment instruments correctly. Just what should be the content of training for ROM is considered next.

What should training in ROM comprise?

The early training in Australia, described above, focused heavily on the 'collection protocol' (the system of rules governing which measures should be applied with which consumers on which occasions) and developing skills in the correct rating of consumers' problems on the provider-completed measures. Given the relatively compressed time available for training, priority was given to trying to ensure that clinicians produced correct ratings at the correct times.

Subsequent experience has shown that this focus was too narrow. Its primary limitation was that it reflected the priorities and needs of those responsible for ROM, rather than those of the clinicians who were doing the collection. There have been numerous calls for initial and additional training to afford more 'clinical utility', i.e. for ROM to be rendered more practically useful to the clinicians themselves.

Clinicians interviewed by Crocker and Rissel (1998) wanted more practical applications of health outcome measures, and Hodges et al. (2001) listed providing ongoing training in how to use data among their strategies for increasing information utilization. Garland et al. (2003) reported that many respondents requested more training and information on how to use interpretation of the scores in practice. The clinicians studied by Callaly et al. (2006) said that they wanted more sophisticated support to help them to understand the meaning and possible use of outcome measure ratings.

Long and Dixon (1996) identified three related but distinct desirable criteria for routinely used measures: feasibility of use, clinical utility and acceptability. Whereas these are sometimes regarded as interchangeable, we contend that it is more helpful to keep them separate. Feasibility is concerned with how practicable a measure is, e.g. not too long, and acceptability is concerned with whether users like it, but clinical utility relates to whether it assists the users in their work. Brief measures may be quite feasible, but if they are not useful they will be seen as less acceptable because they take up time that could be better spent. As a consequence, recent efforts have been made to make ROM more clinically useful.

One strand of such effort has been to assist users to understand what the measures mean. Early assumptions that the meanings of ROM scores are self-evident have proved unwarranted. Of 15 respondents to a structured interview following HoNOS training in the UK, nearly half did not give positive responses to the question 'Do you feel that you understand the HoNOS data?' (Milne et al., 2001, Figure 4).

In Australia, reference and 'normative' information in the form of tables and graphs, as produced by AMHOCN, is frequently presented in basic training sessions, and trainees are shown how to compare the ratings of a given consumer with the reference data, and how to draw conclusions about how 'abnormal' or how typical such a rating is for a consumer of given characteristics, such as age, gender and diagnosis, at a given collection occasion (admission, review or discharge) in a given setting (hospital or community). Somewhat more complicated is assisting users to draw valid conclusions from scores from repeat assessments. Approaches to inferring whether changes in scores represent 'reliable' or 'clinically significant' change require a degree of technical sophistication, and are presented in the chapter on assessing change (Chapter 20), but the challenge in training is to present such methods in a way that is valid yet sufficiently straightforward for the average user to be able to use with confidence in day-to-day practice.

Another strand in promoting clinical utility is to show how to link the measurements to clinical decision-making. The work of Lambert and colleagues (2001) has demonstrated that a simple system of coloured dots on the client's file showing whether progress was on or off track was the kind of feedback that assisted therapists to adjust their practice in the following session. Stewart (2008) in New Zealand has developed a system for use in team meetings whereby initial questions of HoNOS scores are whether the consumer's level of severity is appropriate for the service. Other materials have been developed in Australia to expose staff to using the measures in case presentations and as part of clinical reviews. These ways of using ROM scores make them (more) clinically useful, and are beginning to be included into training.

One of the purposes to which ROM can be put is for clinicians and consumers to discuss their respective ratings with each other, sometimes in the context of collaboratively developing a service plan. There is abundant evidence that clinician and consumer perceptions of the consumer's problems are often quite different (e.g. Hansson et al., 2001, Trauer and Callaly, 2002), but staff get little if any guidance on how to discuss differing points of view with clients in a constructive fashion. We have some unpublished, anecdotal, evidence that some clinicians avoid discussing ratings with consumers for a variety of reasons; some fear that it will upset the consumer, or it may damage the therapeutic relationship, or that the whole exercise will be too difficult and confusing for consumers.

In order to build clinicians' competence and confidence, a training role-play exercise has been developed. The exercise is in two parts. The first part involves participants in training forming groups of three. One plays a consumer, the other a clinician and the third is an observer. The clinician offers the consumer self-assessment measure to the consumer. The observer watches for certain behaviours related to offering the consumer self-assessment measure. This exercise highlights the clinical skills necessary to introduce a consumer self-assessment measure into clinical practice. Some clinicians seem to manage this role play quite easily, but others struggle. It is clear that not all clinicians have thought about how to build a consumer self-assessment measure into the assessment and the therapy process. The second part of the activity is just as important as the offering; here roles are exchanged and the task is for the clinician to now provide feedback to the consumer on what the completed measure is telling the clinician, what has changed from previous collection and what might be the future direction of treatment or therapy. Again, the observer watches for certain behaviours and provides constructive feedback after the role play.

This training exercise almost always exposes a lack of understanding of the measure on the part of the clinicians; they are unsure of how the measure is scored, what certain ratings may be, and feel uncomfortable in their discussions with the consumer about how to talk about change using a set of standard measures. Although these role plays may be challenging, the training sessions are almost always positively evaluated, with many participants feeling that all staff should receive this type of training. A more formal evaluation of this training has shown that these sessions are able to change staff attitudes towards routine outcome measurement, in particular the use of consumer self-assessment measures and the process of providing feedback on the completed measures to consumers (Willis et al., 2009).

In ROM systems that rely heavily on clinician-completed measures, as in Australia, there is evidence that consumers and carers are often unaware of the collection (Guthrie et al., 2008), and sometimes the clinician-oriented instruments are criticized for their negative wording and lack of 'recovery' focus (Happell, 2008a). In response to this, there have been initiatives to involve consumers and carers directly in training and in the design, development and production of training materials that promote consumer perspectives (Black et al., 2009).

What information technology is required?

When ROM is introduced across a large system, an information technology (IT) system is required in order to upload data as they are collected, hold them securely and make them available in a timely fashion and in suitable formats to those who need to use them. Well-designed, reliable and responsive IT infrastructure is essential to ROM (Percevic et al., 2004) and lack of suitable IT has been implicated in limited participation in ROM (Aoun et al., 2002).

Suitable IT systems are a necessary but not sufficient condition for successful ROM implementation. Even when IT systems for ROM are in place, the attitudes and skills of the workforce in using it can be an obstacle. As mentioned above, the mental health workforce is ageing, and some sections of that workforce dislike using computers (Ward et al., 2008). Furthermore, some clinical staff have resisted the idea that they should be involved in 'data entry' on the grounds that it takes them away from their core activities, namely clinical practice. This resistance has resulted in some expansion of the clerical and administrative positions to undertake either the process of data entry or the printing of reports, or even to sit with consumers to complete their self-assessment measures.

Many of the reports produced by ROM IT systems in Australia show aggregated results and are designed primarily for team leaders and service managers. These reports can give them useful information on the symptom and disability profiles of the consumers in the services they manage. Without specific explanation and training in what the scales measure, how and when they are applied and what the averages mean, these local managers can sometimes have difficulty in fully comprehending their reports. Whereas managers usually ensured that their staff attended training, they typically did not attend themselves, which left them at a disadvantage. It can be embarrassing for a manager to have to admit that they understand ROM reports less well than the staff they manage.

The implication for training seems clear. Everyone who is expected to use OMs in some way is entitled to receive the training they require, and the training should cover all aspects of use and match as closely as possible the on-the-job experience of using ROM.

Does training have to be repeated, and if so, how often?

Given the ongoing nature of ROM and the risk of 'rater drift' (Ventura et al., 1993), it seems advisable for involved staff to have repeated practice. Vatnaland et al. (2007) concluded that a 'continually updated educational program' was required in order to ensure reliable clinical use of the Global Assessment of Functioning Scale (GAF, Goldman et al., 1992), widely used as an outcome measure in Norway (see Chapter 9 in this book).

Adams et al. (2000), noting unusually low HoNOS scores in the consumers on an acute psychiatric ward, called for 'required and repeated training which gives staff experience of observing problems throughout the response range' (p. 198). Callaly et al. (2006) reported that 'The most frequent observation from clinicians in relation to making outcome measures more useful to them in clinical practice was that more training, particularly refresher training, is needed' (abstract), and many of those trained by Milne et al. (2001) favoured periodic refresher training. While there is general consensus that training should be repeated, what is not at all clear is how frequently this should occur.

Conclusions

The complexity of the mental health workforce and the differing roles and responsibilities have posed significant challenges to the development of training materials and the subsequent implementation process. It is possible to provide training in the measures and information on the use of routine outcome measurement. The process of implementation has made clear that implementating routine outcome measurement requires much more than simply training in the administration and scoring of the instruments. Clinicians and managers have to be shown the utility of the measures to meet a variety of different needs within services.

Future issues in workforce development include numerical literacy. As we have seen from some of the attitudes of staff, there are concerns regarding the quantification of the human condition. However, increasingly clinicians and service managers will be presented with ROM-based information; their training will in large part determine what they make of this material and how they use it to support clinical practice and improvement in service quality. The requisite skills cannot be assumed to be pre-existing, and need to be developed and maintained; a process that closely mirrors the broader agenda of moving toward evidence-based practice.

Finally, in Australia plans are afoot to place ROM training on a more formal basis. The development of courses through which clinicians (and others) can study ROM in some depth and come away with a recognized qualification can serve several purposes, one of which is acknowledging that ROM is a serious enterprise about which there is a lot to learn.

Acknowledgement

The authors would like to thank Jane Pirkis for advice on this chapter.

References

Adams, M., Palmer, A., O'Brien, J. T. and Crook, W. (2000). Health of the nation outcome scales for psychiatry: are they valid. *Journal of Mental Health*, **9**, 193–8.

Aoun, S., Pennebaker, D. and Janca, A. (2002). Outcome measurement in rural mental health: a field trial of rooming-in models. *Australian Journal of Rural Health*, **10**, 302–7.

Black, J., Lewis, T., McIntosh, P., et al. (2009). It's not that bad: the views of consumers and carers about routine outcome measurement in mental health. *Australian Health Review*, **33**, 93–9.

Brooks, R. (2000). The reliability and validity of the Health of the Nation Outcome Scales: validation in relation to patient derived measures. *Australian and New Zealand Journal of Psychiatry*, **34**, 504–11.

Callaly, T., Hyland, M., Coombs, T. and Trauer, T. (2006). Routine outcome measurement in public mental health – results of a clinician survey. *Australian Health Review*, **30**, 164–73.

Coombs, T., Trauer, T. and Eagar, K. (2002). Training in mental health outcome measurement: evaluation of the Victorian experience. *Australian Health Review*, **25**, 74–82.

Crocker, T. and Rissel, C. (1998). Knowledge of and attitudes to the health outcomes approach among community mental health professionals. *Australian Health Review*, **21**, 111–26.

Eagar, K., Buckingham, B., Coombs, T., et al. (2000). *Outcome Measurement in Adult Area Mental Health Services: Implementation Resource Manual*. Melbourne: Department of Human Services Victoria.

Eagar, K., Buckingham, B., Coombs, T., et al. (2001a). *Final Report on the Implementation of Outcome Measurement In Adult Area Mental Health Services in Victoria*. Wollongong.

Eagar, K., Buckingham, B., Coombs, T., et al. (2001b). *Victorian Mental Health Outcomes Measurement Strategy Framework For Agency-Level Standard Reports*. Wollongong.

Ecob, R., Croudace, T. J., White, I. R., et al. (2004). Multilevel investigation of variation in HoNOS ratings by mental health professionals: a naturalistic study of consecutive referrals. *International Journal* of Methods in Psychiatric Research, **13**, 152–64.

Garland, A. F., Kruse, M. and Aarons, G. A. (2003). Clinicians and outcome measurement: what's the use? *Journal of Behavioral Health Services & Research*, **30**, 393–405.

Goldman, H. H., Skodol, A. E. and Lave, T. R. (1992). Revising Axis V for DSM-IV: a review of measures of social functioning. *American Journal of Psychiatry*, **149**, 1148–56.

Gough, K. and Happell, B. (2007). We can't find the solution until we know the problem: understanding the mental health nursing labour force. *Australasian Psychiatry*, **15**, 109–14.

Graham, C., Coombs, T., Buckingham, W., et al. (2001). *Consumer Perspectives of Future Directions for Outcome Self-Assessment*. Report of the Consumer Consultation Project, Wollongong.

Guthrie, D., McIntosh, M., Callaly, T., Trauer, T. and Coombs, T. (2008). Consumer attitudes towards the use of routine outcome measures in a public mental health service: a consumer-driven study. *International Journal of Mental Health Nursing*, **17**, 92–7.

Hansson, L., Vinding, H. R, Mackeprang, T., et al. (2001). Comparison of key worker and patient assessment of needs in schizophrenic patients living in the community: a Nordic multicentre study. *Acta Psychiatrica Scandinavica*, **103**, 45–51.

Happell, B. (2008a). Determining the effectiveness of mental health services from a consumer perspective. Part 2: barriers to recovery and principles for evaluation. *International Journal of Mental Health Nursing*, **17**, 123–30.

Happell, B. (2008b). Putting all the pieces together: exploring workforce issues in mental health nursing. *Contemporary Nurse*, **29**, 43–52.

Hodges, S., Woodbridge, M. and Huang, L. N. (2001). Creating useful information in data-rich environments.In M. Hernandez and S. Hodges, eds., *Developing Outcome Strategies in Children's Mental Health*. Baltimore, MD: Paul H. Brookes.

James, M. and Mitchell, D. (2004). Measuring health and social functioning using HoNOS. In M. Harrison, D. Howard and D. Mitchell, eds., *Acute Mental Health Nursing: From Acute Concerns to the Capable Practitioner*. Thousand Oaks, CA: Sage.

Lambert, M. J., Hansen, N. B. and Finch, A. E. (2001). Patient focused research: using patient outcome data to enhance treatment effects. *Journal of Consulting and Clinical Psychology*, **69**, 159–72.

Long, A. F. and Dixon, P. (1996). Monitoring outcomes in routine practice: defining appropriate measurement criteria. *Journal of Evaluation in Clinical Practice*, **2**, 71–8.

Milne, D., Reichelt, K. and Wood, E. (2001). Implementing HoNOS: an eight stage approach. *Clinical Psychology and Psychotherapy*, **8**, 106–16.

Office of Health Economics (2008). NHS Outcomes, Performance and Productivity.

Percevic, R., Lambert, M. J. and Kordy, H. (2004). Computer-supported monitoring of patient treatment response. *Journal of Clinical Psychology*, **69**, 285–99.

Pring, W. (1998). The measurement of suffering. *Victorian Branch RANZCP Newsletter*, 2–4.

Productivity Commission (2005). Australia's Health Workforce. Canberra.

Rock, D. and Preston, N. (2001). HoNOS: is there any point in training clinicians? *Journal of Psychiatric and Mental Health Nursing*, **8**, 405–9.

Stewart, M. (2008). Making the HoNOS(CA) clinically useful: a strategy for making HonOS, HoNOSCA, and HoNOS65+ useful to the clinical team. *Australian and New Zealand Journal of Psychiatry*, **42**, A5.

Trauer, T. and Callaly, T. (2002). Concordance between mentally ill clients and their case managers using the Health of the Nation Outcome Scales (HoNOS). *Australasian Psychiatry*, **10**, 24–8.

Trauer, T., Coombs, T. and Eagar, K. (2002). Training in routine mental health outcome assessment: the Victorian experience. *Australian Health Review*, **25**, 122–8.

Vatnaland, T., Vatnaland, J., Friis, S. and Opjordsmoen, S. (2007). Are GAF scores reliable in routine clinical use? *Acta Psychiatrica Scandinavica*, **115**, 326–30.

Ventura, J., Green, M. F., Shaner, A. and Liberman, R. P. (1993). Training and quality assurance with the Brief Psychiatric Rating Scale: 'the drift busters'. *International Journal of Methods in Psychiatric Research*, **3**, 221–44.

Ward, R., Stevens, C., Brentnall, P. and Briddon, J. (2008). The attitudes of health care staff to information technology: a comprehensive review of the research literature. *Health Information and Libraries Journal*, **25**, 81–97.

Willis, A., Deane, F. P. and Coombs, T. (2009). Improving clinicians' attitudes toward providing feedback on routine outcome assessments. *International Journal of Mental Health Nursing*, **18**, 211–15.

Wing, J. K., Beevor, A. S., Curtis, R. H., et al. (1998). Health of the Nation Outcome Scales (HoNOS). Research and development. *British Journal of Psychiatry*, **172**, 11–18.

Woltmann, E. M., Whitley, R., McHugo, G. J., et al. (2008). The role of staff turnover in the implementation of evidence-based practices in mental health care. *Psychiatric Services*, **59**, 732–7.

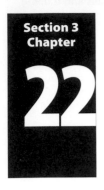

Current Issues in Outcome Measurement

A review of instruments in outcome measurement

Tom Trauer

In this chapter I present a review of instruments commonly employed in outcome measurement (OM). This will involve considering the domains that are assessed, the types of instruments used, and some consideration of how scales are or can be used in combination. Extra attention is devoted to the Health of the Nation Outcome Scales (HoNOS), given its wide use. I shall not attempt to catalogue and describe all the leading instruments in OM since there already exist a number of texts that do that, such as Sederer and Dickey (1996), Schmidt et al. (2000), Tansella and Thornicroft (2001), IsHak et al. (2002) and an Outcomes Compendium produced by the National Institute for Mental Health in England (2008).

Areas of coverage

Since routine outcome measurement (ROM) aims to assess all consumers within a service in a systematic and comparable fashion, the instruments tend to focus on broad ranges of problems, rather than solely on the problems associated with specific mental health syndromes. Naturally, this broad coverage comes at a price, which is some lack of depth. The general requirement that instruments be quite brief also contributes to what has sometimes been described as superficiality. Nevertheless, such instruments as have been used can be grouped into areas or domains.

Some have written on what areas should be encompassed by OMs. Rosenblatt and Attkisson (1993) identified four such areas: clinical status, functional status, life satisfaction and fulfilment, and safety and welfare. Following an extensive systematic review, Slade (2002b) identified 16 outcome domains that could be further grouped into seven 'emergent categories', namely well-being, cognition/emotion, behaviour, physical health, interpersonal, society and services. When consumers are consulted directly on this question they tend to produce similar lists. Those asked by Graham et al. (2001) listed quality of life, functioning, physical health and health risks, relationships, illness symptoms, coping and recovering from illness, and satisfaction with service quality, and a similar list, but with the additions of connection to culture, hope, empowerment and spirituality, was compiled from consumers in New Zealand by Gordon et al. (2004).

While all of these areas will be relevant to various stakeholders, OM in practice has tended to operationalize only some of them. This review will be organized around symptom severity, personal functioning, quality of life, perceived needs and recovery; it will not cover satisfaction with services, which is often regarded as a service outcome rather than a personal outcome.

(a) Symptom severity

When outcome is defined as the effect of an intervention on health status, and that intervention is a form of treatment, it is natural to resort to a measure of illness or symptom severity.

The most widely used such instrument is the Health of the Nation Outcome Scales (Wing et al., 1998), although certain other instruments, such as the Clinical Global Impression Scale (CGI, Guy, 1976), have also been reported in an OM context (Berk et al., 2008).

The HoNOS for adults and its related measures for children and adolescents (HoNOSCA, Gowers et al., 1999b) and for older persons (HoNOS65+, Burns et al., 1999b) have become something of a standard in several countries. It was developed specifically 'to quantify and thus potentially measure progress toward a Health of the Nation target, set by the Department of Health, "to improve significantly the health and social functioning of mentally ill people"' (Wing et al., 1998, p. 11).

The HoNOS and HoNOS65+ have 12 items/scales, while the HoNOSCA has 15, the last two of which are informational and can be omitted from computation of the total score. All versions are completed by the clinician, who is expected to have received some training in their use, including the use of the glossaries (Burns et al., 1999a, Gowers et al., 1999a, Wing et al., 1999). The three HoNOS forms produce total scores and four subscales scores, namely behaviour, impairment, symptoms and social, although the robustness of these subscales has been questioned (Harnett et al., 2005) and alternative subscale structures have been proposed (Trauer, 1999, Newnham et al., 2009).

Members of the HoNOS family are referred to frequently and in many different contexts throughout this book, so we shall not attempt a comprehensive review of their literature here. There are a number of studies reporting their psychometric properties, many of which were reviewed by Pirkis et al. (2005), who described common repeated findings of generally good validity and sensitivity to change, weak relationships with consumer-rated measures, and fair to moderate estimates of reliability. Some HoNOS users have found mixed qualities: for example Bonsack et al. (2002), using a French version, reported good acceptance by clinicians, separation of patient groups and sensitivity in inpatient settings, but susceptibility to measurement errors and low sensitivity to change in outpatient settings where problem severity was milder.

While much of the HoNOS literature is concerned with technical aspects of the instrument and descriptions of small-scale local applications, some of the more recent papers have been about the interpretation of scores and its use at the clinical interface. For example, Burgess et al. (2008) surveyed HoNOS 'experts' in Australia who confirmed that a score of 2 on any item constituted the threshold for clinical significance, and all items were of generally equal importance in the judgement of overall clinical severity, even though some could be expected to change more than others over the course of treatment.

The HoNOS is clearly focused on clinicians' evaluations of problems associated with moderate to severe mental illness. As Jacobs (2007, p. 75) noted: 'HoNOS is rooted very much in a medical model of mental health problems. There is seen to be a big discontinuity with HoNOS between what users perceive to be important aspects of their care and what clinicians perceive to be important. HoNOS therefore potentially under-represents the user's perspective'. In fact, there has been some experience with consumer-rated versions. Trauer and Callaly (2002) used the experimental self-rated version (HoNOS-SR, College Research Unit, 1996) and found that (a) consumers' ratings were significantly higher (worse) than those of their case manager ratings on four the 12 HoNOS items, and significantly lower on one, (b) overall agreement levels were slight to moderate, but particularly low for the depressed mood item, and (c) case managers tended to overestimate the actual degree of similarity between their own ratings and those of their consumers. Stewart (2009) developed consumer and significant-other versions of HoNOS which he used with consumers of an early intervention for psychosis. Unlike Trauer and Callaly, he found that agreement levels between them and with the clinicians were generally good, a finding he attributed to the close working relationships in that service that might have led to better shared understandings and more similar ratings. Also, the response format was adapted for the non-clinicians, and this may have made the rating task easier for them.

The version of HoNOS in use throughout adult services in Australia first appeared in the mid-1990s (College Research Unit, 1996). Since that time it has been widely used, and there have been numerous reports of perceived limitations and suggestions for improvements. An early review identified problems with the reliability of certain items, but advised against local modification, because that would lead to non-standardized use (Trauer, 1998). A more substantial later review (Trauer and Buckingham, 2006) addressed (a) issues relating to certain individual items, (b) choices regarding computation of summary scores when some items are left unrated and (c) the need to maintain standardization if modifications were to be embarked upon. A distinction was drawn between minor changes, which may leave certain problems uncorrected but would retain the essential nature of the current version of HoNOS, and major change that would have the potential to correct more problems, but could lead to the de facto creation of a new instrument. They also recommended that any revision be coordinated between the major users and the copyright owner, and warned against local modifications, however seemingly desirable at the local level, on the grounds that uncontrolled diversification would ultimately be to the detriment of all. Despite the widespread use and interest in the HoNOS, there are certain things that it is not. James and Mitchell (2004) warned that it is not a structured interview, nor a measure of future risk, nor, in isolation, a decision-making tool.

Another instrument designed to assess the severity of mental health problems is the Threshold Assessment Grid (TAG, Slade et al., 2000), a brief measure in which the clinician rates seven domains: intentional and unintentional self-harm, risk from others and to others, survival (amenities, resources or living skills), psychological (distressing problems with thinking or feeling) and social (problems with relationships and activities). Companion papers have described its psychometric properties (Slade et al., 2002) and its feasibility and suitability for routine OM (Slade et al., 2001). Other measures, discussed more extensively elsewhere in this book, are the CORE-OM (Evans et al., 2002, Barkham et al., 2005, 2006, Leach et al., 2005), a self-report instrument with domains of subjective well-being, symptoms, function and risk, and the OQ-45 (Lambert et al., 2001, 2004).

(b) Personal functioning

It has long been recognized that symptom severity and the level of personal functioning are two quite distinct domains that are only somewhat related and need to be assessed separately. In fact, it is part of the recovery philosophy that persons with mental illness can lead functional lives in the face of quite severe symptoms. Fossey and Harvey (2001) have provided a conceptual review of functioning as it related to outcome measurement. They noted the central role of functioning in good outcomes, the conceptual and definitional issues surrounding functioning, and some of the approaches that have been taken to its formal assessment. Reviews of assessment methods of functioning in mental health and rehabilitation include Wallace (1986), Wiersma (1996) and Scott and Lehman (1998). Mausbach et al. (2009) have provided a recent review of eight measures of 'functional recovery' that may have value as outcome measures.

The most extensively used instrument for assessing functioning in routine OM is the Life Skills Profile (LSP), which now exists in three formats. The original scale (Rosen et al., 1989), comprising 39 items, was subsequently shortened to 16 for use in a mental health casemix study (Buckingham et al., 1998), and later some of the omitted items were reinstated into a 20-item version (Rosen et al., 2001). The versions are described and a bibliography of publications and applications is presented, in Rosen et al. (2006). The 16-item version of the LSP (LSP-16) is a mandatory element of the Australian National Outcomes and Casemix Collection (NOCC, Department of Health and Ageing, 2003) in community and residential (but not acute inpatient) services for adults and older persons.

The LSP is not the only instrument to have been used to assess disability and functional status in consumers of mental health services. The World Health Organization Short Disability Assessment Schedule (WHODAS), based on the International Classification of Impairments, Disabilities and Handicaps-2) (ICIDH-2, World Health Organization, 1998) has been used by Aoun et al. (2002) and Chopra et al. (2004). In New Zealand, a review of functioning instruments (Lutchman et al., 2007), undertaken to assist the choice of which to implement, recommended the Personal and Social Performance Scale (PSP, Morosini et al., 2000) for adults and older persons, and the Children's Global Assessment Scale (CGAS, Schaffer et al., 1983) for children. Interestingly, apart from the initial paper in 2000, the whole of the published literature on the PSP (as at 2009) dates from 2007 and concerns the assessment of patients diagnosed with schizophrenia (e.g. Burns and Patrick, 2007, Juckel and Morosini, 2008).

Another instrument that has been used is the Global Assessment of Functioning (GAF, Jones et al., 1995). As reported by Söderberg et al. (2005), the GAF is widely used as an OM in Sweden, where they found that despite reasonable agreements between raters of clinical vignettes, 'the measurement error is too large for assessment of change for an individual patient, in which case it might be necessary to use several raters. If raters are positively inclined to use rating instruments, measurement errors are minimized and reliability is maximized' (abstract). A Norwegian study (Vatnaland et al., 2007) found that while scores assigned by raters in research situations were reliable, those assigned by raters in routine clinical situations fell below acceptable levels of reliability.

(c) Quality of life

At an early stage, it was made clear that 'outcome studies should focus not only on clinical symptomatology but also on patients' social, interpersonal and occupational adjustment as well as on factors that, taken together, shape the quality of life (QOL)' (Mirin and Namerow, 1991). Equally, it has been suggested that 'clinical and social variables predict no more than 30% of the variance in an individual's quality of life' (Slade, 2002a, abstract). Also, Speer and Newman (1996, p. 124) noted that results from outcome evaluations based on QOL in adults with persistent and severe mental illness in the community are modest, suggesting that adjustment of expectations is called for.

Katschnig (2006) has addressed the issues in assessing QOL in persons with a mental illness. He noted in particular the 'affective fallacy', citing evidence that people based their judgements of how happy and satisfied they are with their lives in general on their momentary affective state. Thus depressed people typically regard their well-being, social functioning and living conditions as worse than they appear to independent observers, and even than their own views after recovery; and the opposite effect has been observed in mania (p. 8). He noted too that 'Many persons suffering from long-term mental disorders report themselves satisfied with life conditions that would be regarded as inadequate by external standards. It has been repeatedly observed that such patients adapt their standards downwards . . . '

(pp. 11–12). Given the short-term effects of affective state and longer-term effects of adaptation to one's situation, he recommended that judgements of QOL need to incorporate three elements: subjective well-being, functioning in social roles and contextual (environmental) factors. In order to avoid obtaining misleading results, multiple assessments, by the patient, a family member or friend and a professional, should be conducted. Since subjective well-being is so closely related to affective state, he also recommended that QOL assessments should routinely include assessments of psychopathology, which should be taken into account in the interpretation.

There exist a large number of scales and questionnaires to assess QOL and subjective well-being, which are well reviewed by Lehman (2006) and van Nieuwenhuizen (2006). However, Jacobs (2007, pp. 18–19) noted that there is a lack of consensus around the service user and carer measures of quality of life and satisfaction.

(d) Perceived needs

Like QOL, needs assessment is a very large field that cannot be covered comprehensively here. At the outset, it is important to distinguish between personal needs and needs for care, the former being a consumer-level attribute that could be the basis for routine OM, while the latter is a service- or system-level judgement that is not necessarily related to the consumer's health status; indeed Roth and Crane-Ross (2002) found that level of service provision was unrelated to consumers' perceptions of need.

The most widely used instrument for assessment of needs in mental health settings is the Camberwell Assessment of Need (CAN, Phelan et al., 1995) which is available in several forms (Slade et al., 1999c). The CAN comprises 22 areas of life, such as accommodation, self-care and company, each of which is rated as no need (no problem in that area), a met need (not a problem because of the help received), or unmet need (a problem despite the help received). A particularly valuable feature of the CAN is that it is available in formats that can be completed by the clinician and by the consumer, affording them the capacity of directly comparing their judgements. Apart from being a basis for dialogue and care planning, the most important output from a CAN assessment is the count of unmet needs.

Reviewing a year of literature, Noble and Douglas (2004) concluded that clinical outcomes are predicted by patients' perceptions that services have met their needs, and there are numerous reports of the association between fewer unmet needs and better QOL (Slade et al., 1999b, 2004) and that reduction in unmet needs, especially as rated by the consumer, precedes improvement in QOL (Slade et al., 2005), suggesting a causal relationship. Junghan et al. (2007) have suggested that the relationship between patient-rated unmet need and quality of life is mediated by improved therapeutic alliance.

Other CAN research has shown that, in consumers with severe mental illnesses, clinicians typically identify more areas of unmet need than consumers (Hansson et al., 2001, Ochoa et al., 2003, Trauer and Tobias, 2004). Some studies have tracked the level of met and unmet needs from the point of intake to a service (e.g. Drukker et al., 2008). Several studies have examined the association between scores on the CAN and the HoNOS: Issakidis and Teesson (1999) found generally low agreement levels between clinicians and clients on need ratings and non-significant correlation between numbers of unmet needs rated by clients and HoNOS scores, rated by clinicians. Gallagher and Teesson (2000) concluded that both instruments were promising contenders for routine use, and Slade et al. (1999a) noted that the information from the CAN and HoNOS are quite distinct, with the former being better for tracking change over time and the latter better for indicating whether treatment should be commenced or continued.

Wennstrom and Wiesel (2006) found that CAN summary scores did not vary greatly over time, perhaps limiting their utility as outcomes measures, yet it was effective in detecting changes in need at the individual item level. The chapter by David Smith (Chapter 10) describes the implementation of the CAN across the community mental health services of a Canadian province.

(e) Recovery

Increasingly in recent years, the concept of recovery has become a focus for outcome assessment, despite reservations regarding the compatibility of outcome measurement and the recovery philosophy (Lakeman, 2004, Browne, 2006). As noted by Slade (2009, p. 194), to the extent that recovery is important to consumers, it is important for services to promote it and to evaluate their success in this. Some instruments operate similarly to others discussed in earlier sections, by focussing on assessing recovery at the level of the individual consumer. Other instruments, by contrast, focus on stakeholders' (i.e. clinicians, consumers and carers) perceptions of the service as delivered and the extent to which it aligns with recovery principles.

An early example of such a scale is the Recovery Attitudes Questionnaire (Borkin et al., 2000), which was able to demonstrate differences between professionals, persons with mental disorders, family members and others. Another scale, the Recovery Assessment Scale (RAS, Giffort et al., 1995), was found by Corrigan et al. (2004) to comprise factors of personal confidence and hope, willingness to ask for help, goal and success orientation and reliance on others, and no domination by symptoms, and another measure, the Recovery Process Inventory (RPI, Jerrell et al., 2006), showed conceptual overlap with the RAS. The RAS factors were largely replicated by McNaught et al. (2007), who also found negligible correlations with HoNOS scores, suggesting that a recovery orientation is independent of clinician-assessed severity, but negatively correlated with the consumer-completed K-10 (Kessler et al., 2002), suggesting that, at least cross-sectionally, high levels of psychological distress may be inimical to a recovery orientation.

Resnick et al. (2004), studying a group of consumers with a diagnosis of schizophrenia, also found an inverse relationship between a recovery orientation and severity of psychiatric symptoms (which they characterized as 'a core feature of the biomedical perspective of mental illness'), in particular, depressive symptoms. In a later study using the same data (Resnick et al., 2005), they identified four domains of the recovery orientation: empowerment, hope and optimism, knowledge and life satisfaction.

O'Connell et al. (2005) developed the Recovery Self Assessment (RSA) to 'gauge perceptions of the degree to which programs implement recovery-oriented practices'. Comprising five factors (Life Goals, Involvement, Diversity of Treatment Options, Choice and Individually-Tailored Services), the RSA is a self-reflective tool that can identify areas of strength and opportunities for improvement. The RSA was subsequently used with a sample of hospital workers; the factors were replicated and the expected positive correlations with measures of optimism were found (Salyers et al., 2007b). In a related study, Salyers et al. (2007a) found strong correlations between the (consumer-rated) Illness Management and Recovery scale (IMR, Mueser and Gingerich, 2005) and the previously described RAS. Another instrument targeted at health care staff is the Recovery Knowledge Inventory (RKI, Bedregal et al., 2006), which the authors suggest has value to assess the training needs of staff who 'increasingly are being expected to delivery recovery oriented care'.

In 2003, Andresen et al. proposed a five-stage model for the journey of recovery, the sequential stages being moratorium, awareness, preparation, rebuilding and growth (Andresen et al.,

2003). They subsequently developed an instrument to assess these: the Stages of Recovery Instrument (STORI, Andresen et al., 2006). Further details of this instrument can be found at http://www.uow.edu.au/health/iimh/stori/index.html (last accessed 10 September 2009).

Other relevant instruments, details of which can be found in the Compendium of Recovery Measures by Campbell-Orde et al. (2005), are the Recovery Enhancing Environment/Developing Recovery Enhancing Environment Measure (REE/DREEM) developed by Ridgway, and the Recovery Oriented Systems Indicators Measure (ROSI).

References

Andresen, R., Oades, L. and Caputi, P. (2003). The experience of recovery from schizophrenia: towards an empirically validated stage model. *Australian and New Zealand Journal of Psychiatry*, 37, 586–94.

Andresen, R., Caputi, P. and Oades, L. (2006). Stages of recovery instrument: development of a measure of recovery from serious mental illness. *Australian and New Zealand Journal of Psychiatry*, 40, 972–80.

Aoun, S., Pennebaker, D. and Janca, A. (2002). Outcome measurement in rural mental health: a field trial of rooming-in models. *Australian Journal of Rural Health*, 10, 302–7.

Barkham, M., Gilbert, N., Connell, J., Marshall, C. and Twigg, E. (2005). Suitability and utility of the CORE-OM and CORE-A for assessing severity of presenting problems in psychological therapy services based in primary and secondary care settings. *British Journal of Psychiatry*, 186, 239–46.

Barkham, M., Mellor-Clark, J., Connell, J. and Cahill, J. (2006). A core approach to practice-based evidence: a brief history of the origins and applications of the CORE-OM and CORE System. *Counselling and Psychotherapy Research*, 6, 3–15.

Bedregal, L. E., O'Connell, M. and Davidson, L. (2006). The Recovery Knowledge Inventory: assessment of mental health staff knowledge and attitudes about recovery. *Psychiatric Rehabilitation Journal*, 30, 96–103.

Berk, M., Ng, F., Dodd, S., et al. (2008). The validity of the CGI severity and improvement scales as measures of clinical effectiveness suitable for routine clinical use. *Journal of Evaluation in Clinical Practice*, 14, 979–83.

Bonsack, C., Borgeat, F. and Lesage, A. (2002). Measuring patients problems severity and outcomes in a psychiatric sector: a field study with the French version of the Health of the Nation Outcome Scales (HoNOS-F). *Annales Medico Psychologiques*, 160, 483–8.

Borkin, J. R., Steffen, J. J., Ensfield, L. B., et al. (2000). Recovery Attitudes Questionnaire: development and evaluation. *Psychiatric Rehabilitation Journal*, 24, 95–102.

Browne, G. (2006). Outcome measures: do they fit with a recovery model? *International Journal of Mental Health Nursing*, 15, 153–4.

Buckingham, W., Burgess, P., Solomon, S., Pirkis, J. and Eagar, K. (1998). *Developing a Casemix Classification for Mental Health Services*. Canberra: Department of Health and Ageing.

Burgess, P., Trauer, T., Coombs, T., McKay, R. and Pirkis, J. (2008). What does 'clinical significance' mean in the context of the Health of the Nation Outcome Scales? *Australasian Psychiatry*, 17, 141–8.

Burns, A., Beevor, A., Lelliott, P., et al. (1999a). Health of the Nation Outcome Scales for Elderly People (HoNOS65+): glossary for the HoNOS65+ score sheet. *British Journal of Psychiatry*, 174, 435–8.

Burns, A., Beevor, A., Lelliott, P., et al. (1999b). Health of the Nation Outcome Scales for Elderly People (HoNOS 65+). *British Journal of Psychiatry*, 174, 424–7.

Burns, T. and Patrick, D. (2007). Social functioning as an outcome measure in schizophrenia studies. *Acta Psychiatrica Scandinavica*, 116, 403–18.

Campbell-Orde, T., Chamberlin, J., Carpenter, J. and Leff, H. S. (2005). *Measuring the Promise: A Compendium of Recovery Measures*. Cambridge, MA: Human Service Research Institute.

Chopra, P. K., Couper, J. W. and Herrman, H. (2004). The assessment of patients with long-term psychotic disorders: application of the WHO Disability Assessment Schedule II. *Australian and New Zealand Journal of Psychiatry*, **38**, 753–9.

College Research Unit (1996). *HoNOS: Health of the Nation Outcome Scales: report on research and development July 1993-December 1995*. London: Department of Health.

Corrigan, P. W., Salzer, M., Ralph, R. O., Sangster, Y. and Keck, L. (2004). Examining the factor structure of the recovery assessment scale. *Schizophrenia Bulletin*, **30**, 1035–41.

Department of Health and Ageing (2003). *Mental Health National Outcomes and Casemix Collection: Overview of Clinician-rated and Consumer Self-report Measures, Version 1.50*. Canberra.

Drukker, M., van Dillen, K., Bak, M., et al. (2008). The use of the Camberwell Assessment of Need in treatment: what unmet needs can be met? *Social Psychiatry and Psychiatric Epidemiology*, **43**, 410–17.

Evans, C., Connell, J., Barkham, M., et al. (2002). Towards a standardised brief outcome measure: psychometric properties and utility. *British Journal of Psychiatry*, **180**, 51–60.

Fossey, E. M. and Harvey, C. A. (2001). A conceptual review of functioning: implications for the development of consumer outcome measures. *Australian & New Zealand Journal of Psychiatry*, **35**, 91–8.

Gallagher, J. and Teesson, M. (2000). Measuring disability, need and outcome in Australian community mental health services. *Australian and New Zealand Journal of Psychiatry*, **34**, 850–5.

Gifford, D., Schmook, A., Woody, C., Vollendorf, C. and Gervain, M. (1995). *Construction of a Scale to Measure Consumer Recovery*. Springfield, IL: Illinois Office of Mental Health.

Gordon, S., Ellis, P., Haggerty, C., et al. (2004). *Preliminary work towards the development of a self-assessed measure of consumer outcome*. Auckland: Health Research Council of New Zealand.

Gowers, S. G., Harrington, R. C., Whitton, A., et al. (1999a). Health of the Nation Outcome Scales for Children and Adolescents (HoNOSCA): glossary for the HoNOSCA score sheet. *British Journal of Psychiatry*, **174**, 428–31.

Gowers, S. G., Harrington, R. C., Whitton, A., et al. (1999b). Brief scale for measuring the outcomes of emotional and behavioural disorders in children. Health of the Nation Outcome Scales for Children and Adolescents (HoNOSCA). *British Journal of Psychiatry*, **174**, 413–16.

Graham, C., Coombs, T., Buckingham, W., et al. (2001). *Consumer Perspectives of Future Directions for Outcome Self-Assessment*. Report of the Consumer Consultation Project, Wollongong.

Guy, W. (1976). *ECDEU Assessment Manual for Psychopharmacology – Revised*. Rockville, MD: U.S. Department of Health, Education, and Welfare, Public Health Service, Alcohol, Drug Abuse, and Mental Health Administration, NIMH Psychopharmacology Research Branch, Division of Extramural Research Programs.

Hansson, L., Vinding, H. R., Mackeprang, T., et al. (2001). Comparison of key worker and patient assessment of needs in schizophrenic patients living in the community: a Nordic multicentre study. *Acta Psychiatrica Scandinavica*, **103**, 45–51.

Harnett, P. H., Loxton, N. J., Sadler, T., Hides, L. and Baldwin, A. (2005). The Health of the Nation Outcome Scales for Children and Adolescents in an adolescent in-patient sample. *Australian and New Zealand Journal of Psychiatry*, **39**, 129–35.

IsHak, W., Burt, T. and Sederer, L.(eds.) (2002). *Outcome Measurement in Mental Illness. A Critical Review*. Washington DC: American Psychiatric Press.

Issakidis, C. and Teesson, M. (1999). Measurement of need for care: a trial of the Camberwell Assessment of Need and the Health of the National Outcome Scales.

Australian and New Zealand Journal of Psychiatry, **33**, 754–9.

Jacobs, R. (2007). *Investigating Patient Outcome Measures in Mental Health: research report for the OHE Commission on NHS Productivity*. York: Centre for Health Economics.

James, M. and Mitchell, D. (2004). Measuring health and social functioning using HoNOS. In M. Harrison, D. Howard and D. Mitchell, eds., *Acute Mental Health Nursing: From Acute Concerns to the Capable Practitioner*. Thousand Oaks, CA: Sage.

Jerrell, J. M., Cousins, V. C. and Roberts, K. M. (2006). Psychometrics of the Recovery Process Inventory. *Journal of Behavioral Health Services & Research*, **33**, 464–73.

Jones, S. H., Thornicroft, G., Coffey, M. and Dunn, G. (1995). A brief mental health outcome scale: reliability and validity of the Global Assessment of Functioning (GAF). *British Journal of Psychiatry*, **166**, 654–9.

Juckel, G. and Morosini, P. L. (2008). The new approach: psychosocial functioning as a necessary outcome criterion for therapeutic success in schizophrenia. *Current Opinion in Psychiatry*, **21**, 630–9.

Junghan, U. M., Leese, M., Priebe, S. and Slade, M. (2007). Staff and patient perspectives on unmet need and therapeutic alliance in community mental community mental health services. *British Journal of Psychiatry*, **191**, 543–7.

Katschnig, H. (2006). How useful is the concept of quality of life in psychiatry? In H. Katschnig, H. Freeman and N. Sartorius, eds., *Quality of Life in Mental Disorders*, 2nd edn. Chichester: John Wiley & Sons.

Kessler, R. C., Andrews, G., Colpe, L. J., et al. (2002). Short screening scales to monitor population prevalences and trends in nonspecific psychological distress. *Psychological Medicine*, **32**, 959–76.

Lakeman, R. (2004). Standardized routine outcome measurement: pot holes in the road to recovery. *International Journal of Mental Health Nursing*, **13**, 210–15.

Lambert, M. J., Hansen, N. B. and Finch, A. E. (2001). Patient focused research: using patient outcome data to enhance treatment effects. *Journal of Consulting and Clinical Psychology*, **69**, 159–72.

Lambert, M. J., Morton, J. J., Hatfield, D., et al. (2004). *Administration and Scoring Manual for the Outcome Questionnaire-45*. Salt Lake City: Utah American Professional Credentialing Services.

Leach, C., Lucock, M., Barkham, M., et al. (2005). Assessing risk and emotional disturbance using the CORE-OM and HoNOS outcome measures at the interface between primary and secondary mental healthcare. *Psychiatric Bulletin*, **29**, 419–22.

Lehman, A. F. (2006). Instruments for measuring quality of life in mental disorders. I: up to 1996. In H. Katschnig, H. Freeman and N. Sartorius, eds., *Quality of Life in Mental Disorders*, 2nd edn. Chichester: John Wiley & Sons.

Lutchman, R., Thompson, A., Tait, H., et al. (2007). In search of a standardised comprehensive assessment of functionality. *New Zealand Journal of Occupational Therapy*, **54**, 33–8.

Mausbach, B. T., Moore, R., Bowie, C., Cardenas, V. and Patterson, T. L. (2009). A review of instruments for measuring functional recovery in those diagnosed with psychosis. *Schizophrenia Bulletin*, **35**, 307–18.

McNaught, M., Caputi, P., Oades, L. G. and Deane, F. P. (2007). Testing the validity of the Recovery Assessment Scale using an Australian sample. *Australian and New Zealand Journal of Psychiatry*, **41**, 450–7.

Mirin, S. M. and Namerow, M. J. (1991). Why study treatment outcome? *Hospital and Community Psychiatry*, **42**, 1007–13.

Morosini, P.-L., Magliano, L., Brambilla, L., Ugolini, S. and Pioli, R. (2000). Development, reliability and acceptability of a new version of the DSM-IV Social and Occupational Functioning Assessment Scale (SOFAS) to assess routine social funtioning. *Acta Psychiatrica Scandinavica*, **101**, 323–9.

Mueser, K. T. and Gingerich, S. (2005). Illness Management and Recovery

(IMR) scales. In T. Campbell-Orde, J. J. Chamberlin, J. J. Carpenter and H. S. Leff, eds., *Measuring the Promise: A Compendium of Recovery Measures.* Cambridge, MA: Human Services Research Institute.

National Institute for Mental Health in England (2008). *Outcomes Compendium.* Birmingham: National Institute for Mental Health in England (NIMHE).

Newnham, E. A., Harwood, K. E. and Page, A. C. (2009). The subscale structure and clinical utility of the Health of the Nation Outcome Scale. *Journal of Mental Health,* **18**, 326–34.

Noble, L. M. and Douglas, B. C. (2004). What users and relatives want from mental health services. *Current Opinion in Psychiatry,* **17**, 289–96.

O'Connell, M., Tondora, J., Croog, G., Evans, A. and Davidson, L. (2005). From rhetoric to routine: assessing perceptions of recovery-oriented practices in a state mental health and addiction system. *Psychiatric Rehabilitation Journal,* **28**, 378–86.

Ochoa, S., Haro, J. M., Autonell, J., et al. and the NEDES group (2003). Met and unmet needs of schizophrenia patients in a Spanish sample. *Schizophrenia Bulletin,* **29**, 201–10.

Phelan, M., Slade, M., Thornicroft, G., et al. (1995). The Camberwell Assessment of Need: the validity and reliability of an instrument to assess the needs of people with severe mental illness. *British Journal of Psychiatry,* **167**, 589–95.

Pirkis, J. E., Burgess, P. M., Kirk, P. K., et al. (2005). A review of the psychometric properties of the Health of the Nation Outcome Scales (HoNOS) family of measures. *Health and Quality of Life Outcomes,* **3**, 76.

Resnick, S. G., Rosenheck, R. A. and Lehman, A. F. (2004). An exploratory analysis of correlates of recovery. *Psychiatric Services,* **55**, 540–7.

Resnick, S. G., Fontana, A., Lehman, A. F. and Rosenheck, R. A. (2005). An empirical conceptualization of the recovery orientation. *Schizophrenia Research,* **75**, 119–28.

Rosen, A., Hadzi-Pavlovic, D. and Parker, G. (1989). The Life Skills Profile: a measure assessing function and disability in schizophrenia. *Schizophrenia Bulletin,* **15**, 325–37.

Rosen, A., Trauer, T., Hadzi-Pavlovic, D. and Parker, G. (2001). Development of a brief form of the Life Skills Profile: the LSP-20. *Australian and New Zealand Journal of Psychiatry,* **35**, 677–83.

Rosen, A., Hadzi-Pavlovic, D., Parker, G. and Trauer, T. (2006). *The Life Skills Profile: Background, Items and Scoring for the LSP-39, LSP-20 and the LSP-16,* Sydney, available at: http://www.blackdoginstitute.org.au/docs/LifeSkillsProfile.pdf.

Rosenblatt, A. and Attkisson, C. C. (1993). Assessing outcomes for sufferers of severe mental disorder: a conceptual framework and review. *Evaluation and Program Planning,* **16**, 347–63.

Roth, D. and Crane-Ross, D. (2002). Impact of services, met needs, and service empowerment on consumer outcomes. *Mental Health Services Research,* **4**, 43–56.

Salyers, M. P., Godfrey, J. L., Mueser, K. T. and Labriola, S. (2007a). Measuring illness management outcomes: a psychometric study of clinician and consumer rating scales for illness self management and recovery. *Community Mental Health Journal,* **43**, 459–80.

Salyers, M. P., Tsai, J. and Stultz, T. A. (2007b). Measuring recovery orientation in a hospital setting. *Psychiatric Rehabilitation Journal,* **31**, 131–7.

Schaffer, D., Gould, M. S., Brasic, J., et al. (1983). A children's global assessment scale (CGAS). *Archives of General Psychiatry,* **40**, 1228–31.

Schmidt, L. J., Garratt, A. M. and Fitzpatrick, R. (2000). *Instruments for Mental Health: a Review Report from the Patient-reported Health Instruments Group (formerly the Patient-assessed Health Outcomes Programme) to the Department of Health.* Oxford: National Centre for Health Outcomes Development.

Scott, J. E. and Lehman, A. F. (1998). Social functioning in the community. In K. T. Mueser and N. Tarrier, eds.,

Handbook of Social Functioning in Schizophrenia. Boston: Allyn and Bacon.

Sederer, L. I. and Dickey, B.(eds.) (1996). *Outcomes Assessment in Clinical Practice.* London: Williams & Wilkins.

Slade, M. (2002a). Routine outcome assessment in mental health services. *Psychological Medicine*, **32**, 1339–43.

Slade, M. (2002b). What outcomes to measure in routine mental health services, and how to assess them: a systematic review. *Australian and New Zealand Journal of Psychiatry*, **36**, 743–53.

Slade, M. (2009). *Personal Recovery and Mental Illness,* Cambridge: Cambridge University Press.

Slade, M., Beck, A., Bindman, J., Thornicroft, G. and Wright, S. (1999a). Routine clinical outcome measures for patients with severe mental illness: CANSAS and HoNOS. *British Journal of Psychiatry*, **174**, 404–8.

Slade, M., Leese, M., Taylor, R. and Thornicroft, G. (1999b). The association between needs and quality of life in an epidemiologically representative sample of people with psychosis. *Acta Psychiatrica Scandinavica*, **100**, 149–57.

Slade, M., Thornicroft, G., Loftus, L., Phelan, M. and Wykes, T. (1999c). *CAN: Camberwell Assessment of Need: A Comprehensive Assessment Tool for People with Severe Mental Illness.* London: Gaskell.

Slade, M., Powell, R., Rosen, A. and Strathdee, G. (2000). Threshold Assessment Grid (TAG): the development of a valid and brief scale to assess the severity of mental illness. *Social Psychiatry and Psychiatric Epidemiology*, **35**, 78–85.

Slade, M., Cahill, S., Kelsey, W., et al. (2001). Threshold 3: the feasibility of the Threshold Assessment Grid (TAG) for routine assessment of the severity of mental health problems. *Social Psychiatry & Psychiatric Epidemiology*, **36**, 516–21.

Slade, M., Cahill, S., Kelsey, W., Powell, R. and Strathdee, G. (2002). Threshold 2: the reliability, validity and sensitivity to change of the Threshold Assessment Grid (TAG). *Acta Psychiatrica Scandinavica*, **106**, 453–60.

Slade, M., Leese, M., Ruggeri, M., et al. (2004). Does meeting needs improve quality of life? *Psychotherapy and Psychosomatics*, **73**, 183–9.

Slade, M., Leese, M., Cahill, S., Thornicroft, G. and Kuipers, E. (2005). Patient-rated mental health needs and quality of life improvement. *British Journal of Psychiatry*, **187**, 256–61.

Söderberg, P., Tungström, S. and Armelius, B. Å. (2005). Reliability of global assessment of functioning ratings made by clinical psychiatric staff. *Psychiatric Services*, **56**, 434–8.

Speer, D. C. and Newman, F. L. (1996). Mental health services outcome evaluation. *Clinical Psychology: Science and Practice*, **3**, 105–29.

Stewart, M. (2009). Service user and significant other versions of the Health of the Nation Outcome Scales. *Australasian Psychiatry*, **17**, 156–63.

Tansella, M. and Thornicroft, G.(eds.) (2001). *Mental Health Outcome Measures.* London: Gaskell.

Trauer, T. (1998). The Health of the Nation Outcome Scales in outcome measurement: a critical review. *Australasian Psychiatry*, **6**, 11–14.

Trauer, T. (1999). The subscale structure of the Health of the Nation Outcome Scales (HoNOS). *Journal of Mental Health*, **8**, 499–509.

Trauer, T. and Buckingham, B. (2006). *The Health of the Nation Outcomes Scales (HoNOS), General Adult Version: Towards an Agenda for Future Development, Version 1.0.* Document produced on behalf of the Australian Adult Mental Health Outcomes Expert Group.

Trauer, T. and Callaly, T. (2002). Concordance between mentally ill clients and their case managers using the Health of the Nation Outcome Scales (HoNOS). *Australasian Psychiatry*, **10**, 24–8.

Trauer, T. and Tobias, G. (2004). The Camberwell Assessment of Need and Behaviour and Symptom Identification Scale as routine outcome measures in a psychiatric disability support service. *Community Mental Health Journal*, **40**, 211–21.

van Nieuwenhuizen, C. (2006). Instruments for measuring quality of life in mental disorders II: some new developments. In H. Katschnig, H. Freeman and N. Sartorius, eds., *Quality of Life in Mental Disorders*, 2nd edn. Chichester: John Wiley & Sons.

Vatnaland, T., Vatnaland, J., Friis, S. and Opjordsmoen, S. (2007). Are GAF scores reliable in routine clinical use? *Acta Psychiatrica Scandinavica*, **115**, 326–30.

Wallace, C. J. (1986). Functional assessment in rehabilitation. *Schizophrenia Bulletin*, **12**, 604–30.

Wennstrom, E. and Wiesel, F.-A. (2006). The Camberwell assessment of need as an outcome measure in routine mental health care. *Social Psychiatry and Psychiatric Epidemiology*, **41**, 728–33.

Wiersma, D. (1996). Measuring social disabilities in mental health. *Social Psychiatry and Psychiatric Epidemiology*, **31**, 101–8.

Wing, J., Curtis, R. H. and Beevor, A. (1999). Health of the Nation Outcome Scales (HoNOS): glossary for HoNOS score sheet. *British Journal of Psychiatry*, **174**, 432–4.

Wing, J. K., Beevor, A. S., Curtis, R. H., et al. (1998). Health of the Nation Outcome Scales (HoNOS). Research and development. *British Journal of Psychiatry*, **172**, 11–18.

World Health Organization (1998). *Towards a Common Language for Functioning and Disablement. ICIDH-2 The International Classification of Impairments, Activities, and Participation*. Geneva: World Health Organization.

Current Issues in Outcome Measurement

Some economic and policy considerations for outcome measurement

Rowena Jacobs

Introduction

Patient Reported Outcome Measures (PROMs) are measures of a patient's health status or health-related quality of life and are used to assess the impact of a health care intervention by comparing the patient's self-reported health status at two points in time (e.g. in surgery, before and after an operation). The change in health status provides an indication of the outcome or quality of care delivered.

From April 2009 it has become mandatory for English National Health Service (NHS) acute hospital Trusts to collect PROMs before and after certain elective procedures (unilateral hip replacements, knee replacements, groin hernia and varicose vein surgery) (Department of Health, 2009b). While PROMs are widely employed internationally, this is the first time that PROMs have been collected across an entire health system anywhere in the world. An estimated 250,000 patients will be asked to complete questionnaires before their treatment in the first year (West, 2009). This initiative has enormous significance because it will be the first real test of the scale of benefits which may accrue to patients, the public and providers when evidence from PROMs will be used to assess the outcomes of all providers of these interventions.

As described in other chapters in this book, a wide range of reliable and valid outcome measures have been developed in recent years. Some of these have been developed for particular conditions or treatments (disease-specific measures) while others have been developed to facilitate comparisons between conditions or treatments (generic measures). In the UK PROMs context, both the pre-operative and post-operative PROMs questionnaires consist of a generic health status measure (EQ-5D, which is used to derive a Quality Adjusted Life Year – QALY) and a disease-specific health status measure (e.g. Oxford Hip Score).

It is anticipated that the scope of PROMs will be widened significantly by the English Department of Health (DH) in 2010 and 2011 and the roll-out to mental health services in the future has been explored (Office of Health Economics (OHE), 2008, Jacobs, 2009). The development of PROMs is therefore particularly relevant to mental health services because of the extent to which mental health will be required to follow the footsteps of the acute health services in England in future years in terms of mandatory PROMs.

One outcome measure, HoNOS (the Health of the Nation Outcome Scales), has already been mandated for use by mental healthcare providers in England (Fonagy et al., 2004). HoNOS was developed for people with severe and enduring mental illness and is not a patient-report or self-report measure, but rather is completed by a member of the clinical team. This 12-item outcome measure forms part of the Mental Health Minimum Dataset (MHMDS) which was introduced in April 2003, the collection of which is mandatory. As a minimum, HoNOS is recommended for use for all patients with more complex needs, with at least one measurement taken per year. Despite this, only around a half of all providers complete HoNOS returns in the

MHMDS and coverage is less than 10% among those that do (Jacobs, 2009). In addition, the collection of repeat measures on individual patients is almost non-existent, making measurement of changes in health status impossible and only allowing HoNOS to provide a measure as a snapshot of patient severity or casemix, rather than as an outcome.

It is therefore conceivable that a roll-out of mandatory PROMs to mental health services may entail a renewed emphasis on a measure such as HoNOS as a disease-specific instrument and, in addition, potentially the introduction of a generic health status tool such as EQ-5D, to allow for comparisons across services. The roll-out of PROMs to mental health services is therefore likely to require some adaptations, given the role of the clinician/clinical team in PROMs, since most disease-specific rating scales in psychiatry are completed by clinicians rather than patients.

Health economists tend to be very enthusiastic about initiatives such as PROMs, because of the multitude of uses to which the data can be put, for example, to examine the efficacy of specific treatments, interventions or services. The array of health policy questions which can be answered and the various applications to which health economists or policy analysts might put such data are explained later in this chapter. However, the collection of such data can be a resource-intensive process. In principle, it could potentially save time and money in terms of administering several different instruments to patients, if it were possible to convert one type of measure into another by establishing equivalent scores on each instrument. In addition, if generic measures aren't particularly suited to a clinical area, as is the case in mental health, it seems sensible to explore the conversion of measures. Since clinical teams are likely to have a preference for the use of disease-specific measures rather than generic ones, we describe how we might convert disease-specific measures into generic ones for comparison across services/specialities. We also outline what generic measures are and their applicability to mental health. But first we turn to the evidence for outcome measurement in mental health and the potential uses of outcome data.

The evidence for outcome measurement

While there is consensus that outcomes should be routinely measured, is there any evidence of it actually being effective in improving services in any way?

The overall evidence from various reviews seems to be very little (Gilbody et al., 2003a), or at best mixed (Gilbody et al., 2001). The latter systematic review found only nine studies that looked at the addition of outcome measurement to routine clinical practice in both psychiatric and non-psychiatric settings, with the results showing that routine feedback of instruments had little impact on the identification of mental disorders or longer-term psychosocial functioning. While clinicians welcomed the information imparted from the instruments, they rarely incorporated their results into routine clinical decision-making. Given that routine outcome measurement can be a costly exercise the authors concluded that there was no robust evidence to suggest that it is of benefit in improving psychosocial outcomes in non-psychiatric settings (Gilbody and Whitty, 2002).

Similarly, studies suggest that one-off outcome measurements do very little to shift clinical practice or change clinician behaviour (Ashaye et al., 2003). However, one more recent randomized controlled trial (Slade et al., 2006) on the effectiveness of standardized outcome measurement indicated that monthly outcome monitoring reduced psychiatric admissions markedly. It was not, however, shown to be effective in improving primary outcomes of patient-rated unmet need and quality of life, nor did it improve other subjective secondary outcome measures. Because the study was longitudinal in nature and had more regular outcome measurement for patients (with month on month assessment) it showed that this might prompt earlier intervention by clinicians to avert relapse which would otherwise lead to hospitalization, thus reducing admissions. The intervention therefore reduced psychiatric inpatient days and hence service use costs and proved cost-effective.

More evidence can be found in a six-country European study (Priebe et al., 2002), which examined how service user views could be fed into treatment decisions. The MECCA (More Effective Community Care) trial tested the hypothesis that intervention would lead to better outcomes in terms of quality of life over a 1-year period. A better outcome was assumed to be mediated through more appropriate joint decisions or a more positive therapeutic relationship. Results showed that while the intervention added time to clinical appointments, it did lead to a significant improvement in quality of life.

The key message from these studies appears therefore to be that one-off (or infrequent) outcome measurement seems to have equivocal results in terms of actually improving subjective outcomes, but outcome measurement that is done longitudinally and more regularly using a broad range of measures, ideally collected routinely in databases and backed up by regular monitoring, can significantly improve quality of life and/or reduce psychiatric admissions.

What are the economic and policy applications of routine outcome measurement data?

There are a variety of uses to which outcome data can be put – data can be used locally by clinicians to help inform clinical decision-making and improve patient care. Alternatively, more aggregate data can be used by managers, regulators and commissioners to benchmark providers' performance. The different uses to which the data will be put is an important consideration for the design of any successful routine outcome measurement system. In short, some of the uses are:

(1) informing clinical decision-making
(2) clinical audit
(3) consultant performance review
(4) measuring hospital/provider performance
(5) informing patient choice or GPs (gatekeepers) exercising choice
(6) informing and empowering the commissioning process
(7) evaluating efficacy and cost-effectiveness of new technologies (in research)
(8) productivity measurement
(9) resource allocation
(10) demand management
(11) hospital reimbursement, and
(12) value-based pricing for pharmaceuticals.

While data at a local level may in theory be used to help with clinical audit and patient care, initiatives such as PROMs don't in fact have this in mind as their primary purpose. In fact it is not clear that any mechanisms have been put in place to support clinicians with accessing or using the data, specifically the disease-specific measures which will be most valuable to clinicians. Indeed, it is likely that the PROMs data will go directly from patients to a central clearing house and clinicians will have no involvement with it.

If a measure such as HoNOS were to be used in mental health, clinical teams would of course need to be involved in its completion. Hence, the process of supporting clinicians with the data-collection process and making the feedback of outcomes as clinically useful and relevant as possible becomes crucially important. If clinicians do not see the data from outcome measurement as clinically relevant and timely but rather see it as a form-filling push from managers for higher-level purposes, completion rates will be poor or of a poor quality.

The push for collection of PROMs data for higher-level aggregate purposes has tended to be the main driving force for their introduction. The main rationale is that they can be used to compare hospitals (and possibly clinical teams or individual clinicians) on the basis of how much patients' health improves. They are also intended to help identify where patients are not getting the expected benefits of a healthcare intervention.

In addition, there is interest in using the utility-weighted generic PROMs (QALYs) to determine the relative cost–utility of different interventions to inform commissioning decisions. This will strengthen the commissioning process by offering commissioners the evidence they need to buy the best services based on patient experiences.

Interestingly, the data which have been most widely analysed and used from the PROMs pilot studies (Browne et al., 2007) have been the generic measures (EQ-5D) and not the disease-specific measures, because of the ability to compare across services (Devlin et al., 2009). The greater use of the generic data for higher-level purposes may prove to be a concern for mental health where generic tools do not perform as well.

Measuring health outcomes is a crucial element of assessing productivity. Productivity measurement ideally involves measuring the value of health outputs in relation to the value of health inputs. These are typically measured as quality-adjusted cost-weighted outputs divided by quality-adjusted input factors (e.g. capital, labour) which in turn are adjusted by price deflators. Quality adjustments can include things such as survival rates, waiting times or health outcomes. Not taking account of the quality adjustments in a productivity measure can seriously undermine its accuracy.

The Atkinson Review (2005), which set out the framework for measuring government output in the National Accounts in the UK, recommended a number of improvements in the measurement of productivity as previously undertaken by the Office for National Statistics, notably improvements in the measurement of output and better measurement of aspects of quality of healthcare. The PROMs data will be an important contribution to improving the productivity estimates and these will be used in future in the National Accounts. In particular, to 'quality-adjust' and aggregate outputs from different areas of the healthcare system, for example, orthopaedic surgery and mental health, a generic outcome measure can be used which provides a common currency. This also allows for resource allocation, since it is possible to compare the value in different specialities or different parts of the health service.

The criteria that are deemed to be important for an outcome measure to be included in a productivity index are that it should have wide coverage, should be routinely collected, could readily be linked to activity data, could potentially be converted to a generic outcome measure and should be available as a time-series. Not many instruments in the mental health context in the UK fit this bill (Jacobs, 2009). A likely candidate for inclusion in productivity indices in England would be HoNOS because it has the widest coverage, could potentially be linked to activity data and is available longitudinally (Jacobs, 2009). However, it cannot readily be converted into a generic outcome measure, as we discuss later.

Demand management typically entails different methods to curtail healthcare costs. These can include a range of strategies from financial incentives for providers to greater patient choice. In the UK context, these initiatives are all linked, since there has been the introduction of a new prospective payment system for providers called Payment by Results (PbR) and this has been introduced simultaneously with a policy of patient choice. PbR entails paying hospitals according to the number and complexity of cases treated. Payment by Results is a misnomer since hospitals are paid for the work they do, not (as yet) for the results they achieve. Hospitals are paid a nationally set tariff for NHS activities structured around clinically meaningful groups of diagnoses and treatments known as Healthcare Resource Groups (HRGs). The introduction of patient choice means that patients referred to see a specialist can choose where they will be treated from a list of providers that meet NHS standards on the basis of waiting times, cleanliness, reputation and so on. PbR is critical to the introduction of patient choice, by ensuring that money follows the patient and there is a consistent basis for pricing across the NHS.

PbR will be rolled out to mental health services in the UK in the next few years (Department of Health, 2009c) but, instead of using HRGs to allocate payments, an adaptation of HoNOS has been proposed (called HoNOS PbR or SARN – Summary Assessment of Risk and Need) (Department of Health, 2009c). These instruments allocate service users to 21 clinically meaningful clusters which are similar in terms of care needs and resource requirements. While the clustering is based on clinical and non-clinical need (Self et al., 2008), the 21 clusters are located within three clinical 'superclasses' that are the first step in the classification process: organic disease, psychotic disorders and non-psychotic disorders. Though the care clusters are not based on diagnosis, people with similar diagnoses and levels of symptom severity are likely to be found in the same cluster. These clustering tools essentially maintain the 12 items of HoNOS but add six additional questions on history, engagement, vulnerability and child protection (Department of Health, 2009a). This will allow for the continued collection of HoNOS in the MHMDS. These clustering tools are being evaluated at present and the plan is that they will be rolled out from 2010 onwards for use as currencies and to establish local prices with the potential for national tariffs to be introduced by 2013 (Department of Health, 2009a).

Like PbR, patient choice is another policy where mental health may be required to follow the footsteps of policy initiatives in the acute health sector. Outcome measurement will be the important link between these policies in that it will facilitate patient choice on the basis of actual patient experience; and outcomes can of course be linked to hospital reimbursement (PbR). This has in fact been suggested for the first time in the Next Stage Review Final Report (Darzi, 2008), which indicated the intention to link payments to PROMs.

Outcome measurement can be used in value-based pricing (VBP) of pharmaceuticals. In VBP, the health service would pay pharmaceutical companies based on the *value* of the pharmaceutical to the patient base, rather than on the actual cost of the product, the market price, competitors' prices or the historical price. This may be deemed efficient since pharmaceutical companies will be paid more for treatments that patients value and the health service will not pay for failed drugs.

As mentioned, all of these applications of PROMs data are likely to benefit patients, policy makers, providers, managers, regulators and commissioners. But will they benefit individual clinicians? If indeed clinician-reported outcome measures are used in mental health, as is likely to be the case, then it is vitally important that the data can be used locally by clinicians to help improve quality of care. Outcomes data need to, first and foremost, inform local service delivery (Fonagy et al., 2004), before they can be put to higher-level uses such as benchmarking, provider payments or productivity measurement.

What are generic outcome measures?

By far the most commonly used generic measure is the Short-Form 36 (SF-36, Ware and Sherbourne, 1992). It has 36 standard questions about the individual's health in the last month and these are grouped into eight different dimensions of health, including physical functioning, social functioning and mental health. All items are scored and all items in a given dimension are combined to provide a single score, for example for physical functioning. Responses can also be used to produce two scale scores: a physical component summary (PCS) and a mental component summary (MCS). There is a short version called SF-12 which produces PCS and MCS scores. The SF-36 has been translated into more than 50 languages, it has been the subject of more study than any other instrument and has very strong measurement properties (Fitzpatrick, 2009).

Utility instruments are a type of generic instrument because they have been designed to have the widest applicability. However, their one distinctive feature is that they have been designed specifically to assign overall values (or utilities) to individuals' health states. The overall value is particularly useful in studies of cost-effectiveness of healthcare interventions. It allows researchers to estimate the overall aggregated value of the health states of the samples receiving the healthcare intervention to enable comparisons of costs (Fitzpatrick, 2009). Disease-specific measures do not allow the calculation of the overall value of health states for individuals or aggregations of individuals.

The EuroQol (EQ-5D) is the most widely used utility instrument in Europe (Brooks, 1996). The EQ-5D is a generic measure which covers five dimensions: mobility, self-care, usual activities, pain/discomfort and anxiety/depression. Each dimension has three levels: no problems, moderate problems, extreme problems. The EQ-5D provides a five-dimensional description of health status which can be defined by a five-digit number. For example the health state '11122' indicates no problems in mobility, self-care and usual activities, and moderate pain/discomfort and moderate anxiety/depression. EQ-5D is followed by a visual analogue scale (VAS) similar to a thermometer which ranges from 0 (the worst imaginable health state) to 100 (the best imaginable health state). A single weighted score (value) of the individual's health can be calculated from the five selected responses using weights of values provided by a general population survey. QALY (Quality Adjusted Life Year) weights are based on societal rather than patient values because resource allocation decisions are based on societal preferences (Dolan, 1997). The cost-effectiveness of interventions can therefore be assessed in terms of their cost per QALY.

The applicability of generic measures in mental health

The claim that generic measures are applicable to all interventions and patients has some merit with physical conditions where they have passed psychometric tests of validity and reliability. Generic instruments are, however, generally considered to be less sensitive to changes in patients' health state compared to disease-specific instruments which focus on certain aspects of a given disease and are likely to contain a higher proportion of relevant items for the illness being studied.

For mental health there is evidence that outcome measurement tools such as EQ-5D can be used to detect the impact of conditions such as mild to moderate depression and anxiety. But often generic measures such as SF-36 are not practical with acutely disturbed patients (Kaplan et al., 1998). While the measurement of quality of life is a key concern in mental health services, the QALY has not in fact been widely used as a scale (Bowling, 2001).

A randomized controlled trial (RCT) study by Sherbourne et al. (2001) used SF-12 or SF-36 measures on a group of patients with depression. They argued that there are concerns about the use of utility measures derived from generic health status measures in effectiveness studies for depression.

A study by Gunther et al. (2007) examined whether the EQ-5D could be a valid measure in alcohol-dependent individuals. They compared the EQ-5D against other measures of psychopathology and social functioning. The EQ-5D visual analogue scale (VAS) score and the EQ-5D index showed moderate correlations with other scales. They found some evidence for EQ-5D's validity in the population group, but the EQ-5D showed a ceiling effect.

Evidence on how EQ-5D performs in groups of patients with chronic schizophrenia is more patchy. One study examined the psychometric properties of the EQ-5D in patients with schizophrenic, schizotypal and delusional disorders (Konig et al., 2007). The patients completed the EQ-5D alongside other psychopathology scales and measures of functioning. For almost all EQ-5D dimensions, different response levels were associated with significantly different scores of measures used for comparison. EQ-5D did not correlate well with a disease-specific instrument for schizophrenia. Again the EQ-5D showed a ceiling effect.

Another study found that EQ-5D and its visual analogue scale (VAS) failed to detect changes in a group of patients with chronic schizophrenia (van de Willige et al., 2005). They concluded that the focus on physical components was not suited to the psychiatric context and that generic measures do not capture the impact of severe psychotic and more complex non-psychotic conditions.

Gilbody et al. (2003a, 2003b) reviewed outcome measures used in clinical trials and outcomes research in psychiatry and found that the dominant method of outcomes measurement in randomized trials was the disease-specific psychopathology scales. The use of generic measures is still largely absent. They argue that there is no robust research evidence to support their use as a routine outcome measure in psychiatric settings.

Generic measures may be difficult to apply to mental health patients since they often concentrate on physical functioning and ignore aspects of social functioning. They may have large numbers of irrelevant questions making them unacceptable to respondents and they may therefore also be insensitive to detecting changes in health status. Generic outcome measures are essentially designed to identify health status changes at a population level and the rating scores are often uninterpretable at an individual patient level. While a generic measure may be considered useful for supporting health policy decisions, or for cost-effectiveness analysis, they are not considered sensitive enough or useful enough at the individual patient level.

Can disease-specific outcome measures be converted into generic measures?

As mentioned, for the purposes of resource allocation decisions, cost-effectiveness decisions, productivity measurement and so on, we ideally require a generic outcome measure. However, as mentioned, generic measures are not well suited to mental health. Given that disease-specific measures are therefore more likely to be used, we examine whether they can be converted into generic ones. If this were feasible, it would also save on the cost of data collection.

The issue of conversion to a generic measure is highly problematic in mental health. There are two possible approaches to converting instruments. The first is to find values for the different health states, the second is to map them. We describe each of these approaches with special reference to the case of HoNOS as an example of a commonly used outcome tool.

Valuing HoNOS

Disease-specific instruments in mental health are generally not suitable for valuation using preference elicitation methods given their size and complexity. If one considers the complexity of valuing EQ-5D with five domains and three levels as a dimensionality problem of 3^5 giving approximately 243 items, the equivalent calculation for HoNOS would be 12 domains and five levels (5^{12}), giving over 244 million health states. Even though some health states may be encountered very rarely in practice, there are still too many to create valuations for. Even if one took the 10-item version of HoNOS, this would still amount to finding valuations for approximately 9.7 million items.

An example of a valuation of a HoNOS health state from the 12 domains and five levels (0 – no problem, to 4 – severe) is given in Table 23.1.

Using time-trade-off or other preference elicitation methods, someone would be asked to imagine themselves in this health state for, say, the next 40 years before they die. If they could trade this for full health now, how many years would they be prepared to live in full health to equate to the 40 years in poor health? If they respond, say, 30 years, this would give a utility weight of 30/40 years or 0.75.

It would be very difficult, however, for the general population, whose values are typically used, to imagine what this health state may be like. Some of the problems described are alien to many members of the public and mental health conditions are very difficult to envisage. This may lead to a set of ill-informed values.

The HoNOS statements are also quite complex, with, for example, five levels for dimension six (hallucinations and delusions) and detailed notes accompanying each dimension. Given that the descriptive system for each health state is so complex, this would lead to cognitive overload for respondents.

The main concern remains though that there are far too many health states which require valuations and typically only a small set of respondents are asked to value a subset of health states. The rest of the health states then need to be modelled using various imputation methods, though this leaves a great deal of uncertainty and with 244 million health states is still a near impossible statistical task. Valuing complex disease-specific instruments is not straightforward.

Table 23.1 HoNOS Health State 210103324142

1. Occasional aggressive gestures, pushing or pestering others; threats or verbal aggression; lesser damage to property (e.g. broken cup, window); marked overactivity or agitation [rating of 2]
2. Fleeting thoughts about ending it all but little risk; no self-harm [rating of 1]
3. No problem with drinking or drug-taking [rating of 0]
4. Minor problems with memory or understanding, e.g. forgets names occasionally [rating of 1]
5. No physical health problem [rating of 0]
6. Marked preoccupation with delusions or hallucinations, causing much distress and/or manifested in obviously bizarre behaviour, i.e. moderately severe clinical problem [rating of 3]
7. Depression with inappropriate self-blame, preoccupied with feelings of guilt [rating of 3]
8. Other mental and behavioural problem clinically present, but there are relatively symptom-free intervals and patient/client has a degree of control, i.e. mild level [rating of 2]
9. Severe and distressing social isolation due to inability to communicate socially and/or withdrawal from social relationships [rating of 4]
10. Minor problems with activities of daily living; e.g. untidy, disorganized [rating of 1]
11. Accommodation is unacceptable; e.g. lack of basic necessities, patient is at risk of eviction, or 'roofless', or living conditions are otherwise intolerable, making patient's problems worse [rating of 4]
12. Limited choice of activities; e.g. there is a lack of reasonable tolerance (e.g. unfairly refused entry to public library or baths, etc.); or handicapped by lack of a permanent address; or insufficient carer or professional support; or helpful day setting available but for very limited hours [rating of 2]

Mapping HoNOS

In principle one could consider mapping across from one instrument to another using one of two approaches: judgement or statistical inference. Either approach would allow one to develop a look-up table for a value of HoNOS, giving its equivalent EQ-5D score (called cross-walking). In theory, this could be done by using both EQ-5D and HoNOS together on the same set of respondents and generating equivalent mapped values on either instrument. Ideally it would entail the collection of clinician-rated HoNOS scores, clinician-rated EQ-5D scores and user-rated EQ-5D scores on the same set of patients.

However, there are not many instances where HoNOS and EQ-5D have been used on the same set of patients, even in research studies. There have been isolated examples in the literature, for example two German studies (Gunther et al., 2007, Konig et al., 2007). However, as outlined above, EQ-5D does not always accurately reflect mental health problems for some patient populations.

There are several criticisms around the different methods of mapping for both the judgement and statistical inference approaches, including arbitrariness, and no clear-cut criteria for assessing the performance of the mapping. Performance depends on the degree of overlap in content between the instruments being mapped (Brazier et al., 2007). The degree of overlap between HoNOS and EQ-5D is questionable.

There are therefore immense challenges in mapping from one instrument to another and valuing instruments which are likely to be used in mental health services.

Conclusions

Mental health services are often required to adopt policies that have first been tried out in the acute health sector, though significant adaptations are often required because mental health is seen as difficult and different. The roll-out of PROMs is one example where this is likely to be the case in the future and it would be prudent for mental health services to gear themselves up for this likely eventuality.

There are a number of unresolved issues and challenges for the mandatory application of PROMs (or clinician-rated outcome measures) in mental health. These include the choice of disease-specific and possible generic outcome measures or, in the absence of generic outcome measures, the conversion of disease-specific measures. Generic measures do not seem well suited to mental health and valuation or mapping approaches to convert disease-specific measures are fraught with difficulties. This is a major obstacle at present and will require careful consideration and research effort to resolve.

Other challenges include the design of the routine outcome measurement system, the frequency of data collection, the role and involvement of the clinician and clinical team, the development of timely and useful feedback mechanisms of outcome data to clinical teams and the resourcing and design of information technology (IT) systems to support the easy entry of data and the easy access of feedback for clinical teams. These issues are absolutely imperative to ensure the acceptance of a routine outcome measurement system that is embedded in clinical practice, can provide good-quality data, particularly repeat outcome measures, and can support drives to improve patient care. Linked to the issue of clinically useful outcome data as well as IT data capture is the challenge of what additional patient data can be captured to contextualize or risk-adjust the outcomes data. Changes in health status, or lack thereof, may be the result of factors which cannot be attributed to the healthcare provider. There is little agreement about appropriate risk-adjustment approaches to compare performance of providers (Iezzoni, 2009) and again careful thought and research effort are needed.

Another important consideration for the application of PROMs will be obtaining not only management support for the higher-level drivers of the process and the aggregate service-level uses to which the data could be put, but also management support for the individual clinicians and patient-level data which clinical teams can use. Managers, clinicians and indeed policy-makers, providers and purchasers all require different types of information to make decisions about the outcomes of care. It is important that support is given not just for the aggregate higher-level data. Top-down drives to enforce routine collection will rarely be effective without the resourcing and support of outcome measurement at the clinical level.

Another policy initiative which will be rolled out to mental health in England after having been trialled in the acute health sector is PbR and there has been reference to the linking of PROMs to PbR since this will enable commissioners to purchase not just activity, but improvements in health outcomes. Using a financial incentive such as PbR would indeed ensure that outcome completion rates are high. However, there is a danger of perverse incentives with a clinician-reported outcome measure linked to payment, where clinicians may be tempted to over-report improvements in health status. Very thorough and potentially expensive auditing processes will be required if this route is pursued.

The use of PROMs data for economic and policy-making purposes is ever more likely as the benefits of the outcomes data become more evident. It is therefore important for mental health to get on board with policy developments in the acute health sector such as PbR and PROMs. Otherwise there is a risk of mental health being left out of the picture because commissioners cannot readily see the value for money or patient benefits being obtained compared to other areas of the health service where this is more apparent. There is therefore a risk of budgets being switched and resources being redistributed to other parts of the healthcare system (Elphick, 2007, Fairbairn, 2007). Getting on board with policy initiatives such as routine outcome measurement could help protect mental health funding against pressures to disinvest.

References

Ashaye, O. A., Livingston, G. and Orrell, M. W. (2003). Does standardized needs assessment improve the outcome of psychiatric day hospital care for older people? A randomized controlled trial. *Aging & Mental Health*, **7**, 195–9.

Atkinson, A. (2005). *Atkinson Review: Final Report*. London: HMSO.

Bowling, A. (2001). *Measuring Disease: A Review of Disease-Specific Quality of Life Measurement Scales*. Buckingham: Open University Press.

Brazier, J., Yang, Y. and Tsuchiya, A. (2007). *Review of Methods for Mapping Between Condition Specific Measures onto Generic Measures of Health*. Sheffield: School of Health and Related Research, University of Sheffield.

Brooks, R. (1996). EuroQol: the current state of play. *Health Policy*, **37**, 53–72.

Browne, J., Jamieson, L., Lewsey, J., et al. (2007). *Patients Reported Outcome Measures (PROMS) in Elective Surgery: Report to the Department of Health*. London School of Hygiene & Tropical Medicine, available at: www.lshtm.ac.uk/hsru/research/PROMs-Report-12-Dec-07.pdf.

Darzi, A. (2008). *High Quality Care For All: NHS Next Stage Review Final Report*. London: Department of Health, available at: http://www.dh.gov.uk/en/Publicationsandstatistics/Publications/PublicationsPolicyAndGuidance/DH_085825, retrieved 11 August 2009.

Department of Health (2009a). *Clustering Booklet for use in Mental Health Payment by Results Evaluation Work (July-Dec*

2009), available at: http://www.dh.gov.uk/en/Publicationsandstatistics/Publications/PublicationsPolicyAndGuidance/DH_100818, retrieved 11 August 2009.

Department of Health (2009b). *Guidance on the Routine Collection of Patient Reported Outcome Measures (PROMs): For the NHS in England 2009/10*, available at: http://www.dh.gov.uk/en/Publicationsandstatistics/Publications/PublicationsPolicyAndGuidance/DH_092647, retrieved 11 August 2009.

Department of Health (2009c). *Practical Guide to Preparing for Mental Health Payment by Results*, available at: http://www.dh.gov.uk/en/Managingyourorganisation/Financeandplanning/NHSFinancialReforms/DH_4137762, retrieved 11 August 2009.

Devlin, N. J., Parkin, D. and Browne, J. (2009). *Using the EQ-5D as a Performance Measurement Tool in the NHS. Department of Economics*, Discussion Paper Series No. 09/03, available at: http://www.city.ac.uk/economics/dps/discussion_papers/0903.pdf, retrieved 11 August 2009.

Dolan, P. (1997). Modelling valuations for EuroQol health states. *Medical Care*, **35**, 1096–108.

Elphick, M. (2007). Information-based management of mental health services: a two-stage model for improving funding mechanism and clinical governance. *Psychiatric Bulletin*, **31**, 44–8.

Fairbairn, A. (2007). Payment by results in mental health: the current state of play in England. *Advances in Psychiatric Treatment*, **13**, 3–6.

Fitzpatrick, R. (2009). Patient-reported outcome measures and performance measurement. In P. C. Smith, E. Mossialos, S. Leatherman and I. Papanicolas, eds., *Performance Measurement for Health System Improvement: Experiences, Challenges and Prospects*. Cambridge: Cambridge University Press.

Fonagy, P., Matthews, R. and Pilling, S. (2004). *The Mental Health Outcomes Measurement Initiative: Report from the Chair of the Outcomes Reference Group*. London:

National Collaborating Centre for Mental Health.

Gilbody, S. M. and Whitty, P. (2002). Improving the delivery and organisation of mental health services: beyond the conventional randomised controlled trial. *British Journal of Psychiatry*, **180**, 13–18.

Gilbody, S. M., House, A. O. and Sheldon, T. A. (2001). Routinely administered questionnaires for depression and anxiety: systematic review. *British Medical Journal*, **322**, 406–9.

Gilbody, S. M., House, A. O. and Sheldon, T. A. (2003a). Outcome measures and needs assessment tools for schizophrenia and related disorders. *Cochrane Database of Systematic Reviews*, CD003081.

Gilbody, S. M., House, A. O., Sheldon, T. A. (2003b). *Outcomes Measurement in Psychiatry: A Critical Review of Outcomes Measurement in Psychiatric Research and Practice*. York: Centre for Reviews and Dissemination, available at: http://www.york.ac.uk/inst/crd/CRD-Reports/crdreport24.pdf.

Gunther, O., Roick, C., Angermeyer, M. C. and Konig, H.-H. (2007). The EQ-5D in alcohol dependent patients: relationships among health-related quality of life, psychopathology and social functioning. *Drug and Alcohol Dependence*, **86**, 253–64.

Iezzoni, L. I. (2009). Risk adjustment for performance measurement. In P. C. Smith, E. Mossialos, S. Leatherman and I. Papanicolas, eds., *Performance Measurement for Health System Improvement: Experiences, Challenges and Prospects*. Cambridge: Cambridge University Press.

Jacobs, R. (2009). *Investigating Patient Outcome Measures in Mental Health*. York: Centre for Health Economics, available at http://www.york.ac.uk/inst/che/rp48.pdf.

Kaplan, R. M., Ganiats, T., Sieber, W. and Anderson, J. (1998). The Quality of Well-Being Scale: critical similarities and differences with SF-36. *International Journal for Quality in Health Care*, **10**, 509–20.

Konig, H. H., Roick, C. and Angermeyer, M. C. (2007). Validity of the EQ-5D in assessing and valuing health status in patients with schizophrenic, schizotypal or delusional disorders. *European Psychiatry: The Journal of the Association of European Psychiatrists,* **22**, 177–87.

Office of Health Economics (OHE) (2008). *Report of the Office of Health Economics Commission on NHS Outcomes, Performance and Productivity*, available at: http://www.ohe.org/page/commission.cfm, retrieved 11 August 2009.

Priebe, S., McCabe, R., Bullenkamp, J., et al. (2002). The impact of routine outcome measurement on treatment processes in community mental health care: approach and methods of the MECCA study. *Epidemiologia e Psichiatria Sociale,* **11**, 198–205.

Self, R., Rigby, A., Leggetti, C. and Paxton, R. (2008). Clinical Decision Support Tool: a rational needs-based approach to making clinical decisions. *Journal of Mental Health,* **17**, 33–48.

Sherbourne, C. D., Unutzer, J., Schoenbaum, M., et al. (2001). Can utility-weighted health-related quality-of-life estimates capture health effects of quality improvement for depression? *Medical Care,* **39**, 1246–59.

Slade, M., McCrone, P., Kuipers, E., et al. (2006). Use of standardised outcome measures in adult mental health services:Randomised controlled trial. *British Journal of Psychiatry,* **189**, 330–6.

van de Willige, G., Wiersma, D., Nienhuis, F. J. and Jenner, J. A. (2005). Changes in quality of life in chronic psychiatric patients: a comparison between EuroQol (EQ-5D) and WHOQoL *Quality of Life Research,* **14**, 441–51.

Ware, J. E. and Sherbourne, C. D. (1992). The MOS 36-item Short Form Health Status Survey (SF-36): I. Conceptual framework and item selection. *Medical Care,* **30**, 473–83.

West, D. (2009). NHS PROMs results ready by November. *Health Service Journal,* 6 February, available at: http://www.hsj.co.uk/nhs -PROMs-results-ready-by-november/1984994.article.

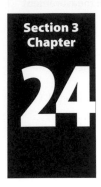

Current Issues in Outcome Measurement

Future directions

Tom Trauer

In this final chapter I shall briefly review the material presented in the foregoing chapters and attempt to draw out some themes relevant to the future of outcome measurement (OM).

Outcome measurement around the world

The first section of this collection comprised accounts of OM from different countries and jurisdictions. I repeat here a point made in the opening chapter: the absence of a country or jurisdiction should not be taken to mean that OM does not happen there at all; the presentations are from settings where there is a reasonable amount of material in the public domain that shows how OM is implemented there. Tom Callaly and Jane Pirkis described the Australian system, Graham Mellsop and Mark Smith the New Zealand approach, Mike Slade the English scene, and Michael Lambert, Jim Healy and Dee Roth, and David Smith described their North American implementations. From continental Europe, Mirella Ruggeri outlined Italian developments, Sylke Andreas, Bernd Puschner, Thomas Becker and Holger Shulz described OM in Germany and Torleif Ruud did similarly for Norway. It is apparent from those presentations that there is great variety in the way the task of OM has been interpreted and implemented in different countries, and one clear conclusion is that there is no one correct way to do it. In some cases OM is centrally organized, while elsewhere there are several relatively autonomous systems. Some are primarily based in service delivery systems while others are more academic in nature. Some rely predominantly on consumer-completed measures, whereas others place greater reliance on clinician-completed scales. It is fair to say that the kind of outcomes systems that a country develops will be determined by many local influences, such as the nature of the health, and mental health, service, the level of interest and support at senior governmental levels, the presence of key individuals and the kinds of economic forces that shape how services are monitored and evaluated.

In trying to discern similarities and differences among the countries reviewed, there seemed to be certain similarities among Australia, New Zealand and England, and among the continental European countries, Germany, Italy and Norway, and among the North American regions, Ontario, Ohio and Utah. One commonality between Australia, New Zealand and England is their strong investment, in both research and practice, in the Health of the Nation Outcome Scales (HoNOS, Wing et al., 1994). This arose because the HoNOS was arguably the first instrument designed for national use as an outcome measure, and was selected as such in Australia, followed shortly thereafter by New Zealand. While the policies in all three countries acknowledge the importance of consumer self-rated measures, the development work, research output and compliance rates are far less for the consumer-completed measures than for the clinician-completed HoNOS. The common threads in the German, Italian and Norwegian implementations are that (a) none is truly national in scope and (b) all have a strong research-based character, with many of the leading figures having senior academic appointments as well as clinical roles. As for the examples of OM in the North American continent, they do all have one feature in common, which may or may not be significant: unlike the Australasian and European systems described, all three have consumer-completed instruments as their central focus.

One of the local influences that will affect the prominence of OM within a country or region is the presence and activity of one or more strong and influential 'champions': these are evident in certain settings and less so in others. Hodges et al. (2001, p. 242) described data champions as 'people within any organization who serve as advocates for appropriate results-based decision-making', Garg et al. (2005) thought that the importance of local champions in facilitating the implementation of decision support systems could not be overestimated, and Jacobs (2007, p. 68) reported that many in the field felt that 'clinical champions enthusiastic about outcome measurement were absolutely essential'. Many of the successes in countries and regions can be traced to the drive and vision of such champions.

At this point one might ask: while champions may be highly desirable, are they necessary and sufficient for OM to be self-sustaining and viable in the long term? And is there not something peculiar about a philosophy based on evidence and data being reliant for its success on the charisma of (usually) one person? History has tended to show, unfortunately, that champions are good at initiating movements, but they are less effective in making them routine. A good example of this is the rise and fall of 'Moral Treatment', which flourished for about two decades in the middle of the nineteenth century in America and was associated with a dramatic increase in discharge rates from mental hospitals, in the absence of any revolutionary discoveries in psychiatric treatment. As Bockoven (1963, p. 20) describes, 'Of the many factors which contributed to the decline and the eventual discard of moral treatment, lack of inspired leadership after the death of its innovators was probably the most important. The founders of moral treatment were shortsighted in not providing for their own successors in numbers adequate to meet the needs of the future'. The relevance to OM is that one limitation arising from excessive reliance on champions is their tendency to neglect succession planning, often related to the personality traits that make them charismatic in the first place. For OM to become a natural part of the clinical landscape, the pioneering work of champions needs to be supplemented by more enduring, and perhaps less conspicuous, contributions. Several authors (e.g. Huffman et al., 2004, James and Mitchell, 2004) have noted the need for 'cultural change', most frequently characterized as an orientation towards evidence-based practice. This may explain to some extent the close link between OM and the research community. We saw that in certain countries the main drivers of OM are clinical academics.

By focusing on large-scale implementations of OM I have inevitably overlooked smaller, more localized, programmes. Such developments may have much to commend them, such as local ownership and tailored design, thus avoiding some of the weaknesses of national programmes, which can tend to have a 'one size fits all' quality. But in this regard bigger may not necessarily be better. Smaller implementations may face certain difficulties, for example, they may fail to attract interest and resources from governments and national bodies because their data are not perceived as contributing to national statistics. Also, they may be frustrated by a lack of external data to compare their own results against. However, if we accept that one main purpose of OM is to inform clinical decision-making, then local stakeholders are more likely to perceive value in a locally designed, developed and owned system. Thus, a smaller system may 'tick more boxes' for stakeholders close to the clinical interface than a large national system.

Outcome measurement in specific groups and settings

Just as there is great variety in how OM is implemented in different countries and regions, there is similar variety when it comes to applying OM to specific groups of service recipients. In the Australian and New Zealand contexts, the major subdivision is into child and adolescent, adult, and older persons, described by Peter Brann, myself, and Rod McKay and Regina McDonald respectively. There has also been some recent impetus for forensic services to be regarded as sufficiently distinct as to merit their own specialized measures (e.g. Sugarman et al., 2009). Although the specific instruments used across these groups vary to some extent (e.g. different forms of the HoNOS are used in child and adolescent, adult and older persons), the overall system of OM is governed by the same protocol (NOCC, Department of Health and Ageing, 2003), which is based on the episode of care, with collections at its beginning and end, and for longer episodes, at intervals between. The division into three main age-defined groups is largely pragmatic and recognizes that, just as ordinary clinical assessment methods are adapted to the specific characteristics of the target group, so should the instruments used in OM differ accordingly.

In addition to the three main age-defined groups, chapters addressed four other groups or settings to which OM has been adapted: indigenous consumers; private hospitals; non-government organizations (NGOs); and drug and alcohol services. Each has its own specific issues and challenges. In relation to indigenous consumers, the main issue was ensuring valid and culturally sensitive assessment. The primary decision, as with any culturally or linguistically different subpopulation, is whether to develop and use specially tailored instruments or to use 'mainstream' measures. As discussed in the chapter by Tricia Nagel and myself, there are advantages and disadvantages to each choice. Fortunately, this choice need not be based on theoretical or ethical grounds alone, since there now exists some empirical evidence to guide future action. In particular, there is now preliminary evidence that mainstream measures can be used by (predominantly) non-indigenous clinicians with indigenous consumers, so long as best practice methods of assessment are adopted.

The implementations of OM in Australian private hospitals and NGOs share some similarities since they both sit outside the mainstream public clinical mental health services. Their relative separateness has given them the freedom to select certain measures specific to their services, although in the event they have also chosen to use some mainstream measures. The private hospitals use the HoNOS, as in the public sector, but use the MHQ-14 as their consumer self-rated measure. The NGO described in the chapter by Glen Tobias uses the BASIS-32, as used in certain Australian public mental health jurisdictions, but also uses the Camberwell Assessment of Need Short Appraisal Schedule (CANSAS), having judged it as particularly appropriate to the kind of consumers that they serve. One feature both sectors share is a much higher completion rate of their measures than in the corresponding public-sector services. The authors of the respective chapters give some clues as to why this might be. In their chapter, Allen Morris-Yates and Andrew Page ascribed the higher completion rates in private hospitals to 'stakeholder involvement, feedback, rebuke and encouragement', while the chapter by Glen Tobias implicated lower case-loads, closer working relationships with consumers who are entirely voluntary, and the perceived practical relevance of the measures, in particular the CANSAS, to the staff who are required to ensure its completion. Interestingly, the Ontario experience as reported by David Smith and Dee Roth, which is also based on the CANSAS, is of few problems with staff compliance.

The review of OM in the drug and alcohol field by Maree Teesson and Mark Deady described a number of specialized instruments that are specifically targeted to substance misuse problems. This raises a question common to OM in all services that focus on subpopulations – should they use 'generic' or 'specific' instruments, since generic measures will allow comparison with other services, while specific measures will allow more targeted and tailored assessment of relevant domains? Broadly, comparison of services will have appeal to those with interests in accountability, value for money and benchmarking, while more relevant assessment will be favoured by clinicians, consumers and carers. This is a theme that I shall return to later.

Current issues in outcome measurement

This section of the book reviewed those issues that had been identified in Chapter 1 as important, namely applications and utility, stakeholder perspectives, the assessment of change, workforce issues, the range of available instruments and the economic aspects of OM.

The chapter on applications and utility identified four main groups of potential beneficiaries of OM: consumers and carers, clinicians, team leaders and managers, and policy makers and funders. The benefits for consumers and carers were listed as promoting dialogue, tracking progress, identifying hidden problems and needs and promoting self-efficacy, empowerment and recovery. For clinicians the list comprised standardized methods for monitoring change, assisting with individual service planning and informing clinical decision-making. Team leaders and managers gained profiling of their services, caseload management and promotion of service quality, while policy makers and funders could expect evidence of effectiveness and a basis for accountability and rational resourcing. Given this impressive list of potential benefits, the question of why some stakeholders in the mental health arena are unconvinced of the value of OM was taken up in the following chapter.

That review concluded that there is a very wide range of sentiment related to OM, ranging from strongly positive to strongly negative, with quite a large section who have mixed feelings. There appeared to be some relationship between one's role in the (mental) health system and one's views about OM, with clinicians being the least impressed and policy makers and funders the most. I noted that no one seriously disputes the philosophical basis of OM; the notions that services should operate in an evidence-based fashion and try to assess as objectively as possible the true progress of consumers have the status of virtually self-evident truths. The literature lists many of the reservations, including dislike of (additional) paperwork, pressure of work (often associated with high case-loads), doubts about the instruments themselves, lack of 'utility', absence of suitable feedback (often associated with inadequate information technology) and vague (but sometimes not so vague) apprehensiveness about the uses to which OM results would be put. Taken individually, each of these factors may be more or less applicable in any individual case, but taken collectively they appear, at least to this observer, to have a common factor – they are all concerns of *clinicians*.

The implication that a sizable sector of the clinician workforce might be lukewarm about OM is of considerable concern, and means that the list of barriers deserves close attention. At the outset, I suggest that some of the objections, such as too much paperwork and pressure of work, are 'general purpose' objections that could be applied to any innovation or change in work practice, and have little inherent connection with OM *per se*. Similarly, doubts about the psychometric properties of instruments are easy to express and difficult to refute, since all mental health measures are imperfect, and an instrument or set of instruments that will satisfy all stakeholders in all circumstances cannot be devised. Indeed, calls for new, improved instruments often neglect to consider the *marginal* benefit of the future measure; that is, will the time and cost of developing the 'better' measure be justified by significant improvement over current measures?

More pertinent to OM are the issues of lack of utility, absence of suitable feedback and apprehensiveness over potential uses. The first two of these appear to be related, in that immediate and understandable feedback seems to be a necessary, but not sufficient, condition for perceived utility. The clearest example of good feedback is the Outcome Questionnaire system described in the chapter by Michael Lambert, where clinicians receive virtually instantaneous feedback of consumers' self-assessments in a format that clearly directs attention to the most important (to the clinician) features. But fast and comprehensible feedback alone does not make the information useful – in Australia there are numerous settings where staff can get quick feedback, yet grumbles about limited utility persist. Closely related to utility is the concept of feasibility of routine OM in mental health, as described by Slade et al. (1999), and which they define as 'the extent to which it is suitable for use on a routine, sustainable and meaningful basis in typical clinical settings, when used in a specific manner and for a specific purpose' (p. 245). Their list of criteria includes such properties as acceptability and value, and it is around these issues that most concerns seem to revolve. A measure is acceptable (to clinicians) when it contributes to the work in hand and does not duplicate known information, and is of value when the benefits of using the assessment outweigh the costs. At a very general level, the 'work in hand' can be conceptualized as minimizing bad outcomes (e.g. symptomatic deterioration, social isolation) and promoting the good (e.g. recovery, social inclusion). Mental health services systems, including their OM systems, tend to be better geared to detecting the former than the latter (Slade, 2009); there are clearly opportunities in the future to rectify this imbalance.

At this point one may ask another rhetorical question: everything else being equal, is a clinician-completed or consumer-completed measure of greater acceptability to the average clinician? In terms of not duplicating already known information, it seems to me that the consumer-completed measure has greater capacity to tell the clinician something that he/she does not already know, compared to the provider-completed measure, which to a large extent simply codifies the clinician's existing information, perceptions and judgements. The consumer measure also shifts the 'burden' of completion away from the busy clinician, a not insignificant consideration when it has been estimated that 'Even simple outcome measurement can add 10% to a clinician's total time spent per patient' (Marks, 1998, p. 282). There is some evidence, too, that clinicians are more comfortable in discussing consumers' views of their health than having to share their own often discordant views (Trauer and Pedwell, 2007).

The same question can now be put, but this time in relation to the average policy maker or funder. At this point it is worth reflecting that policy makers and funders in health are often former (or even current) clinicians, and as such will often share fundamental values with the clinical workforce, with whom their expectations from an OM system will overlap. They will typically be interested in diverse aspects of system performance, including effectiveness and consumer satisfaction. Effectiveness is sometimes conceptualized quite narrowly as symptom reduction or functional improvement. In the Australian system, effectiveness is defined as 'Care, intervention or action achieves desired outcome in an appropriate timeframe' (Information Strategy Committee, 2005, p. 24), which begs the questions of who is doing the desiring and what is desired. Our prototypical policy maker will be interested in service satisfaction, which can really only be obtained from consumers and carers, as well as effectiveness, which could come from consumers/carers or from clinicians, or both. The chapter on the assessment of change presented evidence that clinician and self-evaluations of individual consumers' health status are only weakly related and difficult to reconcile. The two sources have complementary strengths and weakness: under a mandatory collection policy, clinician assessments are likely to be less biased by the selective non-completion by consumers who are too unwell to manage the task, but the necessarily voluntary consumer self-assessments are likely to have greater authenticity, as well as being less tainted by the reality or suspicion of gaming by clinicians. The case for greater reliance on consumer self-assessed outcome is reinforced when one considers that, apart from acute and emergency settings, the progress of many consumers in community care in public mental health services is characterized by small, non-dramatic changes, or even no change at all, from a purely symptomatic point of view. To the extent that modern mental health services subscribe to recovery values, which include leading a satisfying life in the presence of ongoing symptoms and disabilities, routine OM should be as much concerned with how services promote this objective as the narrower traditional clinical outcomes.

Returning to the accounts of OM in different countries and regions, I believe one can discern worse completion rates, and presumably more clinician resistance, where the OM system rests mainly on a clinician-completed measure (primarily HoNOS), and better completion and less resistance where the system is built around consumer-completed instruments (CANSAS, OQ-45, the Ohio Scales). If true, this is hardly likely to be on account of the differing properties of the instruments themselves. The instruments that countries, regions and local services adopt, and subsequently invest most effort in, reflect how they construe their core business. Where the dominant paradigm is biomedical, deficit-oriented approaches might be favoured, while in settings where the consumer/carer voice is stronger, and the culture is more attuned to participatory and 'consumer as expert' models of care, self-report or joint assessment methods will be perceived as more appropriate.

Adopting Slade et al.'s (1999) helpful proposition that for a measure to be acceptable its benefits should outweigh its costs, it was suggested that sometimes its benefits are not readily apparent; what about its costs? The review has suggested that the two main costs for direct care staff are worry about how the results might be used, and time. On the matter of time, one of the most tangible ways that an organization can demonstrate to its workforce that it values something is to ensure that time is set aside for it. Of course, this is rarely done for OM, except for time-limited research projects. As far as *routine* OM is concerned, the expectation is that the activity be blended into normal work practice, a case of not working harder or longer, but working 'smarter'. However, especially when caseloads are high, this can be perceived as unrealistic, or even oppressive, and a likely consequence is tokenistic compliance, resulting in poor quality and quantity of OM data. As to worries about how OM results will be used, this was characterized as fears of vague 'management' motives. Recent developments suggest these concerns are neither vague nor groundless; one leading outcome measure, the HoNOS, is being adapted into the HoNOS-PbR (Payment by Results) in England (Department of Health Mental Health PbR Development, 2009). Elsewhere, a Value Index is proposed (Brown, 2007), whereby the change on a measure is divided by the cost (after making suitable allowance for casemix) which 'as a performance indicator encourages clinicians to strive for better than average outcomes', and will in turn identify 'high value providers' who 'offer a greater return on investment to the health plan and employers for expenditures of behavioral health treatment services'. This of course raises the spectre of gaming, which would be entirely predictable and understandable, and require steps to be taken to safeguard the OM collection system against this threat to validity. This data-quality infrastructure will come with its own additional costs, in terms of money, time and distraction away from the core purposes of OM.

Another current issue that was identified was the assessment of change. It appears that the assessment of change in health, not just in OM, is a dynamic and rapidly changing field. This is both exciting and unsettling, since keeping abreast of developments is time-consuming. Further, some of the time required to keep up involves understanding, and if possible mastering, some fairly complex methods. There are some general principles, however. Even the most powerful and flexible methods will be limited by the quality of the data they are applied to, so attention needs to be continually paid to data issues such as coverage, completion, completeness and even, given the probability of gaming in certain settings, validity. For OMs to be used freely and naturally in everyday mental health practice, all practitioners need some basic grounding in the relevant principles, but only enough to be able to use the results confidently and safely, i.e. without making errors of interpretation, which is surprisingly easy to do. I have suggested that a useful framework in this regard is to distinguish change in the individual case and change in aggregated results, for which related, but different, methods are required. Another idea that will assist users in getting the most from the measures that are collected includes using graphical presentation methods wherever possible. Although I have no firm evidence for it, I suspect that many users of aggregated results will understand them better, and make a closer connection with them, if they are expressed in terms of the fundamental units from which they were derived – i.e. the individual service recipients. For example, rather than express aggregate change in terms of units of the particular instrument used, which generally have no intrinsic meaning, it may be more intuitive to report what proportion of the service recipients changed in various ways, as well as what proportion did not change. This will require the underlying statistical concepts, such as the Reliable Change Index (RCI), to be presented in ways that are adapted to the needs of those who will use them.

Whatever methods of analysing and presenting change information are adopted, they will need to be covered in OM training, and probably periodically thereafter, especially as new methods and procedures are introduced. In the workforce chapter by Tim Coombs and I, it was shown that, at least in the Australian context, training in OM is an evolving art. As greater understanding of the nuances of OM develops, the curriculum for training expands. A distinction can be made between the technical learnings required for OM, such as scoring and interpretation of the numbers on the one hand, and the skills needed to use OM with other people, such as discussing results in clinical meetings or with consumers, on the other. For the former, 'classroom' style training can be inefficient, and greater exploitation of and reliance on computerized and web-based methods are being explored. But for the latter, the opportunities to discuss, ask questions, explore and role-play mean that some level of *in vivo* training may always be required. The latter approaches, being much more labour-intensive, are more costly; it remains an unanswered question what the appropriate balance of methods should be.

The review of instruments covered a large number of instruments in several domains: symptom severity, personal functioning, quality of life, perceived needs and recovery. These domains were chosen on pragmatic grounds – they are by no means the only way to divide the material. Also, not all instruments could be covered, and new ones are emerging all the time. For this reason the commentary on measures is more conceptual than specific.

The comparative ease with which instruments can now be developed, tested, distributed and their results quickly computed and presented is both a blessing and a curse: a blessing because better instruments are being developed, but a curse because the uptake of new measures and the discarding of the old means that one of the great strengths of OM, standardization of how things are measured, is compromised. An increasingly common trend is the modification of existing instruments. Indeed, most of the instruments that have been used in the Australian context (HoNOS, LSP, BASIS (Eisen et al., 1986), K-10 (Andrews and Slade, 2001), CAN (Phelan et al., 1995), MHQ-14 (http://www.pmha.com.au/cdms/home)) are either predecessors or successors of other versions. More often than not, the modification involves abbreviation; this is true of the LSP, BASIS, K-10 and MHQ-14. While the justification for this might be a perceived need for brevity, shorter scales generally capture less information, and reliability is adversely affected. Often, the psychometric properties of the longer version are claimed for the shorter version, but this is hardly ever justified.

Of course, one should not expect that measurement techniques in OM should remain static. The question is: in which direction should changes take us? If reduced 'burden' is the objective, then shorter scales make sense, but if better relevant detail on consumers' problems are desired, then they do not. Also, if additional domains of interest to diverse stakeholders are to be included in what is measured (e.g. recovery), then longer scales might be required.

The last of the foregoing chapters, by Rowena Jacobs, was on economic and policy considerations. It is significant that many of the points made in that chapter echo issues raised elsewhere. Principal among these is that for OM to work at the policy and funder level it must first work at the consumer interface. To repeat, the dangers are of low quantity and quality of OM data. An apt analogy would be that basing complex funding and accountability systems on questionable data is like building a house on sand.

Final observations

In the opening chapter I reviewed the history and principles of OM, and the subsequent chapters have given a flavour of how OM stands at present. Clearly, there are numerous examples of excellent practice, and it has been a privilege and pleasure to assemble them in this compilation. Taking a historical perspective, one may ask how OM is travelling. Thoughtful commentators have identified, alongside the achievements, present and future challenges. These are hardly unexpected, given the complexity of the enterprise – indeed one such commentator noted in relation to OM, perhaps only partly in jest, that 'the first 25 years are the most difficult' (Buckingham, circa 2002, personal communication). If this is even approximately correct, most implementations are still in the more difficult phase. Tim Coombs, who is responsible for training and service development in the Australian Mental Health Outcomes and Classification Network (AMHOCN), has reflected that if he had his time in OM over again, the three things he would do differently were (a) not call it routine outcome measurement, with its connotations of rather tedious data collection, but rather something like systematic assessment, (b) involve consumers and carers from the outset, rather than invite their participation once many of the main decision had been taken, and (c) continue to focus on the reform agenda (Healy et al., 2007). My own feeling is that the most significant present challenge is to ensure that OM does not lose sight of its primary focus, the systematic assessment of consumers' progress for use in assisting them in their journeys.

Acknowledgement

I am most grateful to Mike Slade for comments on an earlier draft of this chapter.

References

Andrews, G. and Slade, T. (2001). Interpreting scores on the Kessler Psychological Distress Scale (K10). *Australian and New Zealand Journal of Public Health*, **25**, 494–7.

Bockoven, J. S. (1963). *Moral Treatment in American Psychiatry*. New York: Springer.

Brown, J. (2007). *Value Index*, available at: https://www.psychoutcomes.org/bin/view/OutcomesMeasurement/ValueIndex, retrieved 19 September 2009.

Department of Health and Ageing (2003). *Mental Health National Outcomes and Casemix Collection: Overview of clinician-rated and consumer self-report measures*, Version 1.50. Canberra.

Department of Health Mental Health PbR Development (2009). *Practical Guide to Preparing for Mental Health Payment by Results*. London: Department of Health.

Eisen, S. V., Grob, M. C. and Klein, A. A. (1986). BASIS: the development of a self-report measure for psychiatric inpatient evaluation. *Psychiatric Hospital*, **17**, 165–71.

Garg, A. X., Adhikari, N. K. J., McDonald, H., et al. (2005). Effects of computerized clinical decision support systems on practitioner performance and patient outcomes – a systematic review. *JAMA*, **293**, 1223–38.

Healy, J., Stapley, K. and Coombs, T. (2007). *Implementation and Development Workshop*. Australasian Mental Health Conference, 2–4 October, Wellington.

Hodges, S., Woodbridge, M. and Huang, L. N. (2001). Creating useful information in data-rich environments. In M. Hernandez and S. Hodges, eds., *Developing Outcome Strategies in Children's Mental Health*. Baltimore, MD: Paul H. Brookes.

Huffman, L. C., Martin, J., Botcheva, L., Williams, S. E. and Dyer-Friedman, J. P. (2004). Practitioners' attitudes toward the use of treatment progress and outcomes data in child mental health services. *Evaluation & the Health Professions*, **27**, 165–88.

Information Strategy Committee, AHMAC National Mental Health Working Group (2005). *Key performance indicators for Australian public mental health services, November 2004*. Commonwealth of Australia.

Jacobs, R. (2007). *Investigating Patient Outcome Measures in Mental Health: research report for the OHE Commission on NHS Productivity*. York: Centre for Health Economics, University of York.

James, M. and Mitchell, D. (2004). Measuring health and social functioning using HoNOS. In M. Harrison, D. Howard and D. Mitchell, eds., *Acute Mental Health Nursing: From Acute Concerns to the Capable Practitioner*. Thousand Oaks, CA: Sage.

Marks, I. (1998). Overcoming obstacles to routine outcome measurement. *British Journal of Psychiatry*, **173**, 281–6.

Phelan, M., Slade, M., Thornicroft, G., et al. (1995). The Camberwell Assessment of Need: the validity and reliability of an instrument to assess the needs of people with severe mental illness. *British Journal of Psychiatry*, **167**, 589–95.

Slade, M. (2009). *Personal Recovery and Mental Illness*. Cambridge: Cambridge University Press.

Slade, M., Thornicroft, G. and Glover, G. (1999). The feasibility of routine outcome measures in mental health. *Social Psychiatry and Psychiatric Epidemiology*, **34**, 243–9.

Sugarman, P., Walker, L. and Dickens, G. (2009). Managing outcome performance in mental health using HoNOS: experience at St Andrew's Healthcare. *Psychiatric Bulletin*, **33**, 285–8.

Trauer, T. and Pedwell, G. (2007). *A Trial of Outcome Measures Reports Designed Specifically for Consumers*. Australasian Mental Health Outcomes Conference, 2–4 October 2007, Wellington, available at: http://www.tepou.co.nz/file/PDF/Powerpoints/Stream-8-Paper-39-Trauer-Pedwell.pps, retrieved 15 September 2009.

Wing, J., Curtis, R. and Beevor, A. (1994). 'Health of the Nation': measuring mental health outcomes. *Psychiatric Bulletin*, **18**, 690–1.

Index

Note abbreviations used: OM for outcome measurement/measures; ROM for routine outcome measurement